Continued Blessings
in all you do!

Sam Christian

III John: 2

Manna*fast* Miracle

How to Lose up to 1000 Pounds

Sam Christian, M.D.
June Christian, Ph.D.

MANNA*fAST* MIRACLE

Sam Christian, MD.

Pond Casé Press with offices in:

- Bowie, Maryland
- Tiffin, Ohio
- London, England
- Toronto, Canada
- Roseau, Dominica
- Capetown, South Africa

Pond Casé Press Books may be bulk purchased for educational, church, or corporate promotional use and for special sales. For information, please write to:
Heartland Nutrition Institute,
478 West Market Street,
Tiffin, OH 44883
Find us online at www.mannafast.org
or call 419 447-9313

The Library of Congress has cataloged the soft cover edition as:
Mannafast Miracle
How to Lose up to 1000 Pounds
Samuel Christian, M.D. _ 1st ed.
p. cm.
1. Nutrition. 2. Quality of Life. 3. Minority health 4. Motivation
Library of Congress Control Number: 2003111218

Cover design by Tim Hartsel
Author's note: Names and details of examples provided in this book have been changed when necessary to respect the confidentiality of the doctor/ patient relationships. This publication is designed to provide accurate and authoritative information with regard to the subject matter covered. It is presented with the understanding that the publisher is not rendering contractual medical advice. If medical or other professional advice is required, please seek the services of your physician or other available healthcare professional.

ISBN 0-9744925-0-7

Printed by BookMasters, Inc. Mansfield, Ohio, USA.

Dedication

To our patients, to whom we are forever indebted,
for sharing their struggles and their strengths.

To our parents, Olive and Oscar Henry,
Alberta and Wendell Christian, who taught us to pray;
for their unconditional love and encouragement over the years.

To our sons, Kwame and Kobie, that they may grow up
in the nurture of and appreciation for the abundant life.

...I will apply nutritional measures
for the benefit of the sick
according to my ability and judgment;
I will keep them from harm and injustice...

From the Oath of Hippocrates
Father of Medicine

Acknowledgements

I believe because my mother first believed. It began before dawn that day on the Nature Island. I was only 12 when she brought me along on a pilgrimage to the *Shrine of La Sallette*. It was there that I saw how hurting people were drawn by the glow of her tireless compassion. Mom taught us how to give back. She instilled in us that there was no greater honor than a life spent ministering to the needs of others.

Later, Parnick and Margaret "Nena' Jennings from Rome, Georgia journeyed as short-term lay missionaries to land unknown to them. They returned with a long-term commitment to medical missions. By faith, they engaged churches in Georgia, Alabama, Tennessee, and North Carolina to share a priceless part in my medical training. This book is a grateful expression of their quietly unfolding story.

To my brother Gabriel Christian, Esq. (*Rain on a Tin Roof*), my sister Esther Christian (*Chance Meeting & Hidden Intentions*), and Judge Irving Andre (*A Passage to Anywhere,* and others, co-author with Gabe of *Death by Fire* and *In Search of Eden* series). Thanks for your guidance and the support of Pond Casé Press. To my other siblings Lawson and Theresa for their chapter reviews, and also to Ivenia Augustus, Frances, Eddie and Katie Delsol, Avonelle Christian, Frazier Jones, Captain Francis Richards, Washway Douglas, Raglan Riviere, Dr. Tompson Fountaine, Dr. Peter St. Jean, Dr. Clayton Shillingford and all my colleagues in the Dominica Academy of Arts and Sciences for their enthusiasm and encouragement.

To all my teachers and professional colleagues for their collective wisdom, confidence, referrals, advice and oversight. To Pastor Dave Serrant of Deliverance Baptist Church and Fr. Reginal LaFleur of St. Alphonsus in Goodwill, Dominica, Maryland's Rev. St. Clair Mitchell of Evangel Assembly / *Strategies to Empower People*, Dr. John Millar and Tiffin University, Pastor Mickey McManus and the congregation of First Baptist Church for their love and encouragement, Fr. Frank Murd and the staff of Tiffin Catholic Schools for their confidence and prayerful support over the years.

To all our nutrition counselors, nurses, psychologists and office staff who have contributed so much to the enduring effectiveness of Heartland Nutrition Institute. Special thanks to Patti Schmitz LPN, Berneita Saum, and Tim & Dorothy Hartsel. Along with others unnamed, their valuable assistance in this project will continue to have a lasting impact on the lives of many.

Introduction

In 1977, an impressive young man from Dominica appeared on the campus of Shorter College. Sam Christian soon endeared himself to the Shorter Community with his friendly smile, wide interests and hard work. In addition to his outstanding academic record, he participated in many extra-curricular activities. He served as president of the International Students Organization, established the soccer program and was active in the Baptist Student Union as well as the Tri Beta Biological Honor Society. Furthermore, he found time to present over sixty missions programs at various churches organized by his mentor, Parnick Jennings. From his early years, he already seemed gifted in persuading others to trust in God's power to change lives.

I am not surprised that Dr. Sam has and gone on to be a successful physician who continues to be involved in missions and church development. May his book, *Mannafast Miracle*, enhance and extend his already impressive health ministry.

Joe R. Baskin, Ph.D.
Professor of Religion,
Shorter College, Rome, Georgia.
Author of *Why I Believe in Jesus Christ.*

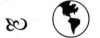

At Tiffin University, we had the privilege of having Dr. June Christian serve as a lecturer in Anatomy and Physiology. Her strong academic background began with a Bachelor's of Science degree from the University of Guyana. June proceeded with her Masters study in thyroid physiology at Auburn University followed by advanced studies in nutrition at Howard University. Her doctoral thesis was on *Iron, Folacin, Vitamin B12 and Zinc Status, and Immune Response in Elderly Subjects in the Metropolitan Washington, D.C. Area.*

June subsequently taught at the University of Delaware. Upon relocating to Ohio, she has been president of the *Heartland Nutrition Institute* associated with Sam's medical practice. Her attention to detail and organizational skills have steadily advanced the much needed faith-based Manna*fast* concept. Her own insights as a scientist and as a mother are invaluable in shaping strategies for reversing childhood obesity.

Introduction

During Sam's twelve-year tour of duty as Battalion Surgeon in the US Army Reserve, he also served as Medical Director of the Morbid Obesity Unit at Windsor Lane Health Care Center in Gibsonburg, Ohio. Under Sam's results-oriented leadership, the facility attracted those most afflicted with complicated obesity from all regions of the country. As patients under his care learned to assume ownership of their present situation, they earned for themselves more spectacular results than they ever hoped for with surgery.

Besides presenting at Tiffin University's *Good Morning World* business breakfast series, Dr. Sam has written newspaper articles and has spoken on related health topics in South Africa, Britain, Germany, Canada and the West Indies. He is a corporate wellness consultant, and a guest expert on numerous radio and television programs. This continued dedication to an approach they truly believe in has led to him being featured on the Discovery and Learning Channels viewed internationally.

John J. Millar, Ph.D.
Vice President for Academic Affairs,
Tiffin University,
Tiffin Ohio

Finding Help

1. **I just can't lose weight.**
   Star Trek's Mr. Spock would say, "That's not logical." The key is your ***Mannameter Score*** in *Jumpstart* (1). *Planes of Progress* (3) and *User's Manual* (7) give the basis for lasting weight-loss success.

2. **I can lose it, but I gain it right back.**
   The secret is in *Stomach Conditioning* (5). Understand the inherent dangers of lo-carb and other quick fixes in *Diet Roller Coaster,* (12)

3 **Those hips and thighs of mine just won't quit.**
   Really? *Move it and Lose it* (6), and *Fluid and Figure* (16) distinguishes between shape and size. It let's us know who is in charge!

4 **I think I'm a stress eater.**
   Eating Disorders (8), explains how to cope with this common tendency. Just popping a pill is not the answer: *Wonder Drugs?* (11).

5 **My weight and my love life are two different things.**
   Get in touch with your feelings and real life challenges in *Keeping it Real* (15), *Fluid and Figure* (16), and *One Love* (20).

6 **I'm thinking of just having the surgery.**
   Get an insider's view: *Surgical Options* (9) examines preparation, risks, benefits and the potential for dreaded, gradual weight regain.

7 **I just want to do what's right.**
   Scripture teaches more about eating for health and happiness than any of today's diet books, bar none. Meditate on *Balanced Nutrition,* (13) *and Faith and Fitness* (10). √ your *VQ's* on p. 30, 98,146, 188 & 234.

8 **I worry about my child's weight.**
   Reversing Childhood Obesity (17) examines strategies to really make sure that no child gets left behind in the quest for fitness.

9. **My weight is my own business.**
   See the impact of our health and lifestyle choices on our loved ones, our companies and our economy. *Health Freedom Ring!* (14), *Corporate Wellness* (18), and *Community Weight Loss* (19).

10. **Anyway, I just love food too much.**
    Join the crowd! *Joy of Eating* (2), *Obesity Epidemic* (4), and *Keeping it Real* (15), may be just what the doctor ordered!

Contents

Now is the Appointed Time.

Some people are simply blessed. They never have to spend a waking moment dwelling on their weight. For many others it is a constant challenge, eating away at self-esteem while relentlessly undermining health. So often, one overhears something like, "I give up. I guess I was just meant to be fat." It is difficult indeed to convince such individuals of the wonderful opportunity for the glory that can be revealed in their lives. I am yet to come across anyone, anywhere, who could not lose at least ten excess pounds in the time it takes to thoughtfully read this book.

Lance Armstrong puts it this way: "The truth is that cancer was the best thing that ever happened to me. I don't know why I got the illness, but it did wonders for me." (*It's Not About the Bike*, Penguin Putnam, NY 2000). Powerful words! Applying the same concept to obesity explains why those who overcome the lean-green natural way are truly among the happiest people I know.

Manna*fast* Miracle is based on detailed knowledge and experience with the latest weight-loss surgical techniques as well as nationally recognized accomplishments with massive non-surgical weight loss. More importantly, it is centered on a keen sense for how people make decisions on the deepest level. Manna*fast* provides breakthrough motivational techniques for sustaining success. Those seduced by quick fixes may scoff at its language of higher consciousness and question its results, but in the end, the results speak for themselves.

Indeed, there is something quite mystical about the moment one begins to do something definite and systematic about their weight. Likewise, the reasons can be frustratingly elusive why certain people persist in harmful behaviors. No doubt, there is someone in your life who fits that bill.

Consider Mandy, vice president of a growing mid-sized company. A sophisticated lady, I could always count on her to share the latest high-tech tips. Much of her office visits were spent dealing with the stress from her father's losing battle with lung cancer. A parent could not wish for a more loving daughter. She agonized with him as he struggled for his last gasps of air. On an intellectual level, Mandy fully understood that cigarettes were directly responsible for her father's demise. She even hated the smell. Yet, she could not bring herself to quit, despite all the warning, coaxing or pleading. I had to learn this sobering medical lesson: with addiction, simply knowing what is right does not always mean doing right.

Unlike nicotine, which when used as advertised produces disease and death, we earn vibrant health when we consume food responsibly. But when it comes to food addictions, *you just ain't seen nothing yet!* It takes a systematic, inspired series of actions to overcome this contradiction. Impressive results are guaranteed once you connect with someone or some group who will never give up on telling you that you can do this!

The Basics

Forget all that talk about metabolism. Obesity is largely a lifestyle disease. Despite the population explosion, today we have far greater access to delicious food so we eat and eat and eat some more. In such a context, nobody loses weight by accident. We have to make a conscious decision to control it. From all my years of surgical and medical treatment of obesity, five basic postulates or principles have emerged. These concepts are daily being validated and refined by researchers and weight challenged individuals alike.

Postulates of Mannafast Gastric Conditioning (MGC)

1. Weight accumulates when the *stomach is stretched* to habitually take in excess calories beyond the body's needs.

2. Diets, self-starvation and other eating disorders inevitably lead to rebound hunger and weight regain.

3. Restriction at the stomach level (by surgical bypass or Manna*fast* gastric conditioning) is *the only sure way to lasting weight control.*

4. Gastric conditioning literally *shrinks the stomach* back to normal through a safe, scientific process of decreasing portion sizes.

5. Understanding *planes of progress* and securing local support from Covenant Groups is essential for effective gastric conditioning.

Manna*fast* Miracle is spiced with stories of people like you who have taken the time to examine their relationship with food. The underlying causes for obesity can be complex and at the same time, unique for each individual. The book is organized in such a way as to facilitate direct navigation to topics of interest, (**Finding Help** across from the Table of Contents). For more interactive step-by-step instructions on actually starting the program, log on to www.mannafast.org. Getting one's body under control is the first step to *getting one's life under control.* The key to achieving that is just a few clicks away.

The basic practical steps are summarized right off the bat in *Jumpstart*. Test your familiarity with 50 selected FITNESS FOODS, in groups of ten, and calculate your Vege-Quotient (VQ). This directly relates to weight control and overall wellness. Five-question chapter REVIEWS focus on the take-home message. They synergize your experiences with the insights of knowledgeable people in your own local network of contacts. The companion *My Miracle* Weight Management Journal ties in with the reviews to serve as a take-off point for discussions at *Covenant Group Meetings*. This is not a place for hearing the same old worn-out facts and pitiful platitudes. It is a place for people who want results. This is a book that demands response, action and accountability every step the way.

Most importantly, you will learn how to use Mannameter LIFESCORE, a true mirror to the soul. It is one of the most powerful motivational tools available. I use it regularly, not only to track my weight, but my overall life performance as well. You too will appreciate that the wisdom gleaned from this unique faith and fitness manual is more than just book knowledge. It empowers ordinary people to become *more effective than today's average health care professional in helping others with their weight.*

Food Control

Imagine a world without food. You can't! Everywhere, people exuberantly celebrate national dishes and regional cuisine. Throughout the ages, God's blessing has been expressed in terms of having abundance of food and freedom from famine. Barns bursting with grain have always been symbols of prosperity and paths to international power. That is where the *Manna* part comes from: Divine Providence; that wonderful nourishment that comes from above, first described in the book of Exodus. We discuss this fundamental relationship with food in Chapter 10, *Faith and Fitness.*

As one studies the rise and fall of empires, a recurring tragic theme comes into sharp focus. Pioneering times are characterized by lean struggle and noble nation-building. Subsequent generations risk acting like spoilt children of hardworking, successful parents. Acquainted only with creature comforts, they revel in an unearned superiority complex, vegetating with excess and abuse. Periodic *fasting* is that essential guardrail that consistently keeps us from plunging into the abyss of destructive self-indulgence. This is the humble gastric discipline, so thoroughly prescribed by the ancients, yet all but forgotten in today's push-button, pill-popping, procedure-possessed society.

An endless parade of suburban vanity diets entices us to "eat all we want and still lose weight." A visitor from outer space would wonder what on earth we are thinking! These diets appeal to an "it's all about me" Hollywood fantasy giving rise to a national pastime of recycling the same old excess poundage. Picture that typical ad with smiling dieters holding up their old trousers twice their size. The public marvels at the too-good-to-true before and after photos. It is left for physicians to see these same individuals years later when their health is eventually ruined by recurring episodes of maladaptive eating.

Begins in the Soul

Alexis De Tocqueville was a great French philosopher who visited the United States two centuries ago. He concluded "America is great because America is good, when America ceases to be good it ceases to be great." I am no expert in theology, but religion as currently practiced in much of western society appears to be floundering, bereft of the motivation necessary to impact health. Indeed, recent statistics suggest that *churchgoers are generally fatter than the general population*. I have a problem with that. We tackle this issue head on in Chapter 10.

Despite all our frailties, failings and fallen nature, within every on of us is that spark of the Divine. According to the Apostle Paul, even the unchurched have faith, though they may strenuously deny it. Standing before intellectuals gathered at the Aeropagus in Athens, the Apostle delivered what is undoubtedly one of the most stirring discourses in the entire Bible. His message was built around the words: "For in Him, we (all) live and move and have our being, as also some of your own poets have said," (Acts 17:28). Mannafast is a record of how different people have moved, oftentimes hesitantly, in a new direction of transforming faith. The miracle is not in some diet, *it is in you!* Manna*fast* brings it out.

In the average household, there are at least a few good cookbooks or magazines, many with healthy recipes. They tend to simply gather dust. Nutrition tips abound in the print and broadcast media, on a wide array of responsible governmental and hospital web sites, on cable channels devoted to food, travel, fitness, and so on. Manna*fast* does not dare to duplicate this excellent body of work. But one thing is clear. Much of what society has been doing to this point just is not working. The population keeps getting larger and sicker. Our job is motivating clients in how to best recruit these terrific resources as part of a personalized, breakthrough weight management plan.

A Journey of a Thousand Miles...

At the rate we are going, the shape of mankind in just 20 years will be truly scary. Much of the population may resemble Jabba the Hutt, that blubbery mass of alien protoplasm in the *Star Wars* trilogy. I don't want to be a part of that problem; I want to be a part of the solution. Obesity is a very serious, but very treatable disease, especially when using the right formula of clinical attention to natural healing and systematic tough love. Professionally, it grew frustrating always trying to shut the door after the horses had bolted from the barn. We have therefore made the conscious decision to devote our energies to a much more thrilling challenge. We are committed to dealing with the obesity well *before* it requires such radical intervention as bariatric surgery or admission to a medical weight-loss facility.

Our patients achieving massive weight loss have been featured on network and cable television. The fact is that losing a thousand pounds (or any amount which feels that way), begins with one step. And you have already taken that step with me. Anyone still capable of performing activities of daily living can safely attain the very same sensational results, *right now,* in the comforts of their own home. Fascinating advances in communication technology make this possible. Truly, the miracle of covenant support now blossoms in clinics, workplaces, seminars, churches, schools and the campfire excitement of community weight loss programs. You will never walk alone. Be assured that by the time you finish this book, others will see a measurable difference in you - both inside and out.

Manna*fast* begins by showing us how to fall in love with one of God's choicest creations - you! This a romance filled with the same kind of heartache and longing, hope and triumph. It moves us from the prevailing practice of disembodied faith to true stewardship of our "temples." For many, losing weight is just a matter of shedding a few pounds to look good on the beach or for that upcoming wedding. Others long oppressed by obesity need a true home run, a Hail Mary pass - it's now or never. They are so ready to say goodbye to traditional diets and hello to a final breakthrough. Manna*fast* will not only move you, it is guaranteed to shake up cherished notions and make you think. In the following pages, you will meet others like Brad, Jessica and Phyllis and discover what went into their miracle. Now it's time to get yours!

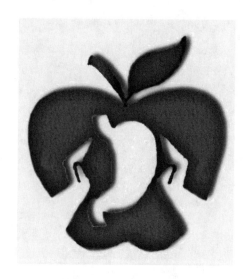

Chapter 1

Jumpstart

What this power is I cannot say; all I know is that it exists and it becomes available only when a man is in that state of mind in which he knows exactly what he wants and is fully determined not to quit until he finds it.

Alexander Graham Bell, inventor of the telephone

Like open-mouthed little birds, we would eagerly await our parents' return from socials. They would discretely smuggle hors d'oeuvres in napkins and bring back the treasure to the nest. The annual cocktail ball at the Governor's House was the best! Hosted at this alabaster mansion surrounded by sun-drenched, swaying palms and manicured lawns, it was by far the most stately building on the island. Directly across the boulevard stood the timeless Fort Young Hotel which catered these events. The hotel itself was a tourist haven perched on the cliffs overlooking the tranquil aquamarine harbor where *Pirates of the Caribbean* would later be filmed. Its glinting brass canons still symbolize the awesome power of its high cuisine.

Food can get you giddy! Peanut butter prunes, finger sandwiches, Mountain Chicken and deviled eggs were our favorites. What a late-night treat that was - with our delicious home-made ginger drink! My Dad's blue-collar firefighter colleagues would badger him to have a Dominican *man's drink* like rum or a shot of whiskey instead of bothering to bring home goodies for the kids. Dad would answer in his lilting, native French patois *"Papa d'enfants pas grand vie."* ("Father of children is not into high life.") So while to his friends, he was always *Papa Zafa,* to us, he more than just brought home the bacon. He always taught us not to bicker among ourselves for first dibs, but to always "Thank God for small mercies."

Who would have thought that "small mercies" would be the basis of my professional treatment of weight problems? Bariatric surgery trained me to impose small portions by cutting stomachs down to size. However, in time, I found a better way. Specifically, through faith, we learn to appreciate "our daily bread" as God's small mercies. Training oneself

1

to stick to small portions is by far a more enlightened approach which actively involves the patient in his own healing.

Needless to say, that is not necessarily the easiest way. Take Brad for example, a 42 year old, married father of three. This self-employed construction worker came to our Tiffin, Ohio office because his tool belt was irritating a growing mole on his hip. He worried whether it was a melanoma like his cousin had. He seemed to carry his burly 253 pounds well on his six foot frame. Incidentally, he complained of a "headache that wouldn't quit," not to mention feeling tired all the time. After finding his blood pressure to be unusual, the nurse rechecked it manually. She was still uncomfortable with her reading and asked me to double-check.

*Pffft, pffft, pffft, pffft, pffft...*the cuff then deflated slowly, *...pshhhhhhhh.* The silver column eased down the glass tube then began dancing much sooner than expected: 230/128! Couldn't be! I too, checked it again - same result. I do not remember ever coming across numbers so high in a walking, talking human being! It was only then he admitted being started on a cocktail of three blood pressure pills by another physician a few years before. However, with two kids in college, Brad never bothered to follow-up since his doctor seemed to care less that the prescription cost over $300 a month. He knew that was dangerous; in fact his father died of a heart attack at age 43!

Well, that mole had to wait and we had to talk. A previous visit to the ER had left him in such a financial hole that he adamantly refused our recommendation to go there. Instead, he consented to take medication in the office and have his pressure monitored for over an hour. We finally impressed upon him that unless he did something really quick, his kids could grow up with the same emptiness that he did.

We got his pressure down to under 200, ordered a stress test and referred him to the cardiologist. Fortunately there was no significant heart damage. We helped Brad with office samples. He had his blood pressure taken by a nurse in his neighborhood, other times at the pharmacy. We eventually got him to invest in his own electronic BP machine. His part of the agreement was to regularly call in the readings to the office. When he lapsed we would check on him. He was a tough nut to crack. It was not until much later that Brad thanked us for helping him

> *Skinless **turkey** breast is a one of the best sources of low-fat protein. The chicken version is an excellent alternative.*

Body Mass Index Table

Height (feet and inches)	Healthy						Overweight					Obese										Extreme obesity												
BMI	19	20	21	22	23	24	25	26	27	28	29	30	31	32	33	34	35	36	37	38	39	40	41	42	43	44	45	46	47	48	49	50	51
												Body weight (pounds)																					
4'10"	91	96	100	105	110	115	119	124	129	134	138	143	148	153	158	162	167	172	177	181	186	191	196	201	205	210	215	220	224	229	234	239	244
4'11"	94	99	104	109	114	119	124	128	133	138	143	148	153	158	163	168	173	178	183	188	193	198	203	208	212	217	222	227	232	237	242	247	252
5'0"	97	102	107	112	118	123	128	133	138	143	148	153	158	163	168	174	179	184	189	194	199	204	209	215	220	225	230	235	240	245	250	255	261
5'1"	100	106	111	116	122	127	132	137	143	148	153	158	164	169	174	180	185	190	195	201	206	211	217	222	227	232	238	243	248	254	259	264	269
5'2"	104	109	115	120	126	131	136	142	147	153	158	164	169	175	180	186	191	196	202	207	213	218	224	229	235	240	246	251	256	262	267	273	278
5'3"	107	113	118	124	130	135	141	146	152	158	163	169	175	180	186	191	197	203	208	214	220	225	231	237	242	248	254	259	265	270	278	282	287
5'4"	110	116	122	128	134	140	145	151	157	163	169	174	180	186	192	197	204	209	215	221	227	232	238	244	250	256	262	267	273	279	285	291	296
5'5"	114	120	126	132	138	144	150	156	162	168	174	180	186	192	198	204	210	216	222	228	234	240	246	252	258	264	270	276	282	288	294	300	306
5'6"	118	124	130	136	142	148	155	161	167	173	179	186	192	198	204	210	216	223	229	235	241	247	253	260	266	272	278	284	291	297	303	309	315
5'7"	121	127	134	140	146	153	159	166	172	178	185	191	198	204	211	217	223	230	236	242	249	255	261	268	274	280	287	293	299	306	312	319	325
5'8"	125	131	138	144	151	158	164	171	177	184	190	197	203	210	216	223	230	236	243	249	256	262	269	276	282	289	295	302	308	315	322	328	335
5'9"	128	135	142	149	155	162	169	176	182	189	196	203	209	216	223	230	236	243	250	257	263	270	277	284	291	297	304	311	318	324	331	338	345
5'10"	132	139	146	153	160	167	174	181	188	195	202	209	216	222	229	236	243	250	257	264	271	278	285	292	299	306	313	320	327	334	341	348	355
5'11"	136	143	150	157	165	172	179	186	193	200	208	215	222	229	236	243	250	257	265	272	279	286	293	301	308	315	322	329	338	343	351	358	365
6'0"	140	147	154	162	169	177	184	191	199	206	213	221	228	235	242	250	258	265	272	279	287	294	302	309	316	324	331	338	346	353	361	368	375
6'1"	144	151	159	166	174	182	189	197	204	212	219	227	235	242	250	257	265	272	280	288	295	302	310	318	325	333	340	348	355	363	371	378	386
6'2"	148	155	163	171	179	186	194	202	210	218	225	233	241	249	256	264	272	280	287	295	303	311	319	326	334	342	350	358	365	373	381	389	396
6'3"	152	160	168	176	184	192	200	208	216	224	232	240	248	256	264	272	279	287	295	303	311	319	327	335	343	351	359	367	375	383	391	399	407
6'4"	156	164	172	180	189	197	205	213	221	230	238	246	254	263	271	279	287	295	304	312	320	328	336	344	353	361	369	377	385	394	402	410	418

give up drinking as many as a dozen beers after work almost every day. He said at first he would actually hide the salad he brought in his lunch box just to avoid comments from his buddies on the worksite. Adding fruit and vegetables was also quite a new thing for him as well. With a regular exercise program, (rather than just relying on manual labor), he managed to reduce his weight to 212 pounds and maintain a reasonably normal blood pressure on only one pill. Brad's remaining headache was how to handle his kids' college education. But he had to learn to tackle first things first. Once we had taken care of him, those things would somehow take care of themselves.

Do the Math!

How many pounds do you need to lose? That is your main goal. Look back at the BMI chart on page 3 and see where you stand. Select your height in the left column. Go across to the column under the BMI of 25. That should be about your healthy weight. For example, a good weigh for someone 5' 6" is under 155. If this person now weighs 205 pounds she is about 50 pounds overweight. As we shall see in Chapter 7 *User Manual,* give and take as much as 10 -15 pounds based on gender, age, frame size and medical history.

If losing weight or maintaining your progress has been frustrating in the past, you are not alone. Here's how this is going to change. First, expect an average initial weight loss of **10 pounds per month.** (This very much depends on starting weight and medical status). It is important that we secure real progress before the body "realizes" and tries to self-sabotage. If weight is the enemy, remove the kid gloves and let's deal with it! Mannafast strengthens your focus so the *cares of this world* won't throw you off track. Massive weight loss calls for massive action!

Tithe Your Excess Weight

Break it up in chunks. Start by tossing just *one tenth* of your excess weight. Come on now; everybody can do that! Give it up as a sacrifice to the Almighty and see how the windows of heaven will open up on your endeavors. Someone 50 pounds overweight pledges to lose 5 pounds. *Just one tenth* - most people will do that before finishing this book! All it takes is an act of the will.

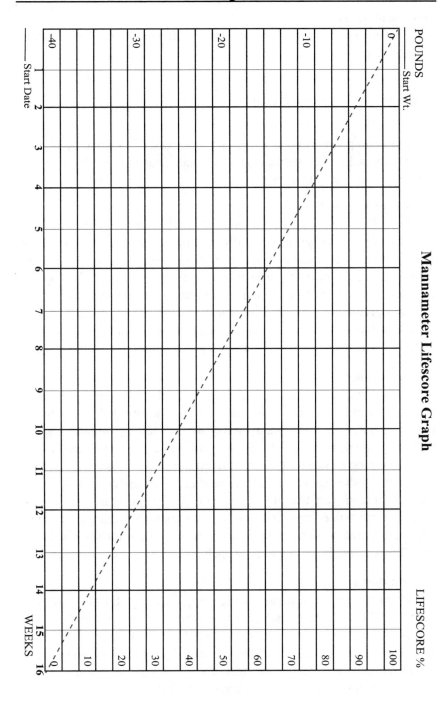

Mannameter Lifescore Graph

POUNDS

LIFESCORE %

WEEKS

Intermediate goal

That is *half of the excess body weight.* Estimate the number of months that will take:

$$\text{Time for the intermediate goal} = \frac{\text{Half of excess weight}}{10 \text{ (pounds per month)}}$$

So, half of 50 pounds excess weight is 25 pounds. Divide that by 10. That is 2.5 months. In other words, the intermediate goal can be obtained within 3 months. Can you picture that?

Start your engines!

Have fun with this and challenge Mannafast to deliver for you. Peg your *weight milestones* to generally celebrated holidays or other dates that have personal meaning. Get hold of a calendar and let's see what's coming up in the next few weeks or months. Birthdays are perhaps the best links - yours or those of your loved ones. Also consider graduations, weddings, reunions, anniversaries, vacations, etc. Do not think of them as deadlines, but as *lifelines!* When that dates comes around, you will tingle with excitement as you remember what you promised yourself today.

Recruit a buddy

A buddy may not necessarily a significant other. Regrettably, a spouse sometimes can be your fitness downfall, part of the family dysfunction that has you where you are. A buddy serves as an external reminder for what the target date does privately. This may not be the person you would want to go shopping or hang out with. However, when it comes to health and fitness, he or she provides gentle inspiration. They are consistent. Surely there is someone like that in your circle of friends, at church or at work! You just have to find them, and then have the courage to bring up the topic. The funny thing is, this person might just be waiting for somebody like you. Rejoice, reinforce, and remind each other that you are worth it.

Write it down.

When building their dream house, people make notes of the features desired. (The architect's budget will provide the reality check). Some supply pictures: I want my kitchen to look like this. I want my bathroom to look *exactly* like this. Let us put the same kind of planning and vision in an even greater project - your health! Pull out a photo of yourself, five, ten, even twenty years ago. Say: I want to be that size again.

1. Jumpstart

Some might think it unrealistic. I used to. So many of my patients have proved me wrong, I have become a believer. You will too. Here's how you track your progress on the Mannameter Lifescore graph on page 5. Ready for step-by-step directions on how this thing works? I will use myself as an example:

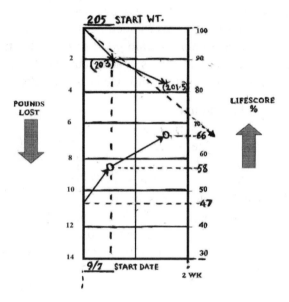

1. Write down the *Start Weight* in the space at the top left corner of the graph. Mine was 205 pounds.

2. Write down the *Start Date* on the lower left. Mine was September 7, (9/7). Each box along the baseline represents one week. Just a 2-week portion of the graph is used in this example.

3. Mark a small "o" on the left axis (sideline) for the first Lifescore. (This is the fascinating percentage score that we will learn how to calculate later in this chapter). Mine was not that great starting off (47%).

4. Write a small "x" on that imaginary vertical date line. Three days later, by 9/10, I was already down to 203 pounds. I wrote an x, two pounds down from my start weight. I then drew a descending, solid *Weight loss* line (**WL**) from the top left upper corner to that x. This gave a clear picture of my weight loss progress.

5. On that new date line, mark an "o" for the new Lifescore. Mine was up (58%). See, I was getting more motivated! I then connected the o's to form the ascending *Lifescore,* (**LS**) line.

7

One week later, I was down another pound and a half (201.5). My Mannameter Lifescore was up to 66% - not impressive numbers compared to several of my clients, but believe me, I felt what they felt. Look at the Mannameter (lifescore/weight loss) graph again on page 5. (You may want to copy or enlarge it and save the original). The sloping dashed line is a guide suggesting that the average person has loses 5 pounds in 2 weeks. Sometimes I was above, sometimes below, but *as long as I kept doing the right things, I kept getting good results.* This tracking device is a fascinating project that shows exactly how well you're doing. The technique itself is easy. Staying motivated is another story.

Get With the Program

Consume fewer calories and move more. That is the secret of weight loss - end of story! Those who try to fool Mother Nature seldom have the last laugh. But there is no

> *You cannot jump across a ten-foot ditch by taking two five-foot hops*

shortage of those willing to try. To do it right, get the ball rolling with these five simple steps. Set a firm foundation as we get into the meat of the matter in the following chapters. If you are already doing any of them, great! We are on our way.

1. *Eat breakfast*

This may not make much sense to those who have been depriving themselves of breakfast, starving themselves to lose weight. Frankly, it took me some time to grasp the concept. Many clients experience a breakthrough by doing just this one simple thing. Actually, the idea is to eat less, more regularly. We are not talking here of a *grand slam* breakfast of two eggs, bacon, hash browns and pancakes with coffee. Start your nutrition makeover today by having something simple and wholesome: rotate between oatmeal, fruit, cereal, granola bar, yogurt, natural juice, soy milk, etc. This keeps up energy levels and reduces your risk of "cheating." It gives the gut something to do, otherwise it will soak up all the calories and fat that next comes down the chute.

By far the best way, in my experience, to start the program is by using a *nutritionally complete supplement shake*. There are several excellent products out there that vary by quality and price. Mannafast.org suggests how to choose those products which provide everything the body needs and none of the excess fat and calories responsible for the weight problem. Those afflicted with eating disorders find it difficult to part with their regular fare, even for a season. They consistently come up with a variety of excuses why they must have "real food." On the other hand, when one is serious about losing weight, he would rather not be confused about "What should I eat now?" With each pound lost, with each chapter mastered, nutritional wisdom is being imprinted on the psyche in a more meaningful and effective manner than ever before. See the major weight loss section, Chapter 5, (*Stomach Conditioning*) for further details.

2. Fill up with fiber

For most of us brought up on fatty foods, the smell of frying bacon will win over fresh fruit every time. However, it lacks fiber and health-promoting nutrients. Though rich in flavor and containing nutrients, it pushes us in the opposite direction of cholesterol control and safe weight loss. Typical lo-carb dieters, hooked on taste, have difficulty accepting that. When change in bowel habits suggests the need for additional fiber, start slowly with any of the over-the-counter products. Too fast and the unaccustomed stomach develops uncomfortable bloating and gas. Patients drift back to highly refined, high fat, high sugar foods after wrongly associating healthy foods with bad effects. Chapter 13, *Balanced Nutrition* explores these issues further.

3. Measure your waist/hip ratio

Chapter 7, *User's Manual* explains how the ratio of waist measurement divided by hip reflects on cardiovascular health.
How to measure:

- Pass a tape measure around the narrowest part of your waist. This would generally be at the belt line, but to be consistent, measure at the level of the navel.

- Then measure the widest part of your hips.

- Divide your waist measurement by your hip measurement.

Write down those numbers. Measure again in one month. You will be pleased at what you have accomplished! Just the waist measurement by itself says a lot about one's health and longevity.

4. *Get up*

It feels so good to get the circulation going. And it's not hard. Try this: Lay the book down. Get up and walk across the room or across the house. Go ahead. If you are not in a position to do that, do some stretches or isometric exercises. For example, clasp your hands in front of your chest. Raise your elbows to the level of your shoulders. Push your hands firmly against each other. Slowly allow the right to push the left hand across to the left shoulder. After about 10 seconds, slowly go the other way. Feel that muscle power beginning to surge through your back, shoulders and forearms. This should take less than a minute. While sitting down, you could also raise your legs and hold them out straight, level with the floor. Slowly you can feel your muscle taking on the strain of gravity. Count 10 seconds. Breathe. You are working out! Isometrically. If it is too much for you to do both legs, do one at a time.

Being faithful in this little exercise will do wonders as we move through the chapters. Every time you pick up this book, take a minute to do your isometrics. Just getting that blood pulsating through your system puts you in the right frame of mind to excel.

5. *Start your Food and Fitness Workbook*

By the end of the month the checkbook has to balance - more or less. It is no different with calories and weight. A simple notebook would do. The companion, *My Miracle Workbook*, does it even better by directing us to the areas that matter. You are guided by the wisdom of the ages as well as the latest scientific and motivational insights. Moreover it provides the opportunity to relate your feelings and events of each day with your *rate* of weight control and fitness improvement. Anything worth doing is worth writing down.

What Makes It Tick?

It takes more than just instructing clients to "eat right and exercise" and consider mission accomplished. The fact is a whole host of subtle factors influence outcomes in everyday life. Consider Jessica's story. She felt lucky to have Dwayne. He brought in a good paycheck and was devoted to his family. So why then was she feeling so irritable and insecure? She felt she could even eat the paint right off the walls that seemed to close in on her every time she tried to shed a few pounds. Once again, she was saddled with a closet full of clothes she could no longer squeeze into. At her aunt's wedding that weekend, she just hated the looks her relatives gave her. Every one kept saying how "well" she looked. But deep down she just knew what they really meant was "Gosh, girl, where you're going with all this weight?!"

Jessica was gushing over the pictures of the family trip to Sea World. The kids had talked her into sitting in the front row so they could get splashed when *Shamu*, the huge killer whale, did his tricks. That crazy cousin of hers just stared at the photo then blurted out that he couldn't tell the difference between her and the whale! "Just kidding," he laughed as he ducked for cover. For Jessica, this was not funny "Ha-ha," that was just plain ridiculous. Right then and there she finally decided this weight had to go.

Phyllis, her "chubby" best friend since grade school, had *the surgery* just four months before. She was always the daring one. In no time Phyllis was weighing less than her. I hate you, I hate you, I hate you, she remembers thinking. She thought back to when Phyllis asked her if she wanted to come along for the very first bariatric consultation. Just out of curiosity she casually replied, "Oki-doki!" At one point, she even interrupted, asking if she too would qualify. The nurse told her she would have to be at least twenty pounds heavier. They listened solemnly to all the risks, "including, but not limited to infection, re-operation and death." There was no way either of us would go for that, Jessica thought. We're too chicken!

Phyllis awkwardly tried to make light of it. While they were waiting for follow-up instructions, she leaned over and whispered to Jessica. "So imagine you were the one going for the operation, and you didn't make it. At the visitation, your loved ones are looking down at you lying there. What would you want them to say about you?"

Jessica did not quite care for such topics. But she was there for her friend, so why not humor her some, she thought. "I hope people would say that I was a good mother, ummm...a loving wife...somebody who knew how to have fun."

"Good answer, honey." Phyllis cooed, giving her a gentle little back rub. "And you?"

Phyllis stroked her chin solemnly; then her eyes sparkled. "Well, I hope they would say...*Look! She is moving!*"

They laughed so hard Jessica had to make a beeline to the lady's room. As she gingerly tiptoed by, some in the waiting room stared her down with that annoyed look. Others smiled curiously as if wishing they could be let in on the joke.

They always had such a good time whenever they got together. Jessica knew that a team of horses could not pull her girlfriend away from a course of action once she had sent her mind to it. For her part, Jessica had started an interesting new program. In fact, she was anxiously waiting to see when Phyllis would first notice...

Available Help

Drama and drum roll does not always herald that mystical hour of decision. Often times it is precipitated by rather mundane incidents unique to individual experience. Some people are spiritually ready to seize that opportunity for personal transformation. Others tragically never get to that point. The spark may come from casual conversation, a radio or TV program, a book shared by a friend or perhaps an online, newspaper or magazine article. Sometimes you can see it coming, but you can never predict for sure when and how inspiration will strike.

Many are at a point where they feel their efforts would be futile without drugs or surgery. While some may have to resort to such measures, subsequent chapters persuade us that it is best to lose weight using safer, more natural methods. *Acupuncture,* for example, is becoming a popular non-invasive intervention to stimulate metabolism and suppress hunger.

Americans first became interested in this ancient art following President Nixon's breakthrough visit to China in 1972. James Reston, a New York Times reporter covering the trip, required an emergency appendectomy in Beijing for which acupuncture anesthesia was used. On his return home he raved in America's leading newspaper on acupuncture's amazing pain relief capabilities. This prompted the FDA and National Institutes of Health to investigate and approve its effectiveness in treating a wide range of illnesses. These include migraines, severe periods, chronic pain, nicotine, alcohol and food addictions etc.

That almost universal fear of needles is the biggest hump to get over. That is perfectly normal. When a phlebotomist approaches me with that rigid needle, I am all good-natured and relaxed. After all, I don't want her to be too tense over having to stick the doctor. However she is trained to know like most patients, this one's toes are probably tightly curled as he prays that she's not a rookie!. Acupuncture needles are different. Since they do not have to be hollow for drawing blood or injecting medicine or IV fluids, acupuncture needles are flexible and much skinnier (like a "cat's whisker"). Neither are they beveled (cutting) but rather actually insert between the cells skin and seldom bleed. I was pleasantly surprised to discover that unlike that so-called "little poke" promised by the typical nurse giving her shots, I barely felt these needles going in.

Acupuncture uses specific points along known "meridians" of the body to enhance the flow of life energy known as *Qi*. This regulates organ function and stimulates natural healing. At first, patients tend to be very curious of acupuncture's role in a comprehensive weight program. They soon come to appreciate the results of this low-risk, low-cost office procedure compared to surgical options (Chapter 9).

Check your motivational pulse

Maintaining a high level of motivation is more important that anything else for successful weight management. Understanding the scientific details of a particular diet does not prevent people from getting bored and simply giving up. Motivation is not some ephemeral quality, hard to hold on to like some vapor, or bobbing for apples. Rather, it is the awareness of the goodness (**Manna**) flowing through your life and mine that can be objectively measured (**meter**). *Mannameter* technology places motivation at your fingertips. It is based directly on one's own self-assessment in ten central aspects of existence. On a scale of 0 to 10, what is your "job satisfaction rating?" Sometimes we feel so exhilarated or emotionally exhausted that there may be a tendency to use extreme scores. Be gentle with yourself. But be fair too. The process will surprise you!

Point System:

1: extremely unhappy	6: somewhat pleased
2: very unhappy	7: moderately pleased
3: moderately unhappy	8: very pleased
4: mildly unhappy	9: extremely pleased
5: average	10: couldn't be better

Now here are the ten main categories:

1. **Faith**: This may involve personal meditation and public worship. However faith certainly is not just about denomination or even religion. Faith is much more universal and goes a lot deeper than that. Chapter 10 describes a faith that directly impacts one's health. It is the core of character. The South Carolina State motto is *Dum Spiro, Spero.* "As long as I breathe, I hope." For every problem in life there is a spiritual response. There is absolutely no conflict between genuine faith and being 100 percent practical and scientific. On a scale of 1 – 10, how active is

your faith today against the negative forces in your life?

2. **Family**: That often goes beyond the traditional "nuclear" family. It may also refer to the extended family, the adopted family, the blended family, etc. Suite-mates in a dorm, work crews on a remote project, colleagues at a camp or conference - can become so close at times as to be considered temporary family. This is the caring community where one finds that sense of belonging and support. That in turn implies certain obligations and responsibilities. Did your actions today contribute to making your "family" more nurturing or more dysfunctional? The amount of *communication* and *quality time* invested helps determine your score.

3. **Fun**: Are you fun to be with? What makes you smile and what makes you laugh? What is your pastime? How do you recreate yourself? Are people drawn to you or do they find you so intolerant and irritable that they have to tiptoe on eggshells around you? How competent are you at processing the inevitable hassles and sad events of life? Would others say you have a sense of humor? Laugh! Sing! Dance! You'll live longer. How do you rate yourself in the enjoyment department?

4. **Exercise**: No diet, drug or surgery can replace the importance of exercise, even when there is a "good excuse." Everybody can do something regardless of their limitation, as discussed in Chapter 6. Only you can do this for you. Fitness gradually improves as you get in tune with your body. Grade yourself according to your efforts and consistency. A confessed couch potato should not be bashful about starting with 0 or 1. That will change!

5. **Weight**: Self-explanatory. How do you *feel* about your weight? Use the BMI chart as a reference. Score yourself according to your weight *progress* on your Mannameter tracking graph. If your weight is where you want it, feel free to rename this category with another that may be more relevant to you such as "Organization" or "To Do List."

6. **Habits**: Here are some free points for you. If you do not smoke, give yourself 3 points right off the bat. Same thing if you do not abuse alcohol or drugs. Subtract points if you are aware of any other high-risk behavior you need to monitor. Be honest with yourself. This is totally private.

7. **Health**: This is a hard concept for the young to grasp unless they have experienced chronically illness in their family. Review the list of generally accepted _Common Screening Tests_ for healthy adults on page 308. If large corporations insist upon these basic health requirements for their executives and essential personnel, why not you? We often trick ourselves into believing we save money by dodging these sometimes unpleasant, time-consuming check-ups. Some of us are in denial, not wanting to discover some dreaded disease. Others figure God will take care of them and shield them from getting sick or that faith will heal them. Sadly, none of us are here forever and each will eventually come down with something. The condition missed now will be much more painful and expensive later. So, how do you rate your health efforts today?

8. **Work**: It is not the particular job you do that defines you as a person. It is how diligent you are about what you do, even if you are between jobs. Are you tardy or reliable? If you work at home, are you proud of your crucial role in supporting the family and molding lives? If you work in the factory, the office or in the service industry, do you get along with your boss, customers, colleagues or those under you? If you are a professional, are you a workaholic or now simply resting on your laurels? Our attitude towards work has considerable impact on our weight and health.

9. **Ministry**: What have you done for _me_ lately? That me refers to the "least of these my brethren" (Matthew 25:40). That means the needy, those unable to repay us, those not blessed with the insight or privileges we enjoy. This is the principle of tithing in the universe; not just our money, but more importantly, _hands-on_ time. To have good stuff coming into one's world and nothing going out, is to become like the Dead Sea, which harbors no life. To be a giving person is to recognize that eternal relationship between service to others and holistic health.

10. **Mood**: You can be sensitive to your feelings without wearing them on your sleeve. Do you feel loved or have the opportunity to love others? Do you allow yourself to be unnecessarily sidetracked and troubled, or do you feel that you are living up to your potential? When we take the time to examine where we are in the grand scheme of things, it may become apparent that we actually are not doing too badly. Give yourself some credit. On the other hand, if your overall _Mannameter Lifescore is_ low,

and you are all happy-happy, then we have to talk. Chapter 8 will show how this is useful in identifying inappropriate mood disorder. Anyway, for now, to what extent is your mood today positive and realistic?
It is time now to check you motivational pulse:

LIFESCORE   Date: ___ / ___ / ___

1	Faith		6	Habits	
2	Family		7	Health	
3	Fun		8	Weight	
4	Work		9	Mood	
5	Exercise		10	Ministry	
				Total Score =	

"How're you doing today?" Fairly routine greeting. It is amazing the kind of feedback we could get if we took time to listen. Occasionally, one hears, "Life sucks!" "I'm having a terrible day!" or "How much time do you have?" - (definitely a low Mannameter score). What does someone with a high score sound like? Well, depending on their level of modesty you may hear, "Just fine, thank you!" "Fantastic!" or "I'm blessed!"

In class, a score above 70 percent is considered satisfactory. It was therefore quite a revelation how often I was cruising well below my best. The mere act of systematically focusing on these ten central aspects of life is a crucial reality check. More importantly, it unleashes a power that defies description. Alexander Graham Bell, quoted at the beginning of this chapter, was fascinated by motivation. We all know the results in his life when he tapped into it. Tracking your Mannameter online using all the bells and whistles really dramatizes your progress. Either way, hard copy or on the computer, monitor you motivational pulse regularly. Then just watch for surging Lifescores and tumbling weight as you plough through the pages of this book!

All reality is twice created ; first in your mind that only you can see,
then physically out there for everyone to behold.
Believe you can do this and most definitely you will achieve it.

1. Jumpstart

REVIEW

1. What do you usually have for breakfast?

2. How long would it take you to *tithe* your weight?

3. What benchmark dates have you chosen for your health goals and why?

4. Who would you consider your *fitness buddy?*

5. How would today's Mannameter Lifescore compare with one you may have done a week ago?

Chapter 2

The Joy of Eating

That every man should eat and drink and enjoy
the good of all his labor. It is the gift of God.

Ecclesiastes 3:12

Food Rocks! Love of good food is among the most wonderfully universal traits of human nature. When the appetite goes, we know a patient is not doing well. But when the *appetite goes out of control*, we know it won't be long before we will have another patient on our hands. Food generates energy for all of life's activities. Food in excess also generates fat - no great revelation. Now that we have jumpstarted our weight management program, let us face up to our relationship with food in order to get a better grip on lasting solutions.

Let the Good Times Roll

"What you're doing for Thanksgiving?" As a foreign student in Georgia, I felt like a lost kid from the islands, quite unprepared for the barrage of questions leading up the meal of the year. A frenetic whirlwind of preparation led up to the big day. Kitchens churned out their best. Each new guest was welcomed with a crescendo of excited chatter. The guys pitched in some before staking out choice seating for the big games on TV. A symphony of sights and sounds overwhelmed my senses: unbelievable aromas - the casseroles and cranberry sauce, corn bread stuffing, honey-glazed ham and the juiciest turkey I had ever seen. My taste buds still quiver and stomach rumbles, just reminiscing on those scrumptious sweet potato and pumpkin pies plus the abundance of other delectable desserts. And when the blessing dragged on a few seconds more, someone hissed "Short prayers, short prayers!" We giggled irreverently. Squinting through one eye, I caught a few others doing the same, peeking through their eyelashes at the sinful spread!

What impressed me most was how no effort is spared for everyone to be somewhere special. The entire nation, including the homeless and strangers, were inviting or being invited, pulled countless miles by an unseen magnet to the great feast. Nothing more typifies the generosity of the American spirit so timelessly captured on Rockwell's canvas.

One may wonder, if this book is about weight loss, why tantalize with all these images about food? It is precisely because few things in life can compete with the joy of eating. We affirm that. The deluge of epicurean delights lingers long after New Year's leftovers. The palate is jaded by the repeated onslaught of tempting treats - parties and goodies at work, church, clubs, his family, her family... By early January, the body is literally begging out for simple, wholesome nourishment.

While the *average* American gains 5 pounds, for those who are struggling, the holiday weight gain is lots more. It represents a sharp spike in stress and comfort eating. The resulting guilt often mars the reason for the season. Despite all the resolutions, the weight gain not only comes to stay but in time invites more. It is only as we honestly analyze our own formative notions about food can we effectively reverse this troubling problem for good. The results we have seen with this positive approach speak for themselves.

No One Plans To Be Fat

The very act of eating predates man's existence. There is broad agreement that before human footprints graced the earth; lower life forms in God's Grand Design were indeed eating for growth and sustenance. Chapter 13, *Balanced Nutrition* will reveal much based on the very biology of these creatures. We therefore should have no remorse tickling our palates with the finest delicacies this world affords. But we also have the responsibility, as an old

> *(God's) witness to us is rain from the heavens and fruitful seasons, filling our hearts with food and gladness.*
>
> Acts 14:7

British saying goes, "not to use our knives and forks to dig our graves." Becoming overweight risks doing just that, as we shall see in greater detail in Chapter 4. *Obesity Epidemic.*

After venturing on the scale for the first time in a couple months, the verdict was that I had bloated up to 25 sluggish pounds above normal. For the first time in two decades I had to punch a couple extra holes in my belt and buy size 36 pants instead of 34's. For the sake of my health, not to mention my reputation, I had to put a stop to that. Failure was not an option. It helped to have a couple athletic sons who would teasingly tug at my love handles and remark, "Hey Pop. That gut's so not cool. It's got to go!"

It was rather sobering to realize that I was just as vulnerable as my patients to weight sneaking up on me. Well meaning friends and family would disarmingly greet my concern with, "Come on Doc; live a little." At the same time, I became keenly aware of this interesting dynamic. Picture that. As the weight drops, one is able to fit again in the older "thin" clothes. But then there is a competing subconscious yearning for the *newer* "fat" clothes. Strategies for dealing with this conflict include burning one's bridges by donating or giving away fat clothes vs. keeping them as trophy reminders of how far one has come.

First Class

Yes we can have the best of both worlds! Can you think of any other human activity that brings more comfort and joy? From weddings to cruises, potlucks, picnics and parties, a delightfully prepared meal represents the peak expression of love and recognition. The power lunch was not the invention of Wall Street. Consider the Old Testament book of Esther. When the king inquired of her petition, this Hebrew queen repeatedly deferred until after she had prepared him an awesome banquet. In that case, fine food greased the wheels to avert a major holocaust plotted by Haman. Remember the exclamation of the ecstatic father when his Prodigal Son came home: "Let us eat and be merry!" (Luke 15:23) Translated today: "Let's party!" Napoleon knew that an army marches on its stomach. Lobbyists routinely treat politicians at the finest restaurants (and more) to entice them to vote in a manner favorable to their special interests.

But in the final analysis, there is no free lunch. Food seizes control in disarming and insidious ways. It lures us by demanding no commitment. The meekest and mildest of us can dominate and ravish food. In times of plenty or in times of stress, food offers itself without objection. It tempts us with its charms to be consumed, ingested, munched, grazed, gobbled and devoured. It stimulates our pleasure centers, leaving us with a sense of satisfaction and fullness.

The stomach governs personality development that in turn eventually determines our weight. We all have our fond foods. Food used as childhood treats and grown-up splurges. At that age, food far and away tops the list of intensely pleasurable bodily sensations. Maturity is expressed in the ability to also find fulfillment in other spheres of life: accomplishment, art, service to others, the thrill of sporting activity, the warmth of companionship and intimacy. As we see in Chapter 8, eating disorders develop when one becomes stuck at some level, or regresses to a juvenile stage of development.

Our upbringing is powerfully influenced by associations with food. Many feel married to certain ethnic staples regardless of nutritive value. Jambalaya, grits with biscuits and gravy, jerk chicken, tamale, strawberries & cream, collard greens, shrimp fried rice, humus, matzoh balls, couscous, corned beef and cabbage, calaloo, shepherd's pie, pancit, poutine, wiener schnitzel, fufu, tandoori chicken, baklava, roti, vegemite, egg drop soup, spaghetti, or escargot all conjure specific cultural profiles. These generate an immediate gut level reaction ranging from, "I've got to have some!" to "Eeeuuu! How could people eat that stuff?!" Some use foods to bolster their identity; others defiantly refuse to be defined by them.

Grandmas everywhere have this thing about their cooking which evokes a kind of visceral emotional response. As a rule of thumb, the state can regulate how fast to drive and where to smoke, but don't mess with people's food. President Bush the First was said to have declared words to the effect. "I never liked broccoli when I was a child. My mother forced me to eat broccoli. Now I am President, nobody is going to make me eat it!"

Food Rewards

Just the mention of certain foods can transport one back into a warm and fuzzy state. A soft-boiled egg does it for me. In those days, use of the word cholesterol was limited to arcane medical literature. Using the baby spoon, Mom would crack open the top of an egg and tenderly peel off the shell. She would then puncture the membrane with a soft plop. Invariably some of the thick, rich, yellow and white substance would dribble over the side of the shell. I remember reaching over to catch the drippings with my finger. I would watch fixated, perhaps impatiently kicking my little feet, as mom would add a pinch of salt and swirl it all around. I knew what came next was a warm, spoonful of the most delightful nourishment ever! That is my childhood picture of mother's love.

What are your childhood memories of being fed? Is it playing with and eating Cheerios from the high chair? Having your meat cut up into tiny bite-sized pieces, or the simple act of fitting you with the bib? How about rewards for going to the dentist, such as a Popsicle or ice cream? Had you ever snuck food up to you room? What were your favorites? One

2. The Joy of Eating

little girl relished a snack of grated coconut 'tablet' baked in sugar. More than just traces of it would be discovered under her pillows and sheets and other secret places in her bedroom.

What kinds of snacks did you get when you first got your allowance or began earning wages? Skittles, Babe Ruths or M&M's? Even before that I remember tightly clutching the grocery list when sent on errands to our little Pottersville (Lotbor) neighborhood shop. Construction and road workers would swagger up to the counter and order a cheese and salami *mastiff*. Ma Thomas, the shopkeeper, would place the designated weights on one side of the old fashioned scales. A pleasant, pungent aroma permeated the air as she cut slices of

> *To me good health is more than just exercise and diet. It is really a point of view and mental attitude about yourself.*
> Angela Landsbury

decreasing sizes from a huge block of cheddar. She gracefully placed it on the waxed paper on the other side. All eyes seemed hypnotically glued on the needle of the scale as it lazily waved this way then the other before balancing dead center.

Ma Thomas would similarly chop chunks of meaty sausage. In the process she would casually snack on any appetizing morsels left over. Oh my, that looked good! How I dreamt of becoming a shopkeeper one day. But my torture was not yet over. Next she would reach for the sharpest of knives and fillet open a hot, fresh-baked, *sub*-sized loaf. She slabbed on generous amounts of golden New Zealand butter that promptly melted. She finally combined the ingredients, wrapped it and completed the transaction. At a time and in a place where people were somewhat more reserved about eating in public, these working men would promptly unwrap their savory meal and wash it down with a tall glass of ice cold *squash* (fresh-squeezed lemonade). I marveled at those big, brawny men towering next to me. That much would feed all my brothers and sisters! And in my little mind I thought, "So that's what it means to be grown up. You can buy whatever you want and wolf it down all up by yourself!"

Think back to some vivid food-related experience in your past. Food is always on our minds from the time we were tiny tots. I distinctly recall the national relief and euphoria when the hostages were eventually freed from the embassy in Iran. I was in medical school in Washington DC and multiplied thousands of people lined the route from the airport. Red, white and blue sprouted everywhere. Schoolchildren watched it live in classrooms, but some lucky ones got a field trip out if it. An intrepid TV reporter approached a bunch of kindergartners, posing the profound question as to why they were out there on that special day. One precious little girl sprang forward excitedly. She tugged the microphone to her slobbering lips and blurted out, "Because the *sausages* are coming home!"

Later in life, food continues to remain high on our agendas. Some may argue that the cutest point in the whole wedding celebration is probably not the slipping on of the ring or the announcement, "You may now kiss the bride." It may be when the couple lovingly feeds each other that cake, even mischievously smearing it on each other's faces. That act recalls the vintage romantic request of all time, when Egyptian queen Cleopatra whispered to her Roman General, "Anthony, peel me a grape."

We have observed in our practice that there are two distinct points when men put on weight. 1: When they get injured (or discontinue strenuous sports or work) and 2: When they get married. Exasperated women trying to get their guys to tone down would exclaim: "Men! You can't live with them and you can't live without them!" Men are programmed with specific no-no's drilled into their subconscious. They first learn to please mom by eating all their food that she labored so hard to prepare. Later, they rave about their date's cooking, even if they have to fake it! At potlucks or when invited over for dinner (at the in-laws), they are suckered into seconds and more so as not to offend the cook. So, while the way to a man's heart is through his stomach, his heart and other organs stand to suffer if that "way" becomes much traveled.

Food Allergies

The palate may love a particular food though the body may be reacting negatively to it. Take the case of the firstborn in a particular family. This was a model child, laughing and cooing, sleeping through the night after a few months. The second child, the exact opposite - a parent's nightmare. Colicky, snotty, sleepless and crying all the time for no obvious reason. That was until the old wise lady of the village suggested switching her to goat's milk. Miracle!

Food allergies affect no more than 7 percent of children and about 5% of adults. Yet one can easily appreciate how this relatively minor malady can contribute to a good deal of child abuse and neglect resulting in borderline personalities. Lactose intolerance is the most common food allergy and is more prevalent in the minority population. Lacking the enzyme to properly digest this sugar in milk, increased gas or diarrhea can develop as undigested lactose reaches the large intestine.

Allergies can be weird. Despite extensive experience in this field, medical science still does not have all the answers. One of my patients was allergic to chocolate, perfume and flowers. Her boyfriend thought it such a pity she was not allergic to jewelry as well! A colleague of proud Irish heritage was allergic to potatoes and cabbage. Another woman would start itching if she even entered a house in which shrimp was being prepared. In November 2005, an allergic 15 year girl from Quebec, Canada, died after reportedly kissing her boyfriend who had consumed a peanut butter sandwich a couple hours earlier.

While some people may be violently allergic, many others may just be marginally intolerant to a particular food. There is a continuum, not all or none. Instead of actually breaking out, they may just become sluggish and retain water. Food industry giants lobby Congress to permit widespread additives to the food supply some of which are harmful to segments of the population. Monosodium glutamate, (MSG) is a notable example. Truth-in labeling laws are often opposed by those with a financial interest. There may be favorite foods that are otherwise "healthy" which maybe slowing

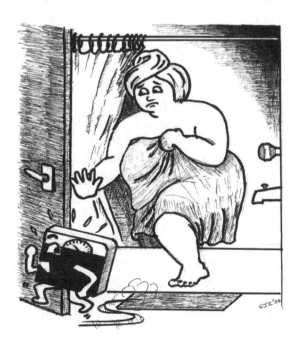

you down and predisposing toward weight gain. Certain blood tests can be helpful in identifying food allergies, but often the search can be tedious and frustrating. Awareness of that possibility must be followed by the discipline to rotate a questionable food out of the diet every couple weeks. Relief of symptoms pinpoints the offending food.

Technology and Body Weight

Herein is the dilemma: How can we "eat, drink and be merry" without causing our waistlines to balloon out of control? We deceive ourselves if we believe that no other nation enjoys food as much as we do. Think again. Yet, obesity is nowhere as prevalent in those countries and their longevity now measurably surpasses ours. This is not some new weird virus or lethal cancer. Obesity is clearly a lifestyle disease which absolutely did not exist 30 years ago anywhere as much as it does today. Continuing clever advances both in pharmaceutical and surgical treatments of obesity, have failed to stem the tide. Why is that so?

The world is changing at warp speed. Just look at cell phone technology. Some of us are old enough to remember the first units, cumbersome clunkers the size of a bread box. And folks felt so hip lugging that around. A pigtail antenna on a Mercedes Benz was a status symbol that the owner had a cell phone. Make way! Today, they are no more than fashion accessories for kids of all social strata. If made any smaller,

> *Don't wait for inspiration. Begin now and the inspiration will come.*

fingers could scarcely press the buttons. Who bothers to remember telephone numbers anymore when it is all programmed in the directories or call logs? Fancier "mobiles" feature organizer functions, text, pix and video messaging, games, MP3's, email, live TV, GPS travel directions, beam credit card payments to vending machines, toll booths and lots more. I think this is a terrific time to be alive! So when we make comparisons to "the way things were", do not for a moment confuse it with a longing for the "good ole days". Rather it is to compare and contrast what we must do to adapt to living in an ultra-modern society.

Such technological advances dramatize how physical activity becoming a stranger to modern life. A generation ago, we got up to change the TV channels, washed our cars by hand, pushed lawn mowers, climbed stairs and walked into restaurants for an occasional meal. Because of automation and labor saving devices today, we are obligated to inject

2. The Joy of Eating

deliberate exercise routines to burn enough calories just to stay even. Added to that, there are all kinds of *statistics showing that we are literally eating up to twice as much.* Why is it so hard to understand where the excess weight comes from?

The abundance of food is the result of great advances in techniques of farming and animal husbandry. However, a couple other factors contribute to today's obesity epidemic. Way back in the industrial revolution, man discovered how to more efficiently separate the wheat from the chaff. Stripped of its natural fiber, flour was then bleached, processed and promoted as the food of refined people. Pastries and pastas, along with alcohol, have grown to dominate the caloric burden in the western diet. But weight problems really began to surface with the exponential growth in the fast food industry. The most popular combos feature meat, milk, cheese and eggs, all from animal sources and high in fat.

Increased Caloric Consumption

Like the perfect storm, another factor joined the sociological changes described above to precipitate this dietary disaster. Consumption of dietary sugar increased 30 pounds per person per year during 1960 to 1980. High Fructose Corn Syrup (HFCS) is cheaper than sugar from cane or beets. Between 1975 and 1985, HFCS market share increased from 4 percent to 33 percent. Much of it is in product like soft drinks. Manufacturers began making a killing as diabetes soared. Soon thereafter, artificial sweeteners joined the party creating its own share of maladies and paradoxical weight gain as described in Chapter 11, *Wonder Drugs.*

Dr. Atkins was right on the money about carbohydrates being a major source of obesity. But beyond that he was dead wrong. No doubt people on the Adkins diet do lose weight. But as we shall see in the history of diets (Chapter 12), promoting fat consumption in place of carbs has devastating consequences. Sadly, the research shows that the doctors themselves who preach this doctrine are not immune. The Framingham study, running now for over 40 years, is considered worldwide as the authority on cholesterol and health. The conclusion is that no one with cholesterol levels less than 150 suffers heart attack, period. So, be clear about what you want; just to lose weight, or more than that - to be healthy.

To summarize:

> Excess carbs + Fiber depletion + Increased animal fat
> + Decreased exercise physical activity
> = Obesity epidemic.

Understanding this hypothesis sets the stage for taking corrective action.

Genetics or Environment?

"The Most Trusted Man in America" Legendary CBS anchor Walter Cronkite trademark sign off from the evening news was, "And that's the way it is... (followed by the date)." Many have come feel the same way about obesity - it's here to stay, get used to it. Conventional wisdom has it that regarding food related dysfunctions, we are simply the product of our genes. The theory goes that we inherited that attraction to high calorie and fatty foods from prehistoric times when famines were frequent. Natural selection suggests that those who survived were the ones better able to store energy as fat. This logic would imply that the future does not look too bright for descendants of those having difficulty coping with today's ready availability of fattening food.

It has been said that one is not responsible for his heritage, but definitely responsible for his personal future and legacy. But using genetics to explain away and excuse obesity is a hopeless strategy. The truth is that even in "large" families; weight is not so much inherited as members share the same attitudes toward food. Identical twins raised in different homes tend to have significantly different weights depending on their diet. The Pima Indians across the Sierra Madre Mountains in Mexico, though poorer, are lean and fit. Pimas across the border on the U.S. reservation are among the fattest people in the world.

We all love to eat. Good food is the well-deserved reward for our labors. The Book of Wisdom introduced this chapter by declaring fine cuisine to be "the gift of God." The popularity and proliferation of cooking shows and celebrity chefs is a wonder of modern civilization. However, the secret of how to overcome our culture of overeating and stay healthy in the face of such gastronomic abundance is truly a spiritual art. The following chapter provides a systematic approach for anyone willing to break that generational curse and experience the joy of accomplishing lasting weight loss success.

I wish above all things that you may prosper
And be in health, even as your soul prospers.

III John: 2

2. The Joy of Eating

1. Give two examples of favorite childhood foods and why they were special to you.

2. What is the main nutrition reason for the obesity epidemic? Is it too much fat, carbohydrates or protein?

3. To what extent is obesity inherited and is there anything that can be done about it?

4. Discuss food allergies you may be familiar with and how it is best managed.

5. Does your lowest *Mannameter* category have anything to do with food?

Calculate your Vege-Quotient (VQ)

In the spaces below, insert a score of based on how often, on average, your eat fruits and vegetables. Just put your best guess as some items are a lot more familiar than others. **Scores**: More than once a week:10. About weekly: 9. Monthly: 5 to 8. few times a year: 3 to 4 Never/few times in your life: 0 to 2.

1. **Apples**   "Keeps the doctor away" heart protector, makes bowels
   _____   more regular, Enhances lung capacity, strengthens joints

2. **Apricots**   High in *lycopene* and antioxidants; aphrodisiac,
   _____   Controls blood pressure, helps dry eyes (contacts), ↓aging

3. **Artichokes** Greco-Roman origin, *choleretic* (increases bile flow to
   _____   treat gallbladder dz.), ↓ cholesterol, Helps blood sugar.

4. **Asparagus** High in protein, vitamins and mineral, low in calories,
   _____   helps fluid retention and rheumatism.

5. **Avocados**   Known to the Aztecs as "fertility fruit." ↓cholesterol
   _____   smoothes skin, stroke protector, ↓ blood pressure.

6. **Bananas**   "Wise man's fruit" High in potassium (replenishes
   _____   athletes), cardioprotective, ↓ blood pressure, ↓diarrhea.

7. **Beans**   Excellent meat substitute, High in fiber & iron, regulates
   _____   bowels, ↓cholesterol, ↓blood sugar, cancer fighter.

8. **Beets**   Contains pigment *Betacyanin*, boosts weight loss and
   _____   detoxifies liver ability, combats hypertension and cancer.

9. **Blueberries** High in antioxidants, memory booster, ↓ aging, cancer
   _____   fighter, heart protector.

10. **Bok choy** Chinese cabbage, used in stir fry, and making *Kimchi*,
    _____   a popular Korean dish.

+ _____ % **TOTAL VQ**

  Now **add your scores**. This percentage indicates how fruit & vegetable "friendly" or "phobic" you are and reflects directly on your health and weight. There are more chances to check your VQ's on pages 98, 188, 234 and 250.

Chapter 3
Planes of Progress

What happens to a dream deferred?
Does it dry up, like a raisin in the sun?

Langston Hughes

"I don't suffer from obesity," George chuckled, "I rather enjoy it!" This retired health professional was a brittle diabetic, twice the size he should be, who stubbornly refused to give up those rich desserts. Eloquent and brazen, he was exceptionally clever at ducking health advice with that good-old-boy kind of charm. Recently diagnosed with sleep apnea, his blood pressure was haywire, his legs massively swollen. Yet, for all he cared, he had a generous prescription plan and surely enough of the right medications would take care of whatever ailed him.

Which diet would work best for this gentleman? None, of course! Most who whine about their weight are simply not emotionally ready to take meaningful action. A blind man could see that George was a train wreck waiting to happen. There was not much I could tell him that he did not already know. The way he saw things, the world was his oyster and I was just a stick-in-the-mud trying to cramp his style. He came to the office at his leisure to tinker with his blood sugar meds, but efforts to persuade him was like trying to sink a battleship with a kid's nerf gun. I prayed for someone else who could better connect with him otherwise only an act of God was going to make any difference in this inevitable story line.

One does not have to be a prophet to see what's coming round the corner. Take cancer for example. Some wonder how physicians can be so presumptuous as to declare "how much time" a particular patient has. Such estimates are based on well-documented statistics. For example, we know that a tumor of a certain type and size usually does its dirty deed in so many months or years. That is influenced by the patient's underlying health, local spread, lymph node involvement and effectiveness of available treatment. This is the science of tumor staging. Yet, Yale surgeon Dr. Bernie Siegel, author of *Love, Medicine and Miracles*, demonstrated that by teaming up

31

with his patients, he was able to instill values of courage and hope. These *Exceptional Cancer Patients* (ECaP) defied the odds and consistently showed superior survival rates. Several had spectacular cures. I highly recommend this book for anyone dealing with cancer.

How are you doing with your weight so far? We are not just talking about another diet. We are going to take care of business for good. I can tell you that at *Heartland Nutrition Institute* we have witnessed equally "miraculous" obesity cures. Like cancer, it must be staged in order to predict how long it is going to take, or even if we are going to make a dent. Height, weight, BMI, waist/hip ratio, etc. are important objective data as discussed in Chapter 7, *User Manual*. Then there is the psychological/spiritual aspect. We cannot weigh or pass a tape measure around that. It is intangible, yet so essential in obtaining lasting results. That is why the word *plane,* rather than stage, is a better fit in this setting. From my years in clinical practice, human beings go through five distinct stages in accomplishing anything. German psychiatrist Dr. Elisabeth Kubler-Ross described a similar analysis of the grief process. Let's see where you fit into this color-coded sequence:

1. Prevent .... (Red):
> Danger zone - A mocking "it won't work" attitude to any encouragement to improve.

2. Ponder .... (Amber):
> Caution. Reflects on the sad state of affairs. Begins to accept the need to change.

3. Plan .... (White):
> Slate wiped clean. Decision made for specific course of action. Battle plans drawn up and written down.

4. Pursue .... (Blue):
> Launch a goal-directed plan. Channels an *ocean* of resources into passionate action.

5. Perseverance (Green):
> Goal zone! Stick-ability. An increasingly rare spiritual gift in a world tuned in to instant gratification.

Some planes may literally take minutes before being check-marked for progress to the next. Others last years, even a lifetime. Old dogs *can*

3. Planes of Progress

learn new tricks. As we saw with Mannameter Lifescore in the previous chapter, *this concept is applicable to any challenge in human endeavor.* When is comes to weight, those who persevere maintain their success by

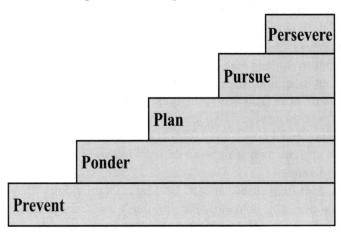

Planes of Progress

analyzing their setbacks and savoring what works for them. Perseverance and perseverance alone results in the abundant life.

1. Prevent

Take smoking for example. One of my patients worked at a drive-through discount tobacco outlet. They had "official" instructions not to sell to people on portable oxygen. Yet she also knew who her best customers were. Approaching vehicles were monitored on the video hook-up. She confessed seeing drivers snatch oxygen nasal cannulas from their faces and stuffing them into glove compartments or perhaps under seats. While she was tickled reporting her on-the-job "war stories," what struck me was the all-consuming power of addiction. And she was not done yet. Ever so often a customer could be seen taking a deep drag on a cigarette through his "trake" (or tracheostomy: a surgical opening in the neck) before pulling up breathlessly to the window. Bear in mind that such customers had their voice box surgically removed because of throat cancer - generally caused by smoking in the first place. Go figure!

New Testament book of Romans declares that all mankind has *fallen short* (Rom. 6:23). The issue therefore with the human condition is not so much that we are all tragically flawed, but many choose to stay that way.

They live in the danger zone - almost hypnotized by the flashing red light. People in the *Prevent* mode are the type who will try to beat the train at the crossing. On some level they are aware of the situation, but they just don't get it. They are not shy to tell of all the diets they have been on and also seem to glory in their convincing explanations for their failures.

Preventers can be quite insistent, even aggressive. They win many battles, but eventually lose the war. And the funny thing is that they feel good about it - at first. With acid wit and ridicule, they disarmingly deflect any offer of help. You see it on stage with self-deprecating comedians poking fun at themselves. Two legendary Johns come to mind, Belushi and Candy. They lived large. They were extraordinarily successful at making us laugh at their own weight while masking their struggles with lethal personal demons.

It is one thing to be amused by Mark Twain's quip "the only way to keep your health is to eat what you don't want, drink what you don't like, and do what you'd rather not." It is quite another thing to build a philosophy of life around it. This attitude is like the proverbial horse that may be brought to the water but cannot be made to drink. Like my patient George at the beginning of the chapter, they are stuck on the *Prevent* plane, spurning efforts by loved ones to get professional help. They may go as far as making an appointment or two before declaring, "See, it doesn't work for me." That is often a final concession to get concerned parties off their backs. They relish the role of being sick and disabled, while harboring deep a fear of success. Once they realize the new demands of being fit and healthy they say, "Uh-uh" and slide back into their comfort zone.

2. Ponder

Dr. Chavez pulled his chair closer and placed his hand gently on the patient's knee. "You know we love you, and we want to see you stick around." He paused, his eyes searching for a response. Doctor's face took on a somber expression of deep concern that the patient had never seen before. "But the way you're going Father, your knees are giving out, your blood pressure is through the roof, you can hardly sleep…I really don't know how much more time you have."

Father Murphy related that encounter with his family physician almost like a conversion experience. It was a story he would use many times in his messages and encouraged me to do so as well, if it could help anyone. "So this is it," the good priest thought. After years of preaching to others, attending to their needs, now he was on the receiving side of a serious lecture.

"You're too young to have knee replacement," Dr Chavez continued. "I've changed all your medicines; I don't know what else to do. You just have to lose this weight. I want you to go see Dr. Christian."

This is the plane where we *Ponder*. It is a time of reflection - coming to grips with the understanding that the current state of affairs is simply unacceptable. Caution! There is not much joy on this plane. It is designated *amber*. Everyone at some point begins to question things, but many never get quite motivated enough to push forward to action.

Not so with Father Murphy. He quickly focused on the task at hand. He cleverly linked his own personal challenge to the central project of his pastorate: major church renovation. Weddings and funerals, christenings, fairs and other special events, all meant visiting with his parishioners around food. A steady stream of irresistible treats always flowed into the rectory; "Cookies, lots of cookies." All these expressions of fondness and appreciation were not helping him one bit. We figured out a *plan*. So up into the pulpit marched Fr. Murphy and laid it on the line. He announced a moratorium on all such goodies. Thanks, but no thanks. Not only that, he solicited pledges from the congregation for every pound he lost. He *pursued* it with a passion.

We monitored his food intake and set up a gradual, personalized exercise program. As his weight plummeted, the contributions skyrocketed. When the public is accustomed to seeing someone as "fat and jolly," there is reluctance to part with the *Santa Syndrome*. Fr. Murphy had to teach parishioners that his sleeker, more vibrant version was just as caring and consecrated. He really had fun with this! An exciting time of health consciousness pervaded the wider community. By the time the money had been raised, Dr. Chavez's patient had shed 145 pounds!

Not many of us are in a position to galvanize such a loyal mass of supporters or to put our lives on hold to be on sensational TV. Rather we can organize *Community Weight Loss as in* chapter 19. In the final analysis, the decision has to be made in the privacy of one's own hearts. The Prodigal Son provides a classic example. It finally dawned on him that he was subsisting on the same slop as the hogs around him. Only then did he *ponder,* what on earth am I doing here?! He shuddered to think of his classmates seeing him in this state. People come to a point when they look at themselves and realize that was not how they pictured their lives would pan out. The estranged son thought of his family. He realized that he was not a kid any more. He knew he could do better. Time was running out.

Those in distress can actually sense the prayers of loved ones. The Prodigal perhaps reflected on words spoken by the prophet: "For I know the thoughts I think toward you, says the Lord, thoughts of peace, and not evil, to give you a future and hope" (Jeremiah. 29:11). It must have been like pulling teeth, but he finally took a deep breath and verbalized his *plan* "I will arise and go to my father" (Luke 15:18).

Do not for a moment think it was either quick or easy. The Gospels provide only an abbreviated account of his recovery. We are left to fill in the blanks. How hard was it to withdraw from all that freedom of not

> *There is a tide in the affairs of men, when taken at its flood, leads to fortune. Omitted, all the voyage of their life is bound in shallows and in miseries.*
>
> Wm. Shakespeare / Julius Ceasar

having to be accountable to anyone? Even in his misery, there surely were those who craved his company. He had acquired certain comfort foods and those are never easy to part with. We see the very same thing happening in the longing for the old times by the Children of Israel (Chapter 10, *Faith and Fitness*). Mindful of that, when you chance upon some inspiration, do not postpone doing what you know you have to do. Strike while the iron is hot!

The debate rages as to whether man is constantly evolving to higher stages of sophistication and ethical behavior. Arguments can be made for both sides, but from where I stand, the picture looks quite the opposite. The things that people do, or allow to happen to them is simply unimaginable! In the richest country in the world, under the shadow of Lady Liberty, countless masses choose bondage in the form of disabling addictions. Abuse of food has reached crisis proportions. It is difficult to measure the loss in productivity from so many good people not living up to their true potential.

In the depressive depths of the *pondering* stage, things tend to be fuzzy. It was only as the Prodigal braced himself and journeyed back to the land of starting over, that he was able to clear his head and realize how shallow his life had become. Unlike Lot's wife, when you make that break, do not look back. Asking yourself some tough questions will help crystallize your vision. What is it that you really want anyway? Your *five top reasons* for losing weight may be among the following.

3. Planes of Progress

- Do you want to **live a healthier, happier life?**
- Do you want to **keep the *Temple* in the best shape possible**?
- Do you want to have **more energy** to fulfill the tasks ahead?
- Do you **want to look younger and more desirable?**
- Would you like to **enjoy outdoor activities** with the (grand)kids?
- Do you want to **fit into most of your clothes again**?
- Do you want some people **eat their words?**
- Would you like **save money on health care costs**?
- Would you like to avoid **embarrassment while traveling?**
- Do you have **an event coming up** - wedding, class reunion, or vacation?

Think. There may be other reasons, but keep it simple. Limit it to your top five. *Write them down,* preferably in your own words. Review your goals (short term, intermediate, long term). If you identified them in *Jumpstart*, by now you must have the confidence to share them with another human being. Mastering this area of your life is the strongest testimony to others: that they too *can* take control of any habit whatsoever that threatens to overwhelm them. What more powerful message could there be than that?

Mindset

The story is told of an old Chinese tattoo artist who was asked why on earth would people permanently inscribed on their bodies words like "Born to lose," "Slut" or other names that would make any parent cringe. "Before tattoo on arm," he replied wisely, "Tattoo on mind!"

The mind is therefore the real battleground. Physical cravings are only symptoms of the real inner problem. Before the pounds can be unloaded, there has to be a change of heart, a deeper conviction in the spirit. "My body is precious. God wants me to be fit and healthy." This has to be my affirmation, my incantation, and my daily prayer. Chapter 10, *Faith and Fitness* describes exactly how we tap into this amazing power.

3. Plan

Sarah was mad. She was 280 pounds when she demanded from the clerk at the health food store "anything you have to make me lose this weight." She had left excitedly with *$355* worth of products. She dumped the now empty containers on to the counter in my exam room. In utter frustration, she wanted me to explain how she could *gain* 5 pounds in the 2 months since that shopping spree!

Some do well navigating the planes from *Prevent* to *Ponder* only to get tripped up because they failed to *Plan* responsibly. Sarah had an impulse, not a plan. The net result is that she got even heavier and even *more* depressed. That is the time to seek professional help. This is the *white* stage. As the Renaissance philosophers would say, clear the mind like a *tabula rasa,* a blank slate. Begin by putting down a plain, new sheet of paper on the table.

"If it was not documented, it did not happen." This is the dictum in the medical profession. The legal environment in which we operate makes this approach necessary. More importantly however, is that documentation is a tool used to monitor clinical pathways and track outcomes. This is especially true in major personal projects that involve large amounts of money and deadlines. Do not waste your breath saying you hate paperwork; you have to *write it down.* The Desiderata encourages you to "enjoy your achievements as well as your *plans.*" Ignore those who may call it daydreaming. As Les Brown would say, "Shoot for the moon. Even if you miss, you'll fall among the stars."

Remember that good-looking photo of yourself from years ago when you were in great shape? When I ask patients to bring in such pictures, they are brimming with pride to show how elegant they once looked. I make a photocopy for their charts and urge them to put it in a conspicuous place. I earn my keep to the extent that I convince them that is still "the real you." They can regain much of that physical charm by consistently focusing on that goal.

Setting Goals that Stick

Be *specific:*

I will keep my calories to (1200, 1500, or 1800).
I will exercise____minutes,____times a week.
I will get and provide support
...by sharing with_____ (buddy)
...by scheduling an appointment with a health professional.
...by meeting with _____ (group) once a week.

Do not be wishy-washy. "I just want to look good" is not a valid goal. Sure, you know what it means but you have to spell it out to your unconscious. Tell it exactly what you want and it will find ways to make it happen. Give it too much wriggle room and it will have you wandering in the wilderness for a lot longer than you deserve.

Set a time frame

3. Planes of Progress

Refer once again to the Do the Math section. What are your goals for today, for this week, this month, and this year?

Make it measurable

Track what you do. Be totally honest. Use the Mannameter graph to monitor your progress compared to how similar people perform. If you are doing all the right things and things are not working out as expected, recruit the help of your physician, dietician or other knowledgeable health advisor. The answer is in there somewhere.

Is it realistic?

Can people really lose a thousand pounds without surgery? Can they only do it in a facility? What size frame am I? Sure, certain medical problems can slow your progress and add unwanted pounds, but that should never be an excuse for being morbidly overweight. I have control over what I eat. If others can do it, why not me?

At the same time, do not beat yourself up thinking that it is entirely your fault. It is more than just a matter of being weak-willed or having a terrible metabolism. Understand the nature of our economy. Millions of dollars are being spent this very moment on how to best push your hot buttons. You are being continually bombarded with subliminal messages cleverly designed to make you continue just the way you are. If you get healthy, somebody is going to lose money. Major business interests stake their very existence on the profits generated by obesity.

Clean house

The church tends to overemphasize the character of Jesus as meek and mild, gentle and suffering. There is another aspect to his personality revealed in John 2:14-15:

> *In the temple courts He found men trading cattle, sheep and doves and others sitting at tables exchanging money. So He made a whip of cords, and drove all from the temple area, both sheep and cattle; He scattered the coins of the moneychangers and overturned their tables..."Get these out of there! How dare you turn my Father's house into a marketplace!*

Jesus was not wimpy about the temple and neither should we. There comes a time when we have to take a stand and toss out the junk. If our temples (our bodies) are in disarray, it's time for to let it rip. Serious about your weight? Let me hear that once again, *with feeling!*

Failing to plan is planning to fail. My observation is that people

39

starting a weight management program before Thanksgiving and Christmas clearly outperform those starting at other times of the year. Perhaps it is because they demonstrate character in the face of endless treats. If you have to do it, you have to do it. Period! Being almost persuaded and waiting for a convenient time is just a sneaky way of copping out on your destiny. You have considered the options and you have settled on a plan of action. Now let's roll!

4. Pursue

There was a time when our lives were consumed with mediocrity, and stalling, (Prevent). Then, for whatever reason we realized something was missing, (Ponder). We decided what we wanted and how to get it (Plan). Now we must *pursue* it with passion. No more daydreaming and what-ifs. We want to see movement. We want to see results.

Observe a gentleman whose car has stalled on a busy highway. He pulls over to the side and checks under the hood. He comes to the conclusion that this car needs a real mechanic. He puts a call into AAA, and in the meantime, decides to push the vehicle to a safer shoulder of the road just 10 yards ahead. He tries to flag down help but there are no takers. With the driver's side window rolled down to steer, he tries to push the car along. It does not budge. He heaves harder. It rocks forward, but no go.

He knows he has to do this. Where he stopped is just too dangerous with cars whizzing past around the curve. He pauses, takes a few deep breaths and gives it all he has. At last, the car begins to roll, just a little bit. He keeps pushing real hard to keep it on a roll. At this point, he is no longer straining as he develops momentum. Just then, another car stops and three wrestler-types jump out. They offer to help and without waiting for an answer they all easily propel the car to safety. The driver thanks them and assures them that everything is under control. As they drive off, he wonders how much easier it would have been if they were there from the start.

The study of physics teaches us the concept of *inertia*. That is the force that keeps things at rest (or in a state of constant motion), unless acted upon by a greater outside force. This means the stalled car is quite happy to stay exactly where it is, thank you. In its moving days, it generated propulsion from its internal combustion engine. With the engine dead, it required some elbow grease. In fact, it required lots of physical energy in order to get it moving that first inch. The driver did all the hard work up front. Once the car *got moving*, the extra help was just gravy.

In like manner, it can be painfully difficult to get a serious weight management program off the ground. Mind you, we are not talking about some herd mentality, "let-me-try-that-because-everybody's-doing-it" diet. We are talking about a well thought-out, coordinated attack on all fronts to turn things around for good. However, once the initial inertia has been overcome, all of a sudden, it does not look like such a big sacrifice. It takes surprisingly less energy to maintain that momentum. This does not mean we will be immune from pitfalls. In fact, Chapters 15 and 20 detail exactly how to prepare for such bumps in the road.

Knowledge Not Enough

Knowing better does not always mean doing better. Consider the deeply touching story carried by Tiffin Ohio's *Advertiser Tribune*. It was about a young boy home alone while his father was at work. Before his mother unfortunately passed away a couple years before, she had rehearsed with him the steps to take in case of a tornado. The Great Lakes region is given to sudden storms as evidenced by the sinking of the *Edmund Fitzgerald* with loss its entire crew. Somehow, Tiffin was immune. At least, that was according to the old Native American legend which held that the fair city was built on "land of the parting winds." TV Doppler appeared to confirm that as the storms barreled eastward.

Despite the popular notion, when an urgent weather alert beeped on his computer, the boy did exactly what his mother had taught. He covered himself in the bathtub. For whatever reason, the tornado ignored tradition and unleashed a savage path of destruction through the county. The father rushed home. The scattered rubble at his address was the only evidence confirming another great loss. Neighbors however had rescued the boy unscathed, thanks to his knowledge which he *acted* upon.

A health professional may be exceedingly knowledgeable, but this is meaningless without the passion to move patients to action. With all that we know about weight, why is there so little progress? One just has to attend any medical convention to see how many physicians follow their own fitness advice. Some people are too smart for their own good. Simply knowing all kinds of stuff about fats and calories does not make one lean and healthy. Many who have done best on Manna*fast* are humble, trusting, people. Regardless how educated one may be, there comes a time when one has to move from saying, "I know that," to "I'm doing that."

Put Yourself on the Spot

Adolph Hitler, consummately evil as he was, did teach us something about strategy. His Storm Troopers beat up on the smaller countries of Europe before taking on the major powers of France, Britain and Russia. Early string of successes fueled a delusional superiority complex for total world domination. It finally took the combined might of the US-led Allied invasion of Normandy to crush the Nazi's dreaded aura of invincibility.

Likewise, losing weight is like a military campaign. Many good people do not accomplish anything worth talking about in life, not because they lack the ability, but basically because they are timid souls. One must establish a success habit by *securing small victories* at the beginning. If only there was a way to bottle the enthusiasm of the clients who return after just one week and having really lost two or three pounds. The joy is pure and unquenchable because they have new-found confidence. Suddenly, it is reality, not just words. No more "Round and round she goes, where she stops, nobody knows." They have shattered that ridiculous notion and the rest is history.

Once you have committed, you need to go after it *with passion*. It is okay to begin privately by challenging yourself. At some point, as you see definite progress, it helps to declare your intentions, beginning with your loved ones. They are going to ask anyway. You don't want them to wonder if you're coming down with some dreaded disease. Like a public confession of faith, you are putting yourself on the spot. At the same time, be careful not to be offensive. Remember that it took some time for you to navigate through planes of progress to get where you are. Too much of an "in your face" attitude may backfire. Others may see you as imposing on them, work or sacrifices that they are not emotionally ready to shoulder. Be wise and adjust your approach depending on your situation.

Losing weight is an inherently aggressive act. Picture it this way: Someone has lost 50 pounds and all that fat is laid out here on this table (not a pretty sight). Anyway, that would be about the size of a five-year old child! You have been carrying this "child" around with you 24/7. It is a little bit more of a stretch for men to grasp, but you get the picture. That weight loss is equivalent to carving out an alien, parasitic chunk of excess stuff from your body. You are commanded to slay it, and destroy it! Listen to these strong words and remember who said them: "If thy hand or thy foot offends thee, cut it off!" (Matthew 18:8). Same principle. That noxious 50-pound mass it not going to excuse itself politely. It's a living thing, and living things generally do not concede to extermination without a struggle.

Or we can use a kinder, simpler picture. A basic office chair weighs about 15 - 20 pounds. I pick it up and ask a patient who has lost that much to hold it up for me. That's not too bad. The longer they hold it up the heavier it seems to get. Soon, they are begging me to let them put it down. If nothing else dramatizes the burden they have been carrying, this always does.

Get Fired Up

You must henceforth declare to the entire universe that you and those extra pounds have irreconcilable differences. That is going to be contested. This fat would much rather stay where it is. Your mission is to disown, disinherit and dispose of it. If you do not, one of those days when you gingerly step on the scales, we are likely to hear that eerie, haunting voice whispering, "I'm baaack!"

The Gospels described the Lord's anguish in the garden of Gethsemane as he embarked on His passion. He *set His face* toward Jerusalem (Luke 9:51). He was fully aware that a series of not so nice things were about to happen. He had to prepare Himself for the greatest of all challenges imaginable. Likewise, we cannot be casual or nonchalant about massive weight loss. Let our conversation and body language reflect that. I find myself routinely *un-slouching* patients in the office. They look defeated even before starting. *Get set.* Chin up, shoulders back, let's do it! Those who do well develop a stature of confidence and radiate that kind of hope. Much of our job as healthcare providers consists of convincing patients first of all, that vibrant health is really what they want and secondly, they can do this. Once they are focused, it is just a matter of time.

5. Persevere

Christopher Columbus was on this hare-brained mission to find a new route to India. Conventional wisdom had it that sail too far west and risk dropping off the face of the earth. Sounds silly to us today, but in 1492, to even think otherwise could earn you a one-way ticket to the land of crispy critters. Besides burning at the stake, the church authorities in the Dark Ages were also very fond of casting heretics into dungeons, selling them into slavery, tenderizing them in "iron maidens" or chopping off their heads. Watching today's world news reminds us that religious intolerance to new ideas has not changed much over the centuries.

Nevertheless, to any sailor worth his salt, old Chris had already gone off the deep end. As a result, Columbus could only get convicts and derelicts to man his ships. Despite their dead-end lives, they desperately wanted to live. Each time the *Nina, Pinta* and *Santa Maria* crested a big wave, the bottom of their hardened hearts dropped with that sinking feeling. Each time, in sheer, expletive terror, they went, "Oh no! - This is it!" Columbus stared down mutiny from violent men on the verge of freaking out. He bravely stood on his beliefs. He bargained with them. "Give me three more days; if we don't see land, then do with me what you must!"

As they say - the rest is history. Most of us now live where we do because Columbus did not give up. He persevered. In much the same way, everyone afflicted with obesity gets the hare-brain notion that they too shall overcome. Negative forces are everywhere saying "Give it up. You'll always be a fatty." In the Scriptures it took just three days to arise in newness of life. However, experienced coaches and counselors agree that if one is able to maintain a new course for *just three weeks*, the success habit is set. That's all it takes and you'll have it made! We call that *getting over the hump.*

Perseverance is the green plane, symbolizing the abundant life. Stick with a plan for that period of initiation and you will begin doing the right thing automatically. Results begin to become visible for others to see. They notice the changes, they sense your energy. You start getting compliments. Medical conditions improve. You begin reaping the benefits and guess what? People start asking you for advice. Imagine that!

A Harvard University study concluded that there is no medical reason why the average adult should not be able to maintain the weight they attained at age 21. That point represents the time of physical, emotional and perhaps vocational maturation. Everything after that, (including the widely accepted "middle-age spread"), is a generally a result of social conditioning and lifestyle choices.

Remember *your five top reasons for losing weight.* Put that list in conspicuous places: on your bedroom side table right next to the clock, on the mirror over the bathroom sink, on the dresser, in your purse or PDA, Pocket PC, on the refrigerator, dashboard, locker, lunch box, briefcase, desk or computer. It will serve as a reminder and motivator whenever you are struggling or get that sinking feeling that you are about to quit again.

What if when a baby is taking its first steps, it plops down - and stays down!? What if that little toddler says in his mind, "You know what? I'll never get this walking thing together like everybody else has. I give up! I'll just let Mom carry me around the rest of my life." Obviously, you did not say that, and neither did I. We did not learn the negative art of quitting. Each time we fell, we got up again - we were expected to.

The pessimists of this world are just waiting for you to slip up. They just cannot wait to justify their negativity with, "I told you so." When a person comes around with a decision to improve their health, I

> *The greatest glory lies not in never falling, but in rising every time we fall.*
>
> **Nelson Mandela**, President S. Africa

have no doubt that this is God's doing. Philippians 2:13 exhorts, "Being confident of this one thing that *God* who has begun a good work in you *will complete it.*" No baby ever had to figure out how to walk. God took care of that. Trust. Weight loss is not rocket science. Take that step of faith. Soon you will be looking back at the footprints in the sands of time, amazed at how far He has carried you.

Repetition

What is weight-loss failure anyway? Just because one regains a few pounds or has not lost any for two or three months does not equal failure. As long as we keep on doing the right thing, we cannot fail. Chapter 15, *Keeping it Real*, describes how to inoculate oneself from different forms of eating disorders when lonely, disappointed and unhappy. Most of our exceptional clients had to bounce back several times. We had to hammer away at the fundamentals until they got it. After that, they were pretty much unstoppable - and so will you!

We have shown how successful weight management is primarily determined by one's psychological/spiritual state. To thine own self be true. Figuring out where you stand on the *planes of progress* literally makes all the difference in the world. This chapter dealt mainly with the mind. Next, we deal with the body and how it is affected. Remember your Lifescore and weight may fluctuate, but you will be amazed at your overall transformation as you continue to refine the techniques presented here.

When the student is ready,

the teacher appears.

Buddhist proverb

45

REVIEW

1. Compare the staging of cancer to the staging obesity.

2. Which plane of progress do you believe you are currently on?

3. Describe some behaviors of people on the *prevent* plane.

4. Describe someone you admire on the *perseverance* plane.

5. What is your main challenge for moving up on the planes of progress?

Chapter 4
Obesity Epidemic

How easy for those who do not bulge.
to overindulge.

Ogden Nash

W hat is an epidemic anyway? The word harkens back centuries ago to the days of the Bubonic Plague. People were petrified. Each morning they peered out through their blinds, summoned by the sounds of creaking wheels. The grave diggers' shuffling footsteps preceded eerie cries piercing the foggy morning air. "Bring out your dead!" Whose body was it to be piled onto the dreaded death wagon this day? Or could it be they were already dead and their spirits were just looking on?

The terror pushed communal sanity to its limits. Citizens locked themselves in their houses, turned to increasingly desperate magical cures, or fled en masse from the urban areas. Country folk feared city dwellers were Bubonic-plague positive. Commerce ground to a standstill. An entire civilization was threatened. Before it was all over, one third of China's population perished. A couple million a year perished between the years of 1347-51. Interestingly enough, few realize that the Flu Epidemic of 1918 killed more people in one year (20 million) than *The Plague*. Today, the specter of AIDS and Bird Flu are being compared to these epidemics by which all others would be judged.

How was such contagion overcome? Several measures were taken, but it clearly was not the result of some fantastic vaccine or antibiotic breakthrough. Actually, these pestilences were defeated in large part by applying basic sanitation, quarantine and control principles gleaned from wisdom literature of the ancients. Tremendous advances in medicine have given way to proliferation of self-inflicted diseases. Today, the word epidemic is being used to describe the ravages of obesity as well. Will it be overcome by some fantastic drug or sleek operation? Not if history is a guide. It could be that use of the word epidemic is too loose, too sensational or premature? Or could it already be a pandemic, affecting the majority of countries around the world?

A billboard promoting the opening of a California health club raised quite ruckus. Depicting an alien, it was captioned: *When they come, they'll eat the fat ones first!* A large number of weight-challenged people took exception. Picketers with rather expressive placards elicited a great deal of honking support. On a slow news-day, it got a remarkable amount of press. For the most part, the public opinion was that while the billboard was somewhat insensitive, the demonstrators should get a grip. Whatever! This episode however definitely proved two things:

(1) The club got its publicity;

(2) Our problem with weight has clearly reached critical mass.

Once the Healthiest

Without a doubt, USA is # 1! When it comes to the number of Nobel Prize winners, the wealth of our health insurance companies and malpractice attorneys, the technology in our hospitals, and the best physicians and nurses drawn from all over the world, no other country even comes close. How much bang do we get for our buck? Actually, the United States, in the span of a century, has plunged from being the healthiest country in the world to now being *one of the least healthy among developed nations*.

According to the World Health Organization, the US now ranks #24. This assessment was based on limited access to health care among the poor, cigarette smoking, violence and *obesity*. The ten healthiest countries at this time are, in order: Japan, Australia, France, Sweden, Spain, Italy, Greece, Switzerland, Monaco, and Andorra.

One may not fully grasp the impact of the obesity epidemic until actually seeing the dynamic PowerPoint slide show. Go to mannafast-org or to the Centers for Disease Control website (www.cdc.gov) and search for "obesity maps." The alarming speed with which obesity seemingly gobbles up entire regions in the United States gives the visual effect of trying to outrun an avalanche or volcanic pyroclastic flow. The typical reaction when one personally checks out the visual is "Wow! I didn't know it was that bad." Like a freight train totally out of control, obesity seems to mock our puny efforts to stem the tide. This is precisely why it such an accomplishment working to make your corner of the world an oasis of fitness and health.

CDC statistics reveal that in 1900 only 6 percent of the US population was obese. By1960, that was up to a modest 12 percent and no more

4. Obesity Epidemic

than 15 percent by1980. By 2001 the number of obese had shot past 25 percent. The overwhelming majority of the population, 66 percent was overweight! The heaviest states were Louisiana, Alabama and Mississippi. The leanest were Colorado, Massachusetts and Vermont at about 16 and 17 percent respectively. According to *Men's Fitness* magazine the three fittest institutions of higher learning were Brigham Young in Utah, the University of California, Santa Barbara and Boston University. Topping the list of fattest schools: University of Louisiana at Lafayette, followed by University of New Orleans and Mississippi State University. Chapter 14 deals with how shared customs in these geographic areas directly impacts personal weight.

Research of the literature shows that massive obesity, once an oddity is rapidly becoming an everyday occurrence. Perhaps the earliest known narrative is the description of the assassination of King Eglon in Judges 3:14-30. Eglon was described as a rather large man who was oppressing the children of Israel. He was eventually stabbed by Ehud, the left-handed Hebrew undercover agent. The account graphically describes how there was so much abdominal fat that the sword got stuck up to the hilt. The Roman physician Galen later wrote about one Nichomachus of Smyrna who was bed bound from sheer obesity - a historic occurrence. Then there was a Roman senator who required two slaves to *help carry his belly for him* on his way to the forum.

As extreme as these cases may sound, each town in America today harbors an increasing number of citizens bed-bound by obesity. Additions to the so-called 1000 Pound Club have been coming in thick and fast. Perhaps the best known early examples are Jon Minnoch of Bainbridge Island in the state of Washington. He was estimated to be in excess of 1200 pounds and succumbed to medical complications at age 43. The other was Carol Yeager of Flint Michigan weighing in at 1189. Legend has it that her surging weight frustrated her loved ones and seriously affected her moral compass. When her boyfriend quit, she went into a steep decline from which she never recovered. Carol will forever be 34. Interestingly, family members were nowhere as obese. This argues strongly that genetics and metabolism are not nearly as essential factors in a great number of cases.

Sensationalist talk show hosts and diet gurus took advantage of both Minnoch and Yeager. They promised assistance but delivered little. Though our patient featured on the Discovery Channel was possibly the heaviest human recorded, he survived as a result of intensive long-term professional and subsequent community support. The same cannot be said of those made into public spectacles. Ethical concerns ensure that those seeking help from us will have their privacy respected. As stipulated earlier, identifying features of examples referenced in this book are deliberately altered so that these individuals can resume normal lives with their families and friends.

Society is constantly retreating and adapting to the reality of very large people. Health-O-Meter's typical bathroom scale 20 years ago went up to 270 pounds. Newer models now have to go up to 400. Physician offices increasingly have to refer patients to hospitals, farm scales and freight facilities to be weighed. Understanding the pervasive effects of obesity will help us commit to challenge each other to do whatever we can to turn things around.

Conditions Caused By Obesity

Some would have us believe that obesity as simply a lifestyle choice or even a spectacle for entertainment. The stark truth is that obesity causes sickness, the full extent and different manifestations of which is only now becoming clear:

Diabetes

In my speech class, one student chose to demonstrate how she had to care for her diabetes. She calmly stabbed a grapefruit with an insulin syringe. Ask me to name my top images from those college days and this one is right up there. That singular act seared an indelible impression into my psyche. Why? Because our hearts went out to the poor thing, having to poke herself with needles like that, so many times a day. Just the needle part made one classmate sick. We had no way of knowing that *in less than thirty years the number of diabetics would increase ten-fold!* Diabetes is now so common, a similar presentation today would probably elicit yawns of "Tell me something new."

Type II Diabetes is an acquired condition, thought to be the result of a lifetime of dietary indiscretion. 90 percent of Type II diabetics are obese. Just twenty years ago, the disease used to be called "adult onset diabetes," first showing up around age 60. Unfortunately, as described in Chapter 17, Type II Diabetes is now rising sharply among children.

This distinction between Type I and Type II is blurring. Patients are increasingly being diagnosed with double diabetes. The common thread is the ineffective use of insulin; a condition called *insulin resistance*. Adding high blood pressure and high cholesterol to the mix results in *Syndrome*

4. Obesity Epidemic

X. Such individuals are like medical time bombs. Experts believe that for every one child with Type II Diabetes, there could be at least four in the pipeline with Syndrome X. It is scary to imagine that by the time today's innocent, young diabetics reach their 20's and 30's, many will suffer from kidney disease, heart attacks, nerve damage (neuropathy), blindness and amputations.

But from an economic standpoint, it is not all bad. Investors in biotech and pharmaceutical companies are making a killing. Thanks to obesity, diabetes rates are soaring even higher than predicted. 17 million Americans are now diabetic. There are over 800,000 new cases of diabetes annually, *nearly half of them children.* If television ad icon BB King got royalties on every glucometer sold, he could give up singing the Blues. Worldwide, experts estimate that cases of diabetes will triple in the next 15 years to about 320 million! Listen to the "chi-ching!" of cash registers and the sound of quarterly earnings ripping through the roof. This may offer some clue as to why many in positions of influence appear complacent in taming this beast.

Rubin, and others, showed in a 1992 study that the cost of caring for confirmed diabetics was more than *four times greater* than for non-diabetics. Back in 1992, diabetics constituted 4.5 percent of the U.S. population, but accounted for 14.6 percent of total US health care expenditures ($105 billion). As a result, once people accept their diagnosis, they tend to feel that diabetes medication and fancier gadgets will make them well. Weight loss for diabetics can be tricky. Not eating on time risks potentially dangerous hypoglycemic shock (fainting). Yet, insulin, while a godsend, also tends to store excess calories as fat. The vicious cycle of more fat and lack of effective weight management sucks the diabetic down a whirlpool of complications.

The evidence from most researchers is pretty compelling: just 30 minutes of daily exercise and 5 percent weight loss is more effective than medical treatment. 90 percent of overweight diabetics no longer need insulin on the Mannafast program. The vast majority will definitely reduce (or no longer need) diabetic pills once they approach the minimally acceptable medical weight. By so doing, they avoid the drug side effects and terrible micro-vascular complications of the disease detailed above.

Heart and Blood Vessel Disease

Heart disease and stroke account for half of all deaths in the US. It is the nation's #1 killer. A high fat, high cholesterol diet causes arteriosclerosis.

This is inflammation in the vessel wall with hardening and narrowing of the arteries. Spasm of a narrowed artery reduces the flow of blood to the heart. The heart cringes in pain, a sensation known as angina pectoris. Some describe it as tightness, heaviness or "like an elephant sitting on their chest." This crushing pain may extend or radiate to the neck, jaw, or left arm. If a blood clot then forms in the area of an ulcerated plaque, it suddenly cuts off blood supply to part of the pump muscle. Such a heart attack (myocardial infarction) is often associated with a cold sweat and fear of impending doom.

> *Low-fat* **yogurt** *is a great source of protein and calcium for strong bones and a healthy heart. Contains live bacterial cultures of Lactobacilus or Acidophilus which helps with digestion and longevity.*

Things may appear totally normal, the next moment, the ground rushing up to meet one's face. Every year in the United States, a myocardial infarction/heart attack is the first sign of heart disease in about 500,000 people. Tragically, for 150,000 of those, it is also the last sign. We recommend a lipid profile (see pages 104 -106) for all new patients and include a blood count and chemistry profile if necessary. It is always quite revealing how many silent disease conditions we pick up when someone decides it is time to do something about his or her weight.

A similar process occurs in the carotid arteries of the neck that supply blood to the brain. When an ulcerated plaque embolizes (breaks off and carried in the bloodstream), it starves parts of the brain of its blood supply. This is a stroke. It is a major cause of unexplained traffic accidents and people dying suddenly in their sleep. Those who survive usually suffer from speech impairment, loss of use of one side of the body and a range of disabilities of which we are all too familiar. Before the 1990's, strokes occurred mostly in the elderly. Nowadays it occurs with increasing frequency among those in their forties and fifties.

Statistics prove in no uncertain terms that the obese are approximately 6 times more likely to develop heart disease and strokes than those of normal weight. They are *40 times as likely to suffer sudden death*. The poor heart simply poops out from the continuous strain of pumping gallons of blood through so large a body.

The average age of a man having a heart attack is 65.8 years, for a woman 70.4. This statistic confirmed my long-held observation that a disturbing number of males seemed to be punching out soon after retirement. Following a lifetime of hard work these men never get to enjoy

4. Obesity Epidemic

those golden years. Those fortunate enough to experience the warning sign of angina go through the routine of high-tech stress testing, cardiac catheterization and coronary bypass. The price tag for treating the 60 million Americans with heart disease is about half a trillion dollars. People talk adventurously about their heart procedure and the pride taken in cheating death. Researchers writing in the *American Journal of Prevention Medicine* suggest all this could be reduced substantially by simply quitting smoking and turning from a high-fat, overweight, sedentary lifestyle.

Stomach Problems

Obesity is a major cause of Gastro-Esophageal Reflux Disease (GERD). This is more commonly known as heartburn although it has nothing really to do with the heart. The upper opening of the stomach (gastro-esophageal sphincter, which is not far from the heart) does not close well when there is increased pressure from a large amount of abdominal fat. Acid from the stomach backwashes up the esophagus. It burns the lining of this feeding tube causing it to become inflamed and swollen. This is one of the two reasons why the obese have difficulty lying flat. Eating slower and avoiding large meals less than a couple hours before bedtime can help reduce symptoms of reflux.

Heartburn affects almost half of the population. The march of the obesity epidemic contributes to the enormous profitability of heartburn medicines (see Chapter 5) with their side effect of increased hip fractures. It is estimated that up to 15 percent of patients with even occasional heartburn will develop a condition known as *Barrett's esophagus*. This is a change in the lining of the esophagus that can eventually lead to cancer. Obesity also contributes directly to constipation and gallstones, which are solid deposits of cholesterol in the gallbladder.

Breathing Difficulty

Excess weight on the rib cage makes it difficult to expand the lungs or to lie flat. This decreases excursion of the chest causing shortness of breath and *hypoxia,* (not enough oxygen in the bloodstream). It becomes increasingly harder to climb stairs, get in and out of vehicles, pick up the mail, go shopping and perform basic household chores. Such difficulty breathing is called *Pickwickian syndrome*, after jolly overweight character in a Charles Dickens 1837 novel, *The Pickwick Papers.*

Laying flat presses the heavy belly up on the lungs. Spouses may describe such patients as snoring hard and gasping for breath. Before they conquered their weight problem, many of our patients had to sleep semi-upright in the easy chair. As you can imagine, this does little to advance the cause of intimacy, although the spouse left in the bedroom is greatly relieved to finally sleep in peace. This restlessness is called *sleep apnea*, which is diagnosed with a sleep study. It is a major consideration when seeking pre-certification for obesity surgery. Sleep apnea also causes headache, irritability, irregular heart rhythm and eventually cor pulmonale (right heart failure).

"The fat and lazy" syndrome historically arises from the fact that the obese are chronically fatigued due to poor sleep. They suffer from increased daytime sleepiness also known as *narcolepsy*. They fall asleep while at work, during movies, on the phone or even in interpersonal situations. It is difficult to estimate just how many accidents are caused by narcolepsy. Traffic police, emergency room physicians and auto insurance analysts believe that it is probably responsible for a significant percentage of cases where there is no evidence of alcohol, distractions or skid marks.

Depression

Desperate parents brought a 14 year-old boy to the office because he had very specific suicide plans. The other kids called him "lard butt" and never picked him for their teams on the playground. Overweight kids endure cruel remarks and jokes. Referring to an absent student, one teacher jokingly remarked to the class that the child was probably at home eating. With nurturing like that, it is not difficult to understand how these kids begin to despise themselves. According to the National Institutes of Health, heavy children were five times more likely to suffer depression. Their level of sadness and despair is about the same as children undergoing chemotherapy. They are less likely to date. When they do enter relationships, they are more likely to be abused and neglected.

Do depressed people develop obesity from not moving; or do obese patients get depressed over not being able to move well? This is the classic chicken or the egg conundrum. The interplay is quite intricate and probably varies from person to person. What we do know is that the thrill of overcoming obesity translates into reduced need for depression medication. When people get good help with this problem, their excitement knows no bounds. We examine this topic in further detail in Chapter 8, *Eating Disorders*.

Social Stresses

Four out of five overweight individuals blame their weight for less than satisfactory social life and upward mobility. Many healthcare professionals tend to see this as a private matter unless there are "medical" complications. Often times, physicians offer little assistance beyond a condescending, "You should exercise more and try to lose some weight." This is of little help to patients who left literally to the mercy of myriad weight loss schemes vying for their attention. Frustration with weight shows up in all kinds of dysfunctional relationships. Jessica (in *Jumpstart*) could probably attest to that.

Reproductive Distress

Obesity induces hormonal disturbances from painful ovarian cysts and uterine fibroids. This results in a higher infertility incidence of severe menstrual irregularities, infertility, facial hair and acne. It also increases the risk of high blood pressure (eclampsia), gestational diabetes, urinary tract infections, blood clots, prolonged labor, birth defects, stillbirths and likelihood of caesarian delivery.

In the past, stress incontinence was associated with the elderly. Today it is common in the relatively young obese patient, especially after pregnancy. A persistent large belly weakens the pelvic muscles and damages the valve of the bladder. This leads to leakage of urine when coughing, sneezing, or laughing. To avoid interruption in their activities or embarrassing themselves in public, many women resort to absorbent undergarments. Those funny "I've got to go" overactive bladder ads seldom portray obesity as a cause or weight reduction as a solution.

In men, obesity contributes to hypogonadism or reduced testosterone levels and *low sperm count*. This affects secondary sex characteristics like body hair and sex drive. They are more likely to need medication for erectile dysfunction. I generally refer such patients to an urologist for a formal impotence evaluation and a cardiologist to minimize any risk. Often times the patient returns frustrated because the problem turns out to be simply logistical: the belly gets in the way.

Joint Pain

Excess body weight places increased wear and tear on the joints. The obese are also at higher risk for carpal tunnel syndrome and other problems involving nerves in their elbows and wrists. Obesity makes involvement in sports, exercise or even regular work a rather painful affair.

Excess weight makes it difficult for factory workers having to stand all day on hard, concrete floors. This increases the risk for low back pain and arthritis. As a result, the obese unemployment rate is higher and participation in social activities is lower. Idleness leads to even more obesity, which leads to more joint pain and the vicious cycle continues. Joint replacement has much poorer results in the obese. Orthopedic surgeons generally shun operating on severely overweight patients because of escalating risks and premature failure of the arthroplasty.

Weight reduction significantly relieves joint pain. My Mom's case provides a good illustration. Growing up on the island, she hurt her right knee while working on her Pappy's garden in Layou Valley. This turned out to be a "greenstick" fracture that had not been diagnosed or effectively treated. In time, it became progressively more arthritic, painful and out of alignment. Overcompensation on the left also hastened degenerative changes there as well. Bilateral knee replacement was subsequently recommended in the United States. As immigrants with no health insurance, the cost was prohibitive, but the family was ready to make the sacrifice. To improve her overall medical condition, I supervised my Mom in a 35-pound weight reduction. For the first time in over two decades she was less than 200 pounds and felt better than ever. Just that amount of weight loss made such a huge difference in her pain level that knee replacement was safely postponed for 15 wonderful years.

Varicose Veins

The veins carry blood back to the heart. Leg veins are equipped with one-way valves to keep the flow upward. The pressure of a large abdomen may increase the load on these valves. The damaged valves cause venous insufficiency, spider veins, followed by more enlarged, unsightly varicose veins. In early stages, injecting them in the surgeon's office followed by treatment with support stockings often yields excellent results. If allowed to get worse, they may require vein stripping in the operating room. This leaves multiple ¹/2 inch scars on the legs. An important reason to take good care of leg veins is that they might be needed in the future for coronary artery bypass.

Vein problems can be genetic, but also follows pregnancy weight gain. Weakened veins cause edema (swelling) of the lower legs as fluid leaks into the tissues. This predisposes to recurrent skin infections called *cellulitis*. The leg frequently becomes red, hot and painful, later causing fevers and sepsis. Preventive treatment with lymphedema therapy involves elevation, diuretics to treat fluid retention and specialized leg compression wraps.

If the situation is not managed properly, pressure in the lower legs continues to increase causing thickening and darkening of the skin. This deteriorates into large, doughy sacks of fat, a mostly irreversible condition known as *lipodermatosclerosis*. Without definitive care, resistant (venous stasis) ulceration of the skin develops. At that point, treatment involves paste bandages (Unna boots) and possibly additional specialized topical preparations (with or without growth factor from recombinant DNA).

Skin Problems

Obesity causes chronic rashes as the large folds of fat rub against each other and traps moisture. There is a constant battle with yeast or fungal infections, the odor of which makes patients less sociable. Darkish velvety areas develop around the neck and armpits known as *acanthosis nigricans*. This is often associated with skin tags, which are signs of other clinical problems on the horizon.

Skin is elastic, up to a point. Even with impressive weight loss, these rolls do not automatically go away. Instead, they drop down as hanging, floppy sacks that interfere with the patient's increasing mobility. Surgical removal is associated with a tremendous infection rate because of difficulty keeping dressings clean and intact. These procedures are generally not covered by insurers even with very time-consuming efforts by the surgeon to pre-certify. If approved, reimbursement is so low that few surgeons are inclined to take the risk. Television often gives the impression that surgeons can simply re-sculpture the body as if it were really plastic. However, allowing massive weight to accumulate lead to all manner of woe not fully appreciated by the general public.

Cancer

According to the American Cancer Society, one third of all cancer deaths are directly related to diet and inactivity. Even so, less than 1% of the population is aware that obesity is a cancer risk. Statistics demonstrate that one quarter to one third of all deaths in the developed world is due to cancers. That translates in up to 300,000 lives a year could be saved in the US if we get a better handle on obesity.

Findings by Dr. Michelle Holmes of the Harvard Medical School were even more dramatic. Regular walking can increase survival rate of breast cancer by 50%. (*Journal of the American Medical Association* May 2005). This explains why we are not really making a dent in the overall cancer rate despite increasingly more sophisticated technology and expensive drug and surgical treatments. There are over 100 different types of cancer; few more emotionally devastating than breast cancer. It is three times more common in the obese. Overweight men have a higher risk of cancer of the colon and the prostate. Other cancers such as cervix and gallbladder are increased in the overweight. While the causes are diverse, most experts agree that up to three quarters of tumors are preventable. In Chapter 9 we discuss a new controversial cause of cancer related to invasive obesity treatment.

How Did We Get Here?

Consider what impresses refugees most upon surfacing in a developed country. More than all the fascinating modern conveniences and technology, it is at the supermarket that the culture shock truly hits home. They are greeted with gleaming aisles upon aisles of groceries of every kind, so clean and delightfully packaged, a blazing temptation to the palate. This is truly overwhelming.

What a blessing it is to live in a country which has never experienced wide scale hunger! The flip side is the curse of unbridled consumption. In 1980 the average American adult consumed 1854 calories everyday. By the new millennium, that average was up to 2002 calories per day due to increased portion sizes. That additional 148 calories per day translated into an extra 15 pounds per year. We are also told that the average American adult weighed 166 pounds in 1980 and 176 pounds in 2000, a 10-pound increase.

Once again, do the math. If we accept these statistics, what would be the total weight gain of the average American in those 20 years? The increase would be:

20 years x 15 pounds = 300 pounds for 20 years.

Still with me? This is not hard. What that means is that in order to limit the *average* increase to just 10 pounds (166 to 176), the average American had to lose 290 of those pounds over the past 20 years. Let us review: The average American adult, by consuming an extra 148 calories per day, gained 300 pounds in the past 20 years. He has lost 290, and is now 10 pounds heavier, on average.

Now, let us leave the population statistics for the moment and look at it from the point of view of the individual. When someone says I have gained and lost x number of pounds so many times, they are being perfectly accurate. They had to, otherwise they would have increased their weight to 466 pounds (166 in 1980 plus the 300 pounds gained in 20 years). This explains why so many of our patients can range in weight from 400 to 1400 pounds! Can you picture yourself at that weight?

Compare that to the Japanese; the healthiest people in the world. At least, that is the consensus of the vast majority of university professors and international agencies. During the same period of relative prosperity they have managed to *decrease* their caloric intake (not compelled by crop failure, natural disaster or war) by 192 calories per day. Result? 66% of American are overweight, compared to 2% of Japanese! It is not even close.

After the US went nuclear on Japan in 1945, there was a feeling of national euphoria associated with a sense of invincibility and superiority. That was until Sputnik and the Cold War had us practicing ducking into bomb shelters. For three decades we were haunted by the ticking of the doomsday clock. The fall of the Berlin Wall in 1989 signaled the end of the "Evil Empire" and the first Iraq War buried the ghost of Vietnam. There seemed to be no end to the wealth created on Wall Street and Silicon Valley. America went into a feeding frenzy. Even after September 11th sent shock waves throughout the economy and increased our sense of vulnerability, we merrily kept right on bingeing. Continued expenses from War on Terror and the exporting of manufacturing jobs combined to raise poverty rates in the face of unrestrained prosperity in the financial markets. As we analyze how these mega-trends impact our weight, we would do well to consider how countries like Japan have managed to become both more prosperous and leaner/healthier at the same time.

Eating Out, Eating More

The TV crew had come down from Toronto to film the *Discovery Channel's Obesity Epidemic* special at our facilities. After a hard day's work we headed out for dinner at this rustic restaurant overlooking the Sandusky River. Quaint, farming implements from pioneering days adorned the walls of the refurbished water-powered mill to provide a quintessential Midwestern ambiance.

"Is that for me, or *for us*?" Brett's eyes opened wide in mock amazement as the waitress graciously placed the large, heaping trough before him. As narrator, and team leader, he had the knack for expressing with pithy wit things that others were just thinking. We all chuckled, commenting on the size of our platters as well. Although only 4 hours away, it was evident that our Canadian guests had distinctly more European culinary tastes. They seemed satisfied with more reasonable smaller portions. Meals majored in taste, texture and conversation; rather than speed and "value" size meals. Japanese researchers also came to the heartland to investigate our massive patients. Their reaction and conclusions were remarkably similar.

These are the simple facts. In 1950, only 5 percent of American meals were eaten out. In most cases it was a special occasion. Fifty years later, over half of our meals are eaten out; mostly fast food. It has been estimated that 3/4 the American population routinely eats out at least once a month. According to the *Journal of the American Medical Association*, between 1977 and 1996, food portion sizes increased both inside and outside the home by anywhere from 50 to 130 percent!

"Cool!" Some may say, especially if they are easily entertained by events sanctioned by the International Federation of Competitive Eating. The person able to cram down the most hot dogs or hamburgers per minute wins some fabulous trophy, TV bragging rights and maybe even a brand new car! Still wonder where is all this fat coming from? It may not be a vast corporate conspiracy, but let us not be naïve about this. This is America, and mega-trends respond to pure market forces. If the powerful were not profiting from it, the march of obesity would be fizzling, not sizzling.

At the drive through window, an innocent high school voice asks, "Do want fries to go with that?" Or "Would you like to biggie-size/super-size your order for just 35 cents?" Many people deny these offers have any impact on their selections. The fact is that the fast food restaurants know that it works, and works quite well for that matter. Fierce retail price competition is fueled by special incentives to the shift that sells the most combos and biggie sizes.

Widespread loss of food control ravages health. The connection has long been established. Over five hundred years ago William Shakespeare wrote:

> *If music be the food of love, play on,*
> *Give me excess of it, that, surfeiting,*
> *That appetite may sicken and so die.*

> Twelfth Night

Translated into simple, modern English, *excess food sickens and causes death*. Obesity shortens lives. As one patient was frank enough to tell me, "Some people overeat because they have issues. I overeat, because I just love food!" I too, love food. But I love myself more. I know only too well that food can fill and food can kill.

Way back in 1939, McCay, C.M. et al described animal experiments which conclusively confirmed this concept (*Journal of Nutrition*). Rats were separated into two groups. One group was provided the average amount of food. The other group was restricted to somewhat less than average. Overfed rats had a 68 percent higher death rate. Those fed less (but definitely not starved) had 39 percent lower death rate than average. These findings have been consistently duplicated by scientists all over the world. Given our fantastic advances in medicine, the *Caloric Restriction Society* projects a routine lifespan of 120 years for those limiting their food intake to just 75 percent of current consumption. This squares with Manna*fast's* Biblical fasting principles and trends we are seeing in our own practice everyday.

The Bubonic Plague was at a time in history when life was described by Thomas Hobbes as "nasty, brutish and short," (*Leviathan*, 1691). Even the poorest among us are rich compared to the constant threat of starvation hanging over the heads of the exploited masses in ages past. Today, we can all identify with that sense of fortune that comes from having access to more/better food than the next person. Just listen to someone excitedly describing his ravenous assault on the delicious spread at some reception, party, picnic or cruise. Obesity exists because the media has conditioned us to think that we eat normally when in fact quite the opposite is true.

Chapter 7 proves that surgical restriction of food intake results in guaranteed weight loss. Mannafast teaches us how obtain even superior results entirely on our own. To be enlightened about nutrition is to understand that only by systematically shrinking our stomachs to desire less can we avoid feeling deprived. It is so simple, yet so true. Mannafast constantly reminds us to eat just a little less than we're accustomed to or want to, right at this moment. It is natural method liberating us to truly enjoy the goodness of food. Whatever our present condition, we must believe that God's will for our lives is to be blessed with fitness, energy and longevity. This singular pleasure belongs rightly to those who can connect the direct health consequences to how heavy we load our plates

To lengthen thy life,
lessen thy meals

Benjamin Franklin

REVIEW

1. How does obesity affect relationships?

2. What is Syndrome X?

3. Portion sizes have increased by how much over the past 50 years?

4. Name 3 main reasons for current American health ranking compared with other nations?

5. What did Shakespeare write about excess food?

Chapter 5
Stomach Conditioning

With God, all things are possible.

Ohio State Motto

"Tastes great!" chanted on group of fans.
"Less filling!" countered another, about their same favorite beverage. "Tastes great!" "Less filling!" "Tastes great!" "Less filling!" and so it continued, tipsy and titillating, but not really meant to be logical. Much the same can be said of the great diet debate of our times: "Lo carb!" "Low fat!" "Lo carb!" "Lo fat!" Well, by now it is evident that these unending arguments about the ratio of carbs, fats and proteins in popular diets have hardly made a dent in the obesity epidemic. Indeed, my experience as a surgeon suggests that only reduced stomach capacity produces massive, *sustained* weight loss. This is because obesity results from *overall* food intake exceeding energy expenditure for that particular individual, age, gender and lifestyle. Just as putting clean water into dirty a container defeats the purpose, so too, all diets eventually fail if *the stomach itself* is not effectively transformed.

As we explore exactly how the stomach functions, we learn how to make it work for us. The study of obesity confirms that overeating causes the stomach to become stretched and oversized. Cinderella's sisters could not get their feet into her inelastic glass slipper. However, when I forced my big feet into my kid bother's new shoes, he somehow knew it no longer fit the same. The good news is that when it comes to the stomach, there are two ways to reduce this enlargement. At present, the best-known and most obvious way is through weight loss (bariatric) surgery. It is highly effective, but invasive (see Chapter 9, *Surgical Options*). It will soon become clear that the *best way by far*, is through the simple stomach conditioning program. I have had the privilege of managing obesity both ways. I am about to share with you the secret, step by step: How to condition the stomach - literally *shrinking* it to deliver that final, lasting, weight-loss breakthrough!

Who Is In Control Anyway?

Before we start, it is imperative that we firmly establish who is in charge here. You are of course! To embrace gastric (stomach) conditioning is to become what the philosophers call the *prime mover*, the active, original agent of change. With surgery, you are the *patient*. Picture the word. What do you see? A sick, dependent person, passively waiting in a room for the all-knowing, all-powerful physician to do something *to* him. Shakespeare's Hamlet saw you and me differently:

> *What a piece of work is man! How noble in reason!*
> *How infinite in faculty!*
> *In form and moving how express and admirable!*
> *In action how like an angel! In apprehension how like a god!*
> *The beauty of the world! The paragon of animals!*

The human body is so beautiful, so fascinating! Look in the mirror. Right this moment, you may not feel exactly like describing yourself in such majestic, poetic terms. No problem. Just watch how this changes.

From reading my Mom's nursing books cover to cover before age 12, to assisting on harvesting and transplanting hearts during my stint at Beth Israel Hospital in New Jersey, it all makes sense. The body is like a garden. Carefully tended it becomes a joy to behold. Neglected, it gets overrun with bush and bramble. To accomplish massive weight loss, you must hold fast to "whatever the mind of man can conceive and believe it **can** achieve." The ability to grasp this concept has little to do with social status, race, looks, or IQ for that matter. Each of us has equal opportunity.

So, welcome to the land of starting over! From Chapter 3, you arose from the *Prevent* plane with all its excuses. You then launched into the plane of *Planning* and now you are taking off in hot *Pursuit* of your dreams. You have acknowledged that you brought this weight upon yourself over so many years; now *you* are going to get rid of it. Begin this journey with a new stomach, one that you have created yourself!.

Mind over Matter

Let us closely examine what this is and what it is not. First of all, it is not magic. Paranormal events are well documented throughout the Bible and dot the pages of history. Generally, they occur in rare, special or supernatural circumstances. Under normal conditions, much of what passes for mind over matter is mostly hallucination, rip-offs and sleight of hand by con artists. True mind over matter cannot be merchandised. The mind overrules the body. Obesity is the disease of our times. To the

5. Stomach Conditioning

best of my knowledge, what passes for faith healing today has never instantaneously 'healed' a single heavy person.

Let us get more specific. Mind over *outer* matter is largely the pixie dust stuff of legend and film. *I Dream of Genie, Sabrina the Teenage Witch, David Copperfield* and *Harry Potter* can cast spells and magically change things in film and theater. After the award-winning entertainment, we are still who we are. However, the power to control *inner* matter is unquestioned. That is because mind and body are directly connected through a complex system of nerves, vessels, chemotactic factors meridians and energy fields. All we need to do is to find the right handles and buttons and we will know how to run this thing.

The body is endowed with an innate capacity to protect and correct itself. Pupils constrict in bright light. Fainting occurs when blood pressure falls suddenly. The head down or horizontal position diverts blood back to the brain and the individual revives. Commercials would have us believe that wounds would hardly heal unless treated with Neosporin and Band-Aids. While we are privileged to have such useful, sterile products, a laceration healing today or 6000 years ago would look amazingly similar if somehow viewed with time-lapse photography. Students of anatomy and physiology learn that these intricate feedback loops and control mechanisms occur naturally, driven by some profound intrinsic wisdom. Such systems should not be disrupted without just cause. On the other hand, there are numerous situations where aggressive medical intervention is absolute and urgent. The fracture must be set; the abscess must be drained; the cancer must be resected, radiated and or treated with chemotherapy. We are blessed to have trained professionals to intervene in our time of need. But what about the stomach? Sure we can cut on it, but can we actually *condition* it to consume less and produce weight loss?

Stretching and Shrinking

Nurses and doctors learn to suppress natural squeamish reactions for the front-row-seat privilege of beholding the wonders of the human body. For me, perhaps the most dramatic experience is assisting with c-sections. This operation is so routine, yet so unlike any other. It is like an Olympic sprint. All the resources have to be in place. The anesthesiologist 'gets set' with the spinal. The injected sedative is the starter's pistol signaling "Go!" This is no time for false starts.

The pregnant womb is a huge, basketball-sized pod, pulsating with precious human cargo. Through a splash of blood and amniotic fluid, the obstetrician's shiny, sterile instruments and gloved hands deliver the tender baby into this world. That miraculous cry is music to everyone's ears as we pass the bundle of joy into the blanketed arms of the waiting pediatric staff. Attention is immediately directed back to that gaping pelvic incision. Within it, the womb is still ajar like a looted purse and bleeding briskly. It must be speedily repaired. If you blinked, you missed it. In a blur of choreographed movements, we have closed all the layers by the time the baby is wrapped in swaddling clothes and presented to the proud parents.

The proud papa behind the drapes softly kisses mom's forehead. That's his job, comforting the exhausted star of the show. It is mother's womb, the uterus, that incredible crucible of life that provides us with the big lesson here. Before we closed, we had kneaded and massaged it as the anesthesiologist administered Pitocin through the I.V. This drug helped constrict the blood vessels, contracting the uterine muscles. Before our very eyes this turgid, swollen organ has almost magically shrunk down to the size of a cantaloupe. If seeing is believing, there is no way one can again doubt the body's capacity to stretch or shrink. It is a daily phenomenon perhaps taking place this very moment at a hospital near you.

Gastric Anatomy and Physiology

Anatomically, the stomach is divided into four sections based on function. The diagram to the right shows the feeding tube (esophagus), connecting the throat to the upper part of the stomach called the *fundus*. This part of the stomach bulges when filled with food. The middle part of the stomach is called the *body* and the lower part, the *antrum*. The *pylorus* is the outlet region just before the muscular pyloric valve. It controls passage of contents into the small bowel. Its inner surface is covered with large folds called *ruggae*. The lower stomach is more muscular with stronger contracting waves called *peristalsis*. It grinds the food down into smaller particles for the gastric juice to dissolve and digest. These rumbling movements occur about 3 times per minute.

Stomach action or gastric motility is controlled by a complicated network of nerves. There are three main types. First, the brain communicates with the stomach via *sympathetic* and *parasympathetic* *nerves*. Secondly, the bowel communicates with the stomach through the *enteric nerves*. Thirdly, the stomach itself produces *intrinsic factor* and enough acidic gastric juice to fill a soda pop liter bottle each day. (Much of that is re-absorbed lower down). Interplay of diverse hormones such as *gastrin* and *cholecystokinin* signal the upper stomach to relax and enhance contractions in the lower stomach. Much more is yet to be discovered.

General surgeons perform all kinds of operations on the stomach for ulcers, trauma, cancer, and weight loss. I have been called upon to open patients to sew up gastric stab wounds or remove bullets. Then there were Ziploc bags of potent street drugs swallowed by the accused before being busted. Instead of family, cops are in the waiting room to retrieve the evidence. At any time the washing machine action of the stomach could have popped the bag and spill its lethal contents. No pressure!

Patients from the nearby "State Hospital" for the profoundly mentally retarded often eat non-food items, a condition called *pica*. This is an exaggerated presentation of the classic disorder seen in malnourished children who ingest materials like cloth, chalk and flakes of paint or even dirt in a bizarre quest for minerals. Most of the objects they swallow amazingly pass right through. We have had to go after the rest that blocked the gastro-intestinal tract: bobby socks, batteries, bottle caps, coins, ping-pong balls, Hefty trash bags, wash cloths...It is hard to look at these everyday objects the same way after extracting them all slimy and gooey... Too much information! Let us instead just focus on this act of digestion

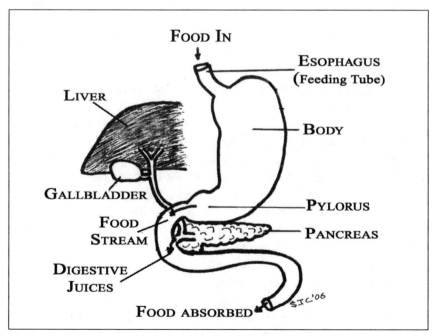

Normal Stomach Anatomy.

67

itself. Such operations can easily lull one into thinking of the stomach as some plain, old sac for dumping food. Detailed study of the stomach enables physicians to determine how best to treat its various diseases. Knowing the stomach up close and personal is to appreciate it as enormously intricate organ, complete and versatile as the brain or heart. It has tremendous capacity to adapt, adjust and correct itself. Upon comparing the diagrams on pages 67 and 132, it would be more accurate to say that the normal stomach anatomy is *disrupted* rather than simply *bypassed* for weight loss. This carries inherent risks not evident at first. In the case of morbid obesity, the stomach itself is innocent. More and more people agree that it is a terrible thing to waste a perfectly working stomach.

Smaller Stomach - The Key Difference

Following any abdominal surgery, the stomach and bowel remain "asleep" for a period of time depending on the extent of the operation. This is called an *ileus*. For a laparoscopic cholecystectomy (gallbladder removal), this may be as little as four to six hours. For a colon resection for tumor or diverticulitis it could be two to four days or even longer. Even in such situations the stomach continues to produce gastric juices, especially when stimulated by smells, sights or even thoughts of food. If enough accumulates before the bowels "wake up" to move things along, the patient may throw up. This is quite painful while having a fresh abdominal incision. To avoid this, the surgeon may insert a naso-gastric tube (through the nose, into the stomach) to decompress or suction out the gastric collection.

Obesity surgery proves that the basis for lasting weight loss is decreased stomach size - no doubt about it. Regardless of what the patient eats afterwards, Adkins, South Beach, Grandma's cooking or junk food, everyone still loses weight and for the most part, keeps it off. Surgical intervention has tremendous appeal, although most people have little idea what all they are getting into. Nevertheless, a smaller stomach feels satisfied with a normal meal. A larger stomach will still growl with hunger pangs and cravings on that same meal because there is still much *empty space* to be filled up. Understanding this concept is essential to appreciating the non-surgical Manna*fast* breakthrough. Here are a couple more points to consider before we begin actually applying these truths.

Patients with advanced diabetes may develop a condition called *gastroparesis*. This literally means "weak stomach" - weak in the sense of poor stomach tone. It has been compromised by the disease and stretched

5. Stomach Conditioning

into a *large, floppy bag*. These patients are in double trouble. Not only do they have to control their carbohydrates to keep the sugar within limits, now they have to struggle with more hunger pangs from having a larger stomach. That is why it is so important to keep weight under control because contracting diabetes causes health problems to snowball.

Common terms long used in medicine supports this concept. *Hypertrophy* refers to increase in size of a body part from excessive use. Weight lifting is an obvious example. *Atrophy,* on the other hand, refers to shrinking of a body part when under-utilized. The legs of a paralyzed person, for example, tend to get smaller. The same applies to organs. With bowel obstruction, the part in front of the blockage stretches. Bowel beyond the blockage shrinks since it is no longer functioning as usual. Surgeons describe this as "proximal dilation and distal collapse." With the stomach, bigger is definitely not better. Shrinking it back to normal size with systematically smaller portions is basically what Manna*fast* is all about. It downsizes the stomach in order to right-size the weight. It is the only non-surgical, weight management approach which currently uses this proven concept of stomach conditioning.

How We Do It

In the Chapter 9, *Surgical Options,* we describe the post-gastrectomy diet, the eating protocol following obesity surgery. It is seriously strict. Failure to follow these instructions, risks ripping the sutures or staples with dire consequences. The consent signed before surgery is very up-front about the severe risks involved. Out of fear of a bad outcome, for the first time, the vast majority complies. There is just too much authority riding on that injunction to do otherwise.

The notion that this thing is "just between me and my surgeon" could not be further from the truth. Besides the surgeon's daily post-op visits, nurses are constantly monitoring the objective recovery. Patients are likely to get daily visits by the dietician and chaplain, not to mention family and friends with ritual flowers and cards. Big money is involved. Risk managers are on call and lawyers are waiting in the wings. The hospital's case manager is hovering around to cut costs and ensure early discharge to maximize profits. The insurance company utilization reviewers are keeping close track of progress as well. The last thing they want is to turn this optional case into a blank check to the healthcare providers. The employer has to plan for this sick leave while co-workers wonder how long they have to cover. One does not have to be a celebrity for the news to eventually leak out that so and so "had the surgery." That, in and of itself, adds another layer of accountability not to mess up this time.

In contrast, here is a Mannafast client. He is losing weight, not as rapidly at first, but in the long run, equally well. That is because the eating plan is similar. The sole difference is what is done to enforce this level of food intake. I made this fascinating discovery while preparing patients for gastric bypass surgery. Patients got to practice that diet beforehand. Some did so well, they began putting off the surgery. This was rather frustrating at first, because, to be perfectly honest, an operation meant more money for me. Yet, I had to confess that these patients were much happier than those who had surgery. I then began promoting the same eating plan - a medically supervised fast, for all comers, including those who did not qualify for surgery. They also had fantastic results – in the end, as good or even better than gastric bypass!

Okay; let's see what's happening here... These patients had in effect, performed the equivalent of major surgery on their own minds and spirits. They were motivated to follow the eating plan, but not by having the fear the *Sword of Damocles* hanging by a thread overhead in the form potential surgical complications. Mannafast clients do not get all the attention and all the fuss, but neither are they in any pain. They are not subject to the financial risks discussed in Chapter 9. They are on their own private schedule, marching to the beat of a very different drummer. *Unlike surgery, we do not turn away Mannafast clients because of serious medical problems, lack the right insurance or because they are too heavy to begin with!*

Start Your Supervised Fast

In common clinical usage, the word *fast* often refers to instructing a patient "to eat or drink nothing after midnight." This is usually before a test or surgery in the morning. Or, it may be a liquid fast as part of a two to three day bowel cleansing before a barium enema or operation on that area. In contrast, a *manna* fast is a spiritually motivated, clinical fast in pursuit of weight control/self-discipline goals. Such fasting is specifically designed not only to overcome domination by our physical and psychological cravings, but to shrink the stomach in the process. There is absolutely no telling just how much can be accomplished when combined with an honest faith component, be that affirmations, meditation or prayer, (*Faith and Fitness*, Chapter 10). Not surprisingly, there are suspicions fostered by concerns that a Manna*fast* may be too uncomfortable or harmful in some way. Be careful not to confuse the Manna*fast* to a hunger strike which is a threat of harming one's body for a cause. On the contrary, Manna*fast* satisfies the body's basic nutritional needs while forcing it to deplete excess fat stores. Neither is it like a traditional diet (Chapater 12). Mannafast is compulsory *balanced* nutrition. It frees us from the whims of the seductive marketplace which appeals to our wanton palates. Mannafast not only reduces weight, but cholesterol as well - while increasing energy and immunity. Its goal therefore is not simply weight loss, but more importantly, improved health.

As you prepare for your fast:
- Complete and submit your medical history (pages 302-305).
- Establish accountability with a buddy or supportive professional.
- Begin basic exercises suggested in Chapter 6.
- Start your food and fitness diary and share in a Covenant group.
- Monitor your progress on the Mannameter Motivational Graph.

Studies show that dieters typically underreport what they actually eat. They tell the nutrition counselor exactly what they think she wants to hear. A food and fitness diary helps us to be true to ourselves by identifying exactly where the excess calories are coming from. We need to get into some *detail* here. How many servings, cups, glasses, ounces, spoonfuls, portion sizes, snacks, lite, low fat, regular or sugar-free, etc.

The easiest way to institute a predictable, effective fast is by using Meal Replacement Supplements, (MRS) for a defined period of time (*Pursuit Phase*). These consist of specially bio-engineered nutritional packets and selected fat-burning foods that facilitate reducing stomach size (Chapter 13). These supplements are designed to provide all the nourishment the body needs and none of the excess fat and calories we are trying to do without. Simply pour the contents in a glass of water, shake or stir and drink. MRS provide a fail-safe start to caloric restriction. This allows time to focus on new balanced nutrition ideas while resetting one's metabolism with a supervised clinical fast.

Overcoming Fasting Excuses

There are those who complain that MRS do not teach people how to eat right. Actually, just the opposite is true. The respect and appreciation for food acquired from fasting is priceless. Before we go any further, let us neutralize some of the more frequent arguments used against fasting.

Taste

Chapter 2 established that we are 100 percent into the joy of eating. Just as the champion cannot experience the thrill of victory without putting in the tough hours of practice, so too for our health and happiness we must give up the idea of getting something for nothing. MRS are not ice cream shakes in the same way vegetables do not have the same

> *At the time, discipline is not joyous but tough; yet afterward it yeilds for those who have passed thru its training, the fruit of peace...*
> Hebrews 12:11

appeal as pizza. MRS are palatable, but it requires you to bring your taste buds under subjection for a designated period of time in order to achieve a higher goal. Once you get into the routine, the battle is half-won.

Feeling Deprived

At first, you will be amazed how food seems to be everywhere and in everything. Although far from starving, the mind with its old habits cries out, "Why me, and how long?" After all, you're an adult and free to eat what you darn well please! Billboard, TV and magazine ads appear bigger and brighter. These images seem to jump right out at you yelling, "Eat me!" One fast-food addict even reported a nightmare in which French fries were beckoning him like fingers and whispering seductively, "Come to Daddy." This too will pass. With every hour you feel stronger, more superior. One has to be mature and hold back from feeling disdain for others who can now be plainly seen as gorging themselves to death. These feelings are replaced with understanding and compassion as you focus on your own success.

But I Like My Treats

Be strong. Exposure to treats and usual foods when starting serious gastric conditioning tends to confuse those with certain food weaknesses. It stimulates flow of digestive juices thus sharpening the perception of physical hunger. This sets the stage for cheating and backsliding.

Miss Chewing Real Food

Mastication, the act of chewing is integral to feelings of satisfaction and stimulation of digestive enzymes. Gum helps. Also, pack baby carrots, grapes, trail mix, celery sticks and other low calorie munchable snacks. Low fat popcorn is a great relaxing snack at the end of the day. It is crunchy, fluffy and satisfies the delicious sense of smell.

Constipation

Bathroom habits vary. Some develop constipation with fasting. Our MRS are high in fiber. Attention to your fruits, vegetables, prune juice, and over-the-counter fiber products are helpful. Before resorting to stool softeners and laxatives, consider a natural alternative such as *Power Pudding*. This is easily made by blending 1/4 cup of bran, 1/2 cup of applesauce, 3/4 cup of prunes, 3 ounces of prune juice. At 1/4 cup serving daily, it is nutritious, tastes okay and most of all cost-effective.

40 Days and 40 Nights

From the first pitter-patter of raindrops, Noah knew it was now or never. Likewise, henceforth, you have all the resources necessary to achieve success. Step out in faith and take charge of the situation. As you commit and prepare to sacrifice, fully expect your belly to pout at first. The body actually goes into a period of withdrawal lasting about 72 hours. The stomach rumbling may be associated with slight hunger headaches, weakness and even a little dizziness. It is expelling old eating habits and poisons from the system. Like demons being cast out, they never go quietly into the night. This great beginning can be compared to labor pains before the prize promised for nine months of eager anticipation.

The Lord declared, "I lay down my life. No one takes it from me. I have the power to lay it down and the power to take it up again." (John 10:17, 18). We have that same power when it comes to food. We do not have to be forced into some harsh circumstance like famine, disaster or abduction in order to experience some measure of deprivation. You will be surprised how rapidly the body adjusts once the message registers that you are serious. Stick with it for that time period required for habits to set in.

For the first time in their lives Manna*fast* clients come to grips with the fact they have been slaves to food. During this time of impressive weight loss, the mind is in peak state for absorbing new, sound nutrition principles. It makes a distinct break with the old times of frustration: losing a couple pounds one month and gaining back more the next. Only those having the courage to deny their appetites for a season know the tremendous storehouse of power that it unlocks. Traditional diets can be compared to trying to tiptoe into the pool. Manna*fast* says "Dive in!"

Timing

More than just the physical weight lost, the fast is designed to unload the burdens of negativity that produced the present reality of obesity. It is therefore essential that we start the fast when relatively free of special real-world obligations or physical concerns such as major business appointments, periods, exams, sporting competition, vacation, etc. You are 100 percent in control. Unlike surgery, you begin at the time and place exclusively of your own choosing while continuing routine work or study as before.

Based on excess weight, plan a Pursuit phase lasting 1 - 4 weeks or more - the time required to install habits. As we saw in Chapter 1, figure on losing up to ten pounds per month. Even those of average weight can benefit greatly from a two or three-day fast to cleanse the system, to focus on a specific need or in support of a loved one. Popular 24-hour sleep-over camps beginning Friday afternoon pack just the right amount of punch to blast off on this great adventure. The experience welds one's commitment to stick with the program while connecting those on a similar quest with local covenant groups.

Bear in mind that metabolic rate may be influenced by several factors including age, gender, depression, previous dieting, etc. We have the technology to electronically determine the exact *caloric requirement for weight maintenance*. But we do not need a machine to tell us what we can deduce intuitively.

Calories needed to maintain weight = present wt. x 10

For example: a 150 pound person needs 1500 calorie diet to maintain weight. To lose weight, must eat less. Decreasing consumption to 1300 would do the trick. However, the idea is not to count calories obsessively. The traditional dieter wants to be spoon-fed. He wants to be told: "Eat this," or "Don't eat that." Mannafast offers a new way, a better way of eating. In time, your food diary will tell. Get a sense of what portions work best. Right there is the most effective tool in your weight loss program. As soon as I notice my weight creeping up, I cut back to one slice of toast for breakfast. Am I thrilled about that? Not really...until I see the results on the scale! Hamburger? Say goodbye to the top of the bun. Take pride in eating less than what the average person would. Unless we change what we have been doing, we will keep getting what we have been getting.

Light Meals

A modest lunch and dinner gives you more time to burn off of the calories you take in. Of course, a heavy lunch causes sluggishness. Each culture seems to have their not-so-flattering name for this phenomenon. This forms the basis for the *siesta* in Spanish countries. Those in charge of the lives of othersProductive people are careful how much they eat to ensure mental alertness during the afternoon. I dare eat a regular lunch if I have important appointments scheduled later in the day. Working people from all walks of life can identify with that. This is one reason why unemployment is such a risk for weight gain. There are no performance consequences to eating large.

By the same token, if you want to lose weight, do not eat a meal less than 2 hours before bedtime. The body is not burning as much energy and the absorbed calories are more likely to be stored as fat. Resistance is low after a long day's work. We therefore need to make responsible eating plans particularly for this time of day. Coming home to labor over domestic issues and kids' homework can be quite draining. No one knows that better than the advertisers. Prime time commercials seductively promote mostly high fat, high calorie comfort treats: the ammunition for all kinds of dysfunctional food behaviors.

Split an Entrée?

Learn to distinguish between real biological hunger and emotional hunger. We are often seduced by external cues. The great fable writer known as Aesop told of the dog about to savor its juicy bone. As he passed a serene pond, he looked down and saw another dog with what seemed like a bigger bone. He dropped his bone to snatch at the more tempting prize. His meal sank into the deep pond and he ended up with nothing.

Forget about psychological hunger for a moment. This dog was plain greedy! I know that I have to find ways to sublimate my own greed if I do not want to end up with nothing in terms of health. Conversation, chores, exercise, hobbies can all take one's mind off food until the craving subsides. Ivan Pavlov was a renowned Russian scientist who conditioned dogs to salivate at the sound of a bell. We can similarly condition our responses to psychological hunger stimuli with healthy foods. In time, we learn respond automatically.

The average person going out to eat generally prefers their appetite to be turbo-charged, especially if someone else is picking up the tab. That is just the opposite for those committed to weight control. They try never to leave home hungry. In so doing, they take authority over fattening menus. They put themselves in control by simply munching on some vegetables and/or fiber supplement or even a glass of water before leaving home.

At this point they can enjoy the social event without stress and go home satisfied without the guilt of having blown their diet.

Remember, every time we eat till uncomfortably full, we do ourselves a major disservice. Sighing with lethargic contentment from a stuffed stomach only stimulates future hunger and weight gain. For this reason, I do not hesitate to split an entree if I am not that hungry. Some may see that as being cheap. I see it as being smart. There is no law that says you cannot ask for a half portion, just an appetizer or a children's order. The food industry intimidates men into proving their manhood with the largest, "Big Buford" type meals and care little for the consequences.

When confronted with a large serving, I immediately ask for a doggie bag. That signals to the person waiting our table, as well as my dinner mates, that I know my limits. Don't even think of trying to coax me into having more. Others at home can share in the fine cuisine. Oftentimes it is forgotten in the refrigerator. As I pitch it, there was a time I would be tempted to regret not having eaten it all when I had the chance. Rather, I rejoice not having to struggle later to get rid of those excess calories.

Eat Slower

From our celebrated eating competitions on TV, to gulping down fast food with one hand on the steering wheel, American dining has been noted for both volume and speed. This is not a recent development. Nearly two centuries ago, Englishman Charles Dickens, after a trans-Atlantic voyage, made the following observation in his book *Martin Chuzzlewit*:

> *"All knives and forks were working away at a rate that was quite alarming; very few words were spoken; and everybody seemed to eat his utmost, in self defense, as if a famine were expected to set in before breakfast-time tomorrow morning..."*

This could easily describe how we eat today. Eating too fast often means eating too much. The hypothalamus portion of the brain and the pituitary gland contain satiety (satisfaction) centers that regulate eating patterns. (Chapter 10 discusses how this area is targeted by various appetite suppression drugs). Digestion breaks carbohydrates down into glucose (sugar molecules) and rising levels stimulate insulin secretion. This signals brain to order the hand to "Stop shoveling it in! I'm full." The process takes about 20 minutes. By eating too fast, the stomach may be already bursting at the seams before the message registers.

5. Stomach Conditioning

Water, Water Everywhere

I was somewhat taken back the first time someone revealed that they drank a dozen cans of soda pop a day. But I was really shocked to realize that this was just the tip of the iceberg. Soda is fun to drink because of the sugar kick and the fizz that tickles the palate. Temple University's Dr. Jie Yang, writing in the *Journal of Dentistry* blamed carbonated drinks for causing "significant, irreversible long-term" damage to the enamel of the teeth. He discouraged soda before bedtime and advocated use of a straw to help reduce dental exposure. More importantly, abuse of sugary beverages is one of the leading causes of today's obesity epidemic. Simply substituting water (not diet pop) therefore has a significant weight loss effect.

The body is composed of more than 60 percent water. The brain, which makes us capable of reason, is even more at 70 percent. Reflect on the wonderful choice we have today to keep ourselves well hydrated. In John 7:38 Jesus proclaimed about those who believe that "Out of their innermost being shall flow rivers of *living water!*" Clearly it is neither rational nor healthy to boast that one does not like drinking water.

At the same time, there can be too much of a good thing. For starters, travelers and busy people do not have the time to interrupt their schedules for unnecessary bathroom breaks. In fact, some deliberately "set the natural alarm clock" by drinking more water at bedtime so that bladder pressure will prompt an early awakening. Instead of simply "forcing fluids," clinicians are increasingly recommending that drinking be guided by thirst. This is especially true for those who have already developed heart and kidney problems, stress incontinence, enlarged prostates or irritable bladders. Physicians routinely inquire about *nocturia,* "How many times do you have to get up at night to urinate?" Certain ailments decrease urine output causing patients to retain fluid and become bloated. Diuretics are then required to get rid of leg swelling to "unload" the heart and lungs. It is counterproductive to pour it in then take medicine to flush it out. *Fluid restriction* is the logical treatment in these situations.

Granted, most people do not drink enough water. However dieters who abuse water do not give their stomachs a chance to tone down. This also contributes to the "floppy bag syndrome." It "biggie sizes" the stomach, the root cause of regaining weight. Forcing down 8 glasses of water a day is highly overrated. This is more a fashion statement pushed by the bottled water industry at the expense the environment and scientific requirements. In 2007, a 28 year California woman took part in a radio station water-drinking competition to win a Nintendo Wii for her kids. The coroner determined she died hours later from brain swelling and water intoxication. Freezing water in your favorite, modest-sized container and sipping on it throughout the day is safer and more considerate. It avoids guzzling and overdosing on a good thing. Few folks I've met are more in love with God's drink than I am. It is my "night cap" and "eye opener," but far be it from me to drown my sense of balance.

Go For It!

The typical dieter complains "My brain is screaming: You're hungry, keep eating." There must be something that screams back louder. "No you're not. Stick to the facts and stay in control!" It's not unlike a hostage situation. The negotiators have done their best trying to resolve this thing, but the bad guys are hell-bent on carrying out their threats. Well, at some point, somebody has to decide enough is enough. Orders to the SWAT team: "We're going in!" Brace for some pain. We're going to storm their barricades with superior, overwhelming force. Guess what? When the dust settles, all those fat hormones analyzed in Chapter 11, the so-called weight set-point and even "metabolism" somehow adjust to the reality of the strong action we have imposed. Mannafast of course, is much gentler, but no less decisive, no less effective.

The Commanding Officer never surrenders control of the mission to the press, family or curious onlookers. The well-being of the hostages is his sole   professional responsibility. Likewise, remember: to reduce calories safely, we must do so ourselves. We affirm that we are "fearfully and wonderfully made." We acknowledge the power of God to transform flesh and set the captives free. We proclaim the potential of our God-given minds to accomplish our dreams. Using natural means to transform the stomach back to normal is pretty straighforward. All we have to do is to guard against interruptions in the process, (Chapter 15). You are embarking on a great adventure! You about to do what the world says cannot be done. If others have discovered that power to condition their stomachs to lose over 1000 pounds - *without surgery* - what's holding you back?

Start by doing the necessary, then the possible,

And suddenly you are doing the impossible.

St. Francis of Assisi

5. Stomach Conditioning

REVIEW

1. Reflect on the time in your life when you felt most hungry. Write down your thoughts and feelings associated with that experience.

2. Select an account of fasting in the Bible. What was the purpose and outcome in that particular situation? Discuss how it relates to today's nutrition concerns.

3. What are the advantages and disadvantages of using a fasting nutritional supplement?

4. How do you calculate the caloric requirement for each individual?

5. What strategies do you use for regulating your intake when eating out?

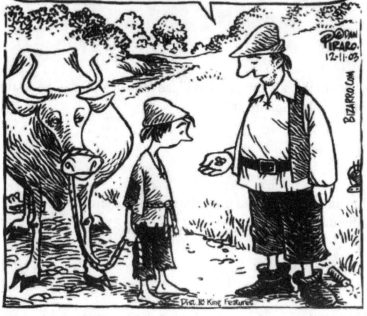

Chapter 6
Move It and Lose It

Run, Forrest, Run.

Forrest Gump

My weight raced from 165 pounds when I entered college to 180 by the end of the first semester. Sounds like the freshman fifteen! Who was to blame? Was it those nice cafeteria servers - always piling my plate high like that and encouraging me to come back for seconds? If truth be told, I had taken a weight training course and it was pure muscle. Really! My fat percentage must have been in the teens. That athletic physique stayed with me until parenthood took over.

Those were the days when Mike Tyson was knocking out opponents sometimes within 10 seconds. As the main draw, he got the lion's share of the prize money. But his opponents picked up a not-too-shabby million for serving as his punching bag. My buddies and I would joke about becoming heavyweights, (190+ pounds). I was certain that by ducking and running around the ring I could at least last longer than that with "Iron Mike." Well in time I did past that milestone, but hardly in the shape as I imagined. Cruising past 205, I found myself having to unbuckle my belt and loosen the top button of my trousers just to be comfortable sitting at my desk. Anyway you cut it, I was up nearly 40 pounds in 25 years. I was not going to put up with that. As I took the bull by the horns, it became apparent that individuals are inspired in different ways. My own experience served as a perfect example of what it takes to get someone just to start moving in the first place.

Physician, Heal Thyself!

Beverly too, came to such a point in her life. Her trusting faith and bubbly personality made quite an impression. She first came to our office for minor surgery. However, while following up she expressed despair with the direction her life was taking.

As your everyday 40-something year-old mother of two teenagers, Beverly was never involved in any organized sports in school. Yet in

81

her skinny school days she described herself oddly as "a zipper turned sideways." She never had to think twice about what she ate. Her husband Rod had a secure middle-management position with a utility company. She had become exactly the kind of devoted housewife she always dreamed of, active in a variety of PTA and church activities. And that was where it all started. Their Sunday School class discussion touched on the temple of the Holy Spirit and what believers were allowing to happen to their bodies. One lady complained about "weighing more than a typical linebacker." At the time Bev said nothing, but realized that the same was true for her.

This is a common affliction. In your mind, you are still that healthy youngster without a care in the world. Then somewhere along life's twists and turns, something happens that shouts you are living a lie. Bev was not opposed to exercise, she just had never committed to it. She went as far as purchasing a health club membership, but going only once did not an athlete make.

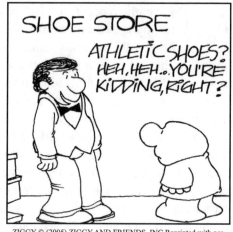

The few commercial diet programs she tried were frustrating experiences. That was when Bev thought it could not hurt having some professional support. She put into practice the same Manna*fast* Eating Plan and exercise recommendations (that I myself was neglecting). First she and Rod began daily walking around the block, and then a mile, and then they began light jogging. Almost on a whim, she had signed up for a 5-K race at the Popcorn Festival in a neighboring town. She was basically thinking in terms of showing up and getting a T-shirt out of it. When she asked my advice preparing for the race, I could hardly imagine her winning first place for her age category. She brought the trophy to our office to celebrate! It was just a tiny little thing. But in all her excitement, it was if her next words would be, "Now I'm going to Disney World!"

What a transformed woman! ...60 pounds less of her than when she first visited our office nine months before. Her euphoria mirrored that of patients bringing in their new babies to the office to share the joy - or proud grandparents showing off precious photos of those little ones they could spoil and send home. Posing for pictures with the staff, she insisted on giving us all the credit, but she was the one who did the work. No diet or drug, no doctor, hospital or insurance company could lay any claim to her priceless accomplishment! Most of all, the way Beverly diligently followed my fitness prescription was quite the inspiration for me to not only talk the talk, but also to walk the walk.

> *The sovereign invigorator of the body is exercise, and of all exercises, walking is the best.*
>
> Thomas Jefferson

Embracing the Future

It has been demonstrated over and over again that exercise is the best predictor of sustained weight loss. You can lose all the weight you want with artificial means, but if you do not *move,* it profits you nothing. The weight eventually comes back, often with a vengeance. And just when walking is being promoted as the answer to the epidemic, here comes the *Segway.* This is a nifty electric scooter with chariot-like wheels on either side. The driver stands on a small platform, steering with an upright handle. Inventor Dean Kamen envisions it as a personal transportation device for zipping through amusement parks, large buildings or touring the city center.

Should the Segway become as commonplace as cell phones, will it join escalators and moving sidewalks in subtracting from our physical activity output? Self-raising recliners and staircase chair-elevators for the privileged elderly will become as standard as the sink garbage disposal for new home buyers. As such *Jetson* conveniences further compound our sedentary trends; the more motivated we must be to inject exercise into our daily lives.

Science fiction writers fifty years ago pictured future generations with personal jet-packs on their backs while Star Wars cars glide effortlessly through the air on clean fuel technology. They imagined the Romeo of the 21st century having the option of actually taking his honey to the moon. The Russian Space Agency currently charges out-of-this-world tourists about $20 million. Toss in an extra 15 and you get a space walk to go with that. But it is no cushy joy ride. Just in case you may be considering it, bear in mind that since the days of Yuri Gagarin and John Glenn, no space traveler has ever returned with leg clots from inactivity. Remarkably, no astronaut, cosmonaut or taikonaut has ever been brought back dead from a *medical* condition. Compulsory in-flight exercises for even these privileged passengers ensure that the space agencies intend to maintain that record. Dick Rutan, aeronautics engineer and first to pilot nonstop around the world, led a team that accomplished the first private "space jet" flight. Backed by maverick British financier, Virgin Airlines' Sir Richard Branson, that incredible trip may soon become in our lifetime as affordable as the now defunct supersonic Concorde. But only the fit will be able to enter the promised land of interplanetary travel.

Exercise Excuses

When we say someone is an "exercise freak," it is as though they have two heads. That remark often reveals a secret envy that the person in question is fit, robust and vibrant. We have all done it - come up with reasons why we don't feel like exercising. Even the handicapped in wheelchairs, those with chronic back pain, arthritis or history of incapacitating injuries can do something. The spectacular recovery of even our heaviest, bed-ridden patients begins with mandatory exercise at some level. Reluctance to exercise is a major hallmark of depression. Once we make an excuse, we tend to convince ourselves it is just for today. More often than not, it turns out to be as long as we can get away with it. Be honest. Have you ever used any of these common excuses?

Too Time-Consuming

Reasons for not doing what we know we ought to do can be as creative as any from the schoolchild failing to turn in his homework. All the presidents in the modern era have set an example of exercise. True, there is a presidential physician whose foremost responsibility is to stay on the Commander-in-Chief's case to keep him in the best possible shape. Anyone busier than the president probably has a good excuse not to exercise. If top executives find time to jog, swim and go biking, then the rest of us would be well advised to do the same. We may not enjoy their perks and privileges, but we have equal right to fitness and health.

Plan the time of day most suitable for you. People work different shifts. Some describe themselves as "day" people or "night" people. Others have no choice but to function whenever called upon. Whenever you catch yourself saying, "I don't have time," say instead, "I haven't *set aside* time." We all have the same 24 hours in each day - same for everybody. Always put exercise near the top of your "to do" list. For a busy mom, that quiet time in the morning may be an ideal opportunity to help focus on plans for the day ahead and work out without interruption.

6. Move It and Lose It

Some do it at lunch. Others take their babies jogging or power walking in an exercise stroller. Trade baby-sitting with friends, use the nursery at the gym, or do whatever it takes to show you are serious about fitness.

Too Expensive

A club membership may be a great investment. But you have to show up! The real benefit to me is the motivation that flows by osmosis from one person to another. Grandma always said, "Birds of a feather flock together." You tend to become like the people you hang out with. If you do are not influencing them, rest assured they are influencing you. The moment you express some hesitation about exercising, the couch potatoes in your life will be happy to supply all the excuses you ever wanted. In that way you become more like them and you don't make them look that bad.

It is estimated that 90 percent of home exercise equipment is no longer in use within one year. After a burst of good intentions, many such units either serve as clothes horses or gather dust en route to the garage sale. When asked the last time they used their equipment, many patients turn away their heads with a weak laugh, bashfully covering their mouths. My instruction: go home and just stand by it, touch it! That begins to take away the aversion or subconscious dislike for exercise. Next time you can get on board. Turn on the switch or check to see if it still works. By now you are that much closer to diving into life as the active, exercising person listed in your New Year's resolution.

Too Tired

One patient presented to the office with a chief complaint of shortness of breath. Sounds fairly routine until further questioning revealed exactly why he came that particular day. He was so short of breath, he couldn't even smoke! That is exactly how it sounds when someone says, "I don't exercise because I have no energy." Only a small number of patients with diagnosed Chronic Fatigue Syndrome, mono, hypothyroidism, depression or fibromyalgia are too tired to exercise. Apart from that, exercise is what stimulates energy.

Too Out of Shape

Okay, so you were not a cheerleader or captain of the football team. That has little bearing on who stays fit later in life. Athletic *talent* is no predictor of longevity. Many big names in high school and college sports try to hide at class reunions, or even not attend. Athletes suffer injuries during their careers. Former sports stars thrive at doing commentary, politics or business. These as the lucky ones. Many blow their millions and lack reliable disability and savings plans. You would not envy them as they later drag around bruised and battered bodies trying to catch up with life as we know it. They tend not to train diligently without a demanding coach, scholarship or glory to motivate them. Once prima donnas, catered to and burning the candle at both ends, years later, athletes are at higher risk for all kinds of addictions, including to food.

How often do we hear of the premature passing of another of our beloved sports heroes? So shake off that inferiority complex and get on with it like Beverly did. Remember, *movement* is one of the characteristics of living things. The less you move, the closer to death. The more you move, the closer to health and lasting weight control.

Too Risky

A few years ago, I happened to be doing my thing in the weight room at the "Y" when a bunch of jocks from Heidelberg College football team took over the place. As these thoroughbreds went through their paces, I found myself thinking, "I can do that!" Whatever they did, I did. It was quite a macho moment. That didn't look too hard. Until the next day when I discovered hurting muscles which I did not even know existed. I should have known better and worked out according to my age and capabilities. The last thing you want to do is to hurt yourself and spend weeks grumbling, "This exercise thing is not for me."

One can get hurt emotionally as well when starting an exercise program. Everyone is self-conscious to some extent. Research shows that women, more so than men, are not particularly thrilled about mirrors in the gym. It tends to discourage those who are very unhappy with their bodies and it is easy to get overwhelmed with how far you have to go. Just hang in there. It is a tough transition, getting into shape, but in time you will reap the rewards.

Too Boring

So exercise is boring compared to what? Exercise gets me excited. As the blood pounds through my veins, it helps me focus. It is somewhat uncomfortable for a while, but I am so refreshed and full of energy when I'm done! Every step I take is another step along the road to vibrant health and lower medical bills. What could be boring about that?

Here are some ideas. Earphones with upbeat music make a world of difference. Mini gadgets like the Ipod make this increasingly more convenient. Talk on the cell phone while exercising. That's like killing two birds (...terrible expression, by the way! How would *you* say it?) Anyway, you know what I mean. Regularity, no intensity, is essential. You only need to be doing more if training for competition. Anyway, imagine the inspirational effect your somewhat heavy breathing would have on the person at the other end of the line. Listen to books on tape. Position your treadmill or exercise bike so you can see the television or out of the window. Some pieces of equipment have magazine stands so that you can browse while exercising. As the circulation surges through the cranium, you feel smarter, stronger. Solutions to problems become clearer. Exercise infuses an amazing can-do spirit giving you the boldness to tackle issues which otherwise would be oppressing you. Have pen and paper handy or even a little recorder to make yourself quick "to do" notes. Exercise will only be boring if you choose to make it so.

Nobody To Do It With

You are an army of one. Start the ball rolling. Someone else is saying the same thing. They will see you conquering your excuses and ask to join in. Problem solved.

> *In males. as weight goes up, sperm count goes down, along with sexual desire.*

Bad Weather

Marvel at those, who like the US Postal Service, let nothing keep them from their appointed tasks. You see them jogging through storms, sleet, sizzling heat or shroud of darkness. I tend to be somewhat more selective. Weather permitting; enjoying the neighborhood and nature outdoors is clearly better. Some are easily distracted by chores when they remain indoors. After all, housework is never done. But when the weather does not cooperate, go to plan B. Find an exercise videotape, use home exercise equipment, step aerobics, exercise bands, push-ups, sit-ups, or whatever. Wherever you live, never let the weather trip you up.

My tropical origins made it difficult at first for me to understand the impact of *Seasonal Affective Disorder* (S.A.D.) The effects of the changing seasons were something I had to get used to. Excitement mounted as my first winter approached. As soon as the temperature dipped below 32 degrees, I placed a glass of water outside my dorm window, in Rome, Georgia. I stayed up most of the night checking to see if it would really, really freeze. I could hardly wait to respond to the letters from home repeatedly asking if I had seen snow yet. I was disappointed that night, but the anticipation climaxed the following afternoon. I finally caught sight of the first few fluffy snowflakes slowly dancing past my window. Shunning the elevator, I skipped down from the fourth floor at Greystone Manor, just bursting to make a fool of myself in the "blizzard." But the students from Florida beat me to it!

For ages people had a sense of the winter blahs, associating it in some way with hibernation in the shorter, darker days. Today the condition is well documented. Symptoms include increased appetite, binge eating of high carbohydrate foods, increased sleep, lethargy, weight gain, and depression up to the point of suicidal thoughts. Why it affects certain people more than others is not clear, but scientists have found increased light exposure to be therapeutic. To the extent that you feel secure no voyeurs and psychopaths are snooping, open the blinds and let the sun shine in.

An increasing number of people go to the mall to walk for exercise when the weather is being contrary. Come to think of it, the atmosphere is perfectly controlled and you are surrounded by lots of pleasant things. Of course, there is a down side. Be strong and avoid stopping to stare at the sales or to visit with acquaintances every few stores. If you are a sworn *shopperholic*, then that could be like putting a kid in a candy shop. Make sure that you have a clear plan. How many rounds am I doing today? Should I lock my wallet or purse in the car so that I would not be tempted to buy?

To quote the legendary Bishop Fulton Sheen, "Each of us makes his own weather, determines the color of the skies in the emotional universe which he inhabits." Manna*fast* weather is always perfect for exercise because it is never about what is physically happening out there.

Hate to sweat

I was sharing with one of my more successful clients how often I was hearing that complaint. "What's wrong with a bath?!" She laughed. The cosmetic counters tout an increasing array of "cleansers." The fact is that there is no greater cleanser than flushing out the pores with a good sweat followed by a rewarding shower. To put it bluntly, sweat is a form of excretion. It gets rid of impurities from the body.

Furthermore, those who sweat have more appeal (maybe not quite at the time they are doing so). They say men have a knee-jerk response to the sight of a toned and slender female physique. Anyway, science more and more is analyzing the opposite response. A study from the University of Pennsylvania found that male perspiration had a surprisingly beneficial effect on women's moods. According to the *Journal of Biology of Reproduction*, it helps reduce stress, induces relaxation and even affects the menstrual cycle.

We examine the different ethnic views on exercise and hair in Chapter 14. It seems that whether they express it or not, women like a man who works hard and plays hard. Some women find excessively muscular men intimidating, but they all generally prefer their men active. As middle age approaches, more women than men are urging their partners to take walks together. No one argues that walking the dog puts it in a better mood, but somehow we are skittish about extending that logic to humans.

> *Only those who want every-thing done for them are bored.*
>
> Rev. Dr. Billy Graham

Stretching For Flexibility

From Richard Simmons to Billy Blanks, Janet Austin to Tony Little to your local health club trainer, you have ample choice of fitness gurus eager and willing to provide details on exercise. My mission is to go deeper and ferret out the reason why good people have trouble getting their feet in gear in the first place.

The very first birth-cry clears amniotic fluid as baby's lungs embraces life in a new environment. Likewise, this morning's yawn opened wide the bosom to the breath of a new day. The natural accompanying stretch draws nutrients into lymphatic channels into the muscles. In this way we transition from a state of rest to be ready for action. The weekend warrior jumping into vigorous exercise *lickety-split* will soon be in full retreat.

With advancing age, it becomes that much more important to stretch. This should be gentle and relaxing, lasting about 30 seconds for each muscle group. Every few days, gently push the envelope and increase your range of motion. Before long, those who used to think themselves stiff are beginning to feel more supple and limber. Observe how people are likely to be called young when they do certain flexible things, like getting down and playing with the kids. It has been well established that physically fit senior citizens maintain their independence much longer than those who spend their retirement in the rocking chair. More importantly, they are less likely to develop Alzheimer's disease, or to cause fatal traffic accidents.

Manna*fast* is built on the firm foundation of creating the spark of inspiration to exercise. It is a spiritual thing that goes beyond the mind-body connection. The average person awakes and growls at the reflection in the bathroom mirror like a grizzly disturbed from hibernation. It is understandable for those suffering from a hangover or poor self-esteem. But waking up with such a sour disposition is quite unbecoming for a child of Promise. Roll back the videotape and let's try that again.

You open your eyes and squint at the clock. Yep. It's that time again. The bargaining starts. "Come on. Just a few more minutes under the covers." You hug the pillow, close your eyes, perhaps trying to recapture some nice dream you vaguely remember. Success for your entire day often hinges right at this point. You had decided before you went to bed that you would transform yourself into a "super wake-upper." Nothing is more beautiful than those who wake up with grace and gratitude.

Push aside the covers. Lying on your back, embrace your knees unto you chest - a somewhat fetal position. Breathe deeply. Slowly stretch out your right leg. Hold it just a few inches off the bed for ten seconds. Feel the muscles tense. Okay. Spread it sideways, back to the middle, then down. Do that with the other leg. Now, if you can, do both legs together. Slowly raise them a few inches of the bed, spread; gently bring them back together again (scissors action). Now slowly, gently, lower them to the bed.

Let's do the upper body - *before* getting out of bed. Again, simple. Interlock your fingers with your palms facing you. As you stretch your arms upward, turn your palms outward, pushing them further from you. Just like that, you are awaking... Sit at the side of the bed. Stretch your arms overhead, back, back, back, like you're doing a West Indian limbo. Don't worry, you won't fall. Well, if you do, it's on this nice, soft bed. But no, no. You're not going *back* to bed. I know you. Come on, you're almost wide awake now. This stretch has stimulated your circulation, recharging the muscles. Now you are actually beginning to *feel* like springing out of bed! See! By the time you walk over to get freshened up, you are already bright-eyed, bushy-tailed and happy to be alive.

Any day above ground is a good day! Whatever the form of your devotions, it centers on the affirmation: "This is the day that the Lord has made. I will rejoice and be glad in it!" (Psalm 139:14). Such creative, early morning calisthenics set the tone for the entire day. Later on, even when spending long hours at the computer terminal or looking at television, do your isometrics and see how much more alert and positive the mind becomes.

We are often conditioned to think that we are not exercising unless wearing sweats and sneakers, headband and earphones. That is simply materialism just wanting you to buy stuff. The trick is to incorporate it in our daily lives. Take advantage of down time: waiting for the elevator, train or cashier. When filling up, you have the choice of staring blankly at the gas price numbers race upward on the pump. Or you can do some heel raises to stretch those lovely calf muscles. The self-conscious will not do that. But you are different. You know that being faithful in these small things equips you to accomplish the loftier goals outlined later.

How Much Exercise?

"The race is not for the swift, nor the battle for the strong" (Ecclesiastes 9:11). It is not about who runs the fastest of the furthest, it is about who walks or runs more regularly as a lifestyle. Certainly most of us need to be doing more, but unless you are a professional athlete, or preparing for *Survivor*, stick with the basics. Be *consistent* and the results will take care of themselves. It has been said that we do not decide our future. We decide our habits and our habits decide our destiny. The Centers for Disease Control and Prevention demonstrate 30 minutes of physical activity at least every other day adds years to any life. Now may be a good time to invest in an affordable pedometer. Set an eventual target of about 10,000 steps a day. Remember there is nothing magical about the gadget. All it does is to remind us that a mile at least every other day will do the trick.

Exercise is the only true fat burner. Weight-bearing exercise strengthens muscles, boosts energy and increases metabolism. It reduces stress and increases bone density thus preventing osteoporosis. Regular physical activity reduces cholesterol, lowering the risk of heart disease, hypertension, diabetes and certain cancers.

Have you ever caught yourself looking jealously at others who have great lean figures and wondering, "Why is it that *they* can eat whatever *they* want and not get fat - and *they* don't have to exercise?" Life appears to be unfair in certain respects. Just look at the fingers on your hand right now. They all have nice knuckles and nails but they are all different lengths and have different purposes. The ring finger is often first in line for jewelry, but is perhaps the weakest. The pinky is the baby and is cute. Finger #3 is the most impulsive, while the index finger has the most sensation and control. You may think of him as short and stumpy, but from a mechanical standpoint, that "opposable thumb" is the most important of all. The thumb has to accept that it is not a princess like the ring finger and vice versa. A woman may be pleasantly plump and may never drafted for the pageant, but that does not mean that she has to be frumpy. We may

91

come in different shapes and sizes, but we all have the same need to stay fit and maintain a reasonable weight.

It is a tragic misconception for genetically thin people to believe they have no need for exercise like other mortals. The fact is that lots of people who look skinny on the outside have bad health habits and store the fat on the inside. Chapter 7, *User's Manual* explains how this inner fat can be just as lethal as someone visibly out of shape. Like the thumb, science shows that it is better to be "thick" and fit than to be thin with flabby flesh.

Exercise and Metabolism

You have heard it said before that dieting decreases metabolism. Built in our genes is a survival mechanism that automatically burns less energy to conserve in the face of an apparent famine. After stored glycogen is used up the body begins to burn not only fat but also muscle. The effect is even more dramatic with surgery which is associated with a higher risk of malnutrition. A good weight loss program is one that can prove it not only sheds fat, but also *increases muscle mass*. Exercise offsets that decreased metabolism resulting from caloric restriction. This is the only safe method of long-term fat burning and maintenance even after the formal weight loss component is over. Without exercise our weight loss trophies are nothing more than fool's gold.

Some argue that exercise increases hunger, some insist on the exact opposite. The best way to understand it is through *shunting*. As with the "fight or flight" reaction, exercise diverts blood away from the internal organs to the muscles as adrenaline kicks in for explosive power. This pumps the body with those "feel good" hormones called *endorphins*. During that time the stomach is in neutral, it has no desire for food. So, to be accurate, in the period during and shortly after exercise, hunger decreases. Later, when blood shunts back to the internal organs; the stomach says, "Feed me! We have to replace the energy we burned!" Someone only interested in weight loss tends to reach for the nearest food, which in today's society is usually junk. Mannafast anticipates that increased appetite and encourages having complex carbohydrates, fruits and vegetables at hand to replenish glucose. Those who know better do not get carried away by the entire lo-carb craze. On the contrary, any good trainer or coach will vouch that their athletes perform better on *carbohydrate loading*. Small wonder that fad diets and surgery appeals to those less inclined to exercise.

Obesity evaporates as people see the light and learn to put one foot in front of the other. Walking and walking alone is enough to do the trick. Experts estimate that anyone can lose 30 pounds a year from just walking a mile a day. It costs next to nothing. It refreshes relationships by providing wholesome opportunity for conversation. Let us examine why it is then, that exercise is such a low priority for many.

Take it Slow

Honestly, have you ever met a weight-challenged person who has been consistently meeting exercise guidelines? We can all do something. Some severely obese patients can scarcely make it to the doctor's office, may not be able to afford physical therapy, or club membership. Regardless of their housing situation, we motivate them to begin their fitness program by simply walking back and forth from one end of the house (or apartment) to the other. Next, walk around the yard if available, or doing "reps" on the steps: At the bottom of the stairs, hang on to the banister or the wall for support and take one step up followed by one step down. It may not be glamorous and does not sound like much, but this improvised "Stairmaster" can give a surprisingly useful work-out. If a stair-step is too high or awkward for starters, purchase a sturdy plastic 4 or 6 inch high "step" for simple step-aerobics. Then you can follow with any of the work-out programs on TV or on video. So far we have not even left the house or invested more than $20.

> *Q: Why do interior designers place the refrigerator and TV in different rooms?*
>
> *A: So that everyone can get a little exercise.*

Once again, it is important to understand that we are dealing with the very basic level here. Mannafast serves as a portal that ushers the willing over the threshold from inactivity and obesity into robust health. Many of our clients were previously bed-bound because of their massive weight. The 1400 pound patient featured on Discovery Channel was *confined to bed for five years*! He literally could only move his hands. Our program got him out of bed, driving and even playing basketball again! It is so incredibly important just to get started. I check the pulse-oximetry of all patients; especially those I suspect are trying to pull the wool over my eyes. Next, I have them count about 20 step-ups on the exam room stool as I monitor how their heart rate. If convenient, I even walk with them through the office corridors and observe their breathing.

In the final analysis, all kinds of activity count. Intensive housework, factory work or waiting tables have a fitness advantage over sitting at a computer 8 hours a day. But "running after kids" is not an exercise program. If domestic responsibilities alone made folks skinny, then housewives would not be so desperate. At the end of the day, you may be tired (bless your heart) from working hard, but you have not *worked out* hard. Burning calories requires somewhat more *uninterrupted* movement, enough to get your pulse up into your target zone for your age. Again, you do not need some fancy chart to tell you when you are putting out enough effort. You are really exercising when you begin to crack a sweat and breathe a little harder. However, do not get so breathless that you cannot keep up a conversation. Exercise is something that only I can do for myself. There is no way around it. If you're not doing *something extra,* you're not yet convinced that your health is worth it.

Aerobic exercise is just the start. If we do not move forward, we most certainly will fall back. Advance to strength training using 3 or 5 pound hand weights to build up well-toned muscle mass. We are in a fight with gravity. It's all going to sag unless we do what we have to do to firm things up. Strength training is the only safe way to further increase metabolic rate. This enables the body to burn calories throughout the day, even when asleep.

Set Reasonable Goals

What's your goal? It could be just keeping up with the kids and grand kids. Or not being totally pooped if forced into a situation of walking long distances on a trip. It is all a mindset. Your goal is good health. Forget about weight for the moment. Simply affirm, "I'm an active person." Record your efforts on the Workbook and or Motivation Lifescore software. Track your progress. Go back from time to time and read previous entries. You will see as clear as day, times that you score high for exercise correspond with good things happening in your life - including weight loss. Treat yourself for your accomplishments. You have earned it. New clothes or "toys" make good rewards. Challenge yourself that if you make an entry in your journal every day for 30 days, you will pamper yourself with such and such.

Studies done at Harvard University proved a 23% increase in obesity and a 14% increase in diabetes for every 2 hours of television watched daily. Another study shows that normal weight individuals watch 3.5 hours of TV compared to overweight individuals who watched 4.6 hours per day.

6. Move It and Lose It

Could that one-hour difference represent some physical activity? Or does it mean that obese individuals, with their higher poverty and depression rates have fewer amenities or diminished capability to perform physical activity? Cable and satellite TV today offer seemingly endless distractions. Tear yourself from the virtual world, watching successful people do their thing. Make yourself a success and let others marvel at how fantastic you look now. Experts demonstrate that if one could limit TV viewing to 1 1/2 and walk at least half an hour a day, it would half ones risk for obesity and diabetes.

Fitness Awards

Let us close this chapter on a high note. Regardless of where they begin, I challenge clients with two important and achievable goals. The first is the President's Council on Physical Fitness Award and next is *Age-Fit*, adapted from the US Army Physical Fitness Test (APFT).

The beauty of the Presidents fitness award is that it simply rewards consistency. It is for everybody. It can be documented from a wide variety of activities as diverse as walking and dancing to archery and kayaking. Simply go online and we will assist you with certification. Few gifts that a parent or grandparent grants a child can surpass the motivation to achieve the Presidential Award. Point them to an organization that will lead them in that wholesome direction. Show your love by giving them incentives to accomplish something that no one can take away. Get the seal of approval from the highest office in the land that they are indeed on the right track.

He who is serious about his health knows a good challenge when he sees one. The APFT is used to screen for admission into, or retention in the US Army. Administering this test was one of my major duties in the Reserves. It simply sets age and gender-specific goals as to the number of push-ups and sit-ups to do in 2 minutes and minimum times for completing a 2 mile run. Frankly, it is not that demanding. It does not qualify you for the Navy Seals, 82nd Airborne, Delta Force or Army Rangers. APFT is just the lowest common denominator that everybody in the military must pass from captain to cook, from high school grads to those approaching the golden years. I have adapted the table for our Mannafast clients (AGE-FIT, next page). The *average* person can attain this basic level of fitness well within a year. And, guess what? You just do not look like the one to pull down the average. So *forward march!*

The consensus of experts after years of research is reflected in the USDA's updated food pyramid (page 197). In addition to advocating

AGE-FIT TABLE			scores for passing at the 60th percentile		
Age	Push-ups*		Sit-ups*	2 Mile Run (in minutes	
	Male	Female	Male & Female	Male	Female
20	42	19	53	15:15	18:54
30	39	17	45	17:00	20:36
40	34	13	38	18:18	22:42
50	25	10	30	19:30	24:00
60	18	8	27	19:54	24:48
*Minimum # of reps in 2 minutes					

decreasing portions of balanced foods, it now strongly affirms exercise as essential to good health and weight control. Our intent at this point is not to offer details of specific routines or training programs. We simply get into our patient heads so that they just feel like leaping off the couch.

Weight loss with fitness is *firm*, not flabby. It thrills me so to receive feedback from patients like Bev announcing that they just left their Age-Fit benchmarks in the dust! Looking at the table may seem impossible for you now. You are about to surprise yourself. Then challenge your loved ones, your workmates and your fellow worshipers to do likewise. Passing this test equips you for God's Army. It means that you now strong and energetic enough to accomplish your life's Mission; you are physically capable of helping your family should some emergency arise. Your health is their best life insurance. Henceforth, whenever you hear the word *fit*, you will say, "Yeah, that's me!" Just keep on moving as God gives you strength and the weight will take care of itself.

> *"The heights by great men reached and kept,*
> *Were not obtained by sudden flight.*
> *But they, while their companions slept,*
> *Were toiling upward in the night."*

Henry Wadsworth Longfellow

6. Move It and Lose It

REVIEW

1. How well do you wake up? Rate yourself on a scale of 1-10

2. How does a yawn and a stretch prepare the body for action?

3. Which exercise excuses have you used most?

4. Give examples of ways in which you can better incorporate physical activity in your regular lifestyle?

5. According to the table to your left, what should be your personal Age-Fit goals? How close are you to achieving them?

Vege-Quotient: Assessment # 2

Scores: More than once a week:10. About weekly: 9. Monthly: 5 to 8.

A few times a year: 3 to 4. Never/few times in your life: 0 to 2

11. **Broccoli**   Cruciferous vegetable high in phytochemicals. ↓breast,
_____   cervical &prostate cancer. Stabilizes blood pressure

12. **Cabbage**   Cruciferous vegetable high in phytochemicals. Promotes
_____   weight loss, Cancer fighter. ↓ peptic ulcers.

13. **Cantaloupe** Nutrient dense and low in calories. has adenosine:
_____   aids the heart. Cancer fighter, Strengthens immune system

14. **Carrots**   Highest in *provitamin* A; Saves eyesight. Assists weight
_____   loss. Regulates bowel. Regular use ↓cancer rate by half.

15.**Cauliflower** Cruciferous vegetable. ↓ breast and prostate cancer.
_____   Strengthens bones. Helps heal bruises.

16. **Cherries** High in melatonin. Helps sleep. Protects the heart. ↓
_____   gout, cancer. DC's cherry blossoms: gift from Japan 1912

17. **Celery**   Contains *coumarins*, enhance white blood cell function.
_____   ↓ migraines, rheumatism, muscular aches & pains.

18. **Chili peppers** Clears sinuses. ↑ sore throat. ↑ immune system.
_____   Prevents clot formation. Boosts immune system.

19. **Citrus**   Fights colds. Strengthens immune systems.
_____   ↓ cancer, hypertension & heart dz. Smoothes skin.

20.**Collard greens** ↑ in Vit B6 and C, and manganese. ↓ cancer. "Soul
_____   food" esp on NY's Day w black-eyed peas and corn bread.

+ _____% **TOTAL VQ**   (VQ #3 on page 188).

Let food be your medicine
Hippocrates

98

Chapter 7

User's Manual

Superior doctors prevent disease.
Mediocre doctors treat the disease before it becomes evident.
Inferior doctors treat full blown disease.

Hwang Ti, 2600 B.C. Nei Ching Oldest Chinese Medical Text

After logging several thousand miles in just seven months, serious transmission problems forced Phil's car back to the dealership. The perky customer service clerk glanced through his records and switched abruptly to her 'all business' mode. "Sorry Sir, but you will have to pay for the repairs."

"What?!" Phil was livid. He was going to take this all the way.

"There's no sign that you did any scheduled maintenance." She clipped, pointing to his purchase agreement. *"The warranty is invalidated."*

Fortunately, her boss cut him some slack. But somehow, the message did not carry over to other areas of Phil's life. This is the same gentleman always looking for wood to knock on when boasting that he had not been to a doctor in almost twenty years! ... Not very wise for someone pushing fifty! Is Phil more the exception than the rule? Or is he like many gentlemen who take better care of their wheels than they do their health? With so many well-meaning adults skipping on check-ups to save on spiraling health costs, wouldn't it be great if humans had an *owner's manual*? What all would it involve anyway?

The World Health Organization defines health as "a state of complete physical, mental and social well being and not simply the absence of disease or infirmity." If we are to heed the ancient Chinese wisdom inscribed above, our emphasis should not only be on diagnosing and treating, but more so *preventing disease,* the best we can. But weight control is just the start. Despite all the fantastic advances in medicine, it is the things that we fail to do which are more likely to take us out. How exactly do we go about staying healthy? Which screenings are more likely to increase our chances for wholeness and happiness?

This chapter helps us focus on the foundation of building a long healthy life. Having reviewed the importance of exercise in the previous chapter, let us now examine the role of weight, cholesterol, and screening tests. Do well in these areas and you will not only be a better patient, but also be equipped to motivate others to take better care of themselves.

Body Composition

Remember Hansel and Gretel? The old, visually-impaired witch forced those abducted kids to stick their fingers out of the cage to check whether they were fat enough to be eaten. What a vivid imagination they had, tricking her by sticking out a bone instead! Anyway, *skin fold thickness* works on the same principle. It is one of the older methods of measuring body fat. Nutritionists and dieticians use special calipers to measure the skin-to-skin thickness, generally at the back of the upper arm.

But in order not to be tricked about patients' true fat content, more sophisticated methods had to be developed. In the past, to accurately measure percentage of body fat, one had to be dunked in a special tank of water. Unlike the popular ball-throwing/trap door set-ups at the county fair, these elaborate units were only available at large research centers. Muscle is denser and therefore weighs more than fat for the same size. Scientists therefore use the relative buoyancy to calculate *Body Fat Analysis* (BFA). Newer technology based on electrical impedance, processes the differential speed of a tiny current through the body. However, BFA can be affected by the level of hydration and fluid retention. Results may vary at different times of a woman's cycle and so it is a good idea to get repeat readings and take the average. This technology is now readily available in bariatric physicians' offices, health clubs, personal trainers and even the more sophisticated home bathroom scales. With harmful weight loss programs being so commonplace, BFA helps differentiate whether the weight loss is actually coming from excess fat rather than from good, lean muscle.

The *Body Mass Index* (BMI) is the most commonly used measure of obesity. Mathematically, the BMI is calculated as the weight (in kilograms) divided by the square of the height (in meters).

$$\frac{\text{Weight (kg)}}{\text{Height (M)}^2} \quad \text{or} \quad \frac{\text{Weight (lb.)} \times 705}{\text{Height (in)} \times \text{Height (in)}}$$

Refer back to the table on page 3. You can also plug your measurements into any of the free online calculators which automatically figure out your BMI. This correlates well with the amount of fat in the body. Obviously, fat in conspicuous places trouble people more - the hips, buttocks and belly. But, it is *central obesity*, fat around the midsection, that carries the highest cardiovascular risk. The fat we cannot see may be even more deadly. For example, NFL linebackers and sumo wrestlers may appear to be simply fat on the outside. But we do know that these highly trained athletes also have large muscle mass. CT scan studies actually show a *lower* amount of fat around the organs (*visceral fat)* than compared to a couch potato of similar weight. These huge athletes therefore suffer less cardiovascular disease (until they stop working out and continue eating like growing boys). Visceral fat accumulation pushes against the diaphragm causing sleep apnea and predispose to high blood pressure and diabetes. As we saw in Chapter 3, abnormal weight has significant health consequences.

B.M.I	Category	Common Description	Mortality
Less than 18.5	Underweight	Thin	1.5
18.5 - 24.9	Healthy	Normal	1
25 - 29.9	Grade I overweight	Overweight	x 1.5
30 - 39.9	Grade II overweight	Obese	x 2
40 plus	Grade III overweight	Morbidly obese	x 3 +

World Health Organization Classification for Body Weight

The above chart shows baseline mortality or death rate for normal BMI between 19 and 25. Significant underweight (BMI less than 18.5) actually increases mortality by at least 50%. It is associated with cancer, AIDS, anorexia and other serious afflictions. (Details in Chapter 8, *Eating Disorders*). In an article in the March 9, 1998, issue of the *Archives of Internal Medicine*, Kaiser Permanente Medical Care Program demonstrated that mortality doubles for the obese, triples for the morbidly obese (BMI over 40) and rises sharply thereafter.

We have grown rather casual with use of the word 'morbid,' but these facts serves as a reminder of its original dire meaning. Society has lucrative roles for big, beefy guys, but not for long. *Heavies* throwing their weight around in childhood and adulthood are rapidly fading from the scene by the time retirement rolls around. By age 80, they are mostly extinct. Next time there is a feature on people making it over 100, observe carefully: are they generally overweight, normal sized or *slightly underweight?*

Manna*fast* Miracle

Where Do You Fit In?

The knee jerk reaction of someone in the *Pessimist* mode is, "Who wants to live to be a hundred anyway?" They conjure images of helpless, confused nursing home residents, all twisted up like pretzels. Actually, healthy centenarians are more often than not quite active and delightful. Their wisdom-laden mind remain as sharp as a tack well into the twilight years. People who live selfishly cannot age gracefully, as is the norm in today's society. Instead of searching for the fountain of youth, *seek the source of lasting health.* Here is another formula giving a slightly different angle on assessing weight:

> Each person 5' 0" should weigh about 122 lb.
> For Women: add 3 lb. for each additional inch.
> For Men: add 4 lb. for each additional inch.

Example:

> Female, 5' 5" - ideal body weight would be:
> *122 + (5 x 3 which is 15) = 137*
>
> Male,   5' 10" - ideal body weight would be:
> *122 + (10 x 4 which is 40) = 162*

To adjust for large or small frame, add or subtract 10 to 15 pounds either way. How does your weight measure up? Check the graph on page 301.

Don't panic now, this is just a rough guide, not something to get all bent out of shape about. In fact, in my opinion, this formula seems to favor the low side of normal. And do not get carried away by the different fancy methods of estimating *frame size*. Some folks are tiny or slight. You can tell intuitively by looking at the hand, shoulder or foot size. Being overweight is one thing, but having a small frame and carrying hundreds of extra pounds makes obesity that much more severe.

Nevertheless, certain vocations, like dance, favor smaller frames. Take for instance the firing of an experienced ballerina, 27 year-old Anastasia Volochkova, perhaps the leading dancer in the world-renowned Russian Bolshoi Theater. Though weighing 110 at 5 feet 7, male partners complained that she had grown too heavy to lift! It took intervention from the highest level of the Kremlin to get her reinstated.

Frame size therefore influences choice of vocation. Cheerleaders, models and actresses know what kind of figure to bring to the audition. On the flip side, if you are interested in the NFL, competing in field events like the shot put, tug-of-war, becoming a bodyguard, or bouncer, being puny is no asset. In such situations involving considerable muscle mass, the BMI is not the best overall indicator of health status. Challenge yourself if you now weigh more than 15 pounds above your maturity weight. Some of our patients have allowed their weight to get so far out of control, *just getting on the BMI chart* is an accomplishment in itself.

Waist Not

BFA, BMI, frame size, are handy in tracking your progress, but the waist is the first to give you the verdict. What is it about the waist which throughout history seems so closely associated with character? Perhaps it represents the most visible sign of a person's level of self-appreciation and health discipline. Society tends to judge women more harshly though they have the greater challenge of maintaining a trim figure after pregnancies, and pelvic surgeries. Yet one of our patients, a regular working woman, had an incredible five (5) c-sections and still maintained incredible shape. She did not allow it to limit her abdominal crunches and overall work out. Sure, part of it was her natural physique, but she also deserved credit for focusing on her health and reaping the rewards.

In Chapter 1, *Jumpstart,* we measured our waist-hip ratio (WHR). Ideally, women should have a ratio of 0.8 or less and men less than 0.95. Apple-shaped individuals have a high

> *Healthy Waist Measurements:*
> *Females: Less than 35"*
> *Males: Less than 40"*

WHR and carry their excess weight around the waist and abdomen. Call them "love handles" and "beer bellies" if you will, but more men fall into this category. *Apples*, however, seem to lose weight faster. This can be a cause of some consternation when we counsel couples beginning a weight management program together. Upon their return for their first follow up visit, the gentleman invariably has lost more weight than the lady. "What's up with that?!" She would complain, going on to describe how much harder she worked on it than him.

Patience, my dear. *Men are from Apples and women are from Pears*, generally speaking. We know that "Pears" carry excess weight around the hips, buttocks and thighs. These are the troublesome "saddlebags", "thunder thighs" and what one frustrated patient bluntly described as a "butt with its own zip code!" While they may find it somewhat more difficult to lose weight at first, the good news is that pears keep it off longer and are less likely to suffer from heart-disease. Knowing this, we can focus on more targeted exercises.

Chloe's Choice

55 year-old Chloe from Arizona became our first "remote client," added to the many real patients sent to us from most states in the union over the years. Her parents resided at the extended care facility in Gibsonburg Ohio where we established the national in-patient morbid obesity unit. She had seen our program on the Discovery Channel; now she was hearing about it directly from her loved ones. Chloe signed up for the supervised fast communicating directly through the Internet, telephone and parcel post. Down 62 pounds in 10 months, hers was a drop in the bucket compared to many of our other patients. Yet, like so many others, she reported that she had tried all the popular diets with only limited and transient results. For the first time in 15 years her waist was less than 33 inches and she really felt good about herself. She was simply ecstatic! Her exact words "This is the best thing that my parents have ever done for me!"

> *The measure of our years is three score and ten; and if through strength we make it to four score, its pride is only trouble and sorrow, for it comes to an end and we are quickly gone.*
>
> (Psalm 90:10)

As responses like Chloe multiplied over the years, we found ourselves moving from operating on the morbidly obese to effecting phenomenal weight loss by getting patients to control their habits. In time, it became more obvious how personal weight is so closely linked with health, productivity, relationships and meaning in life. So we credit Chloe for finally persuaded us to move to the next level: how to effectively *prevent* obesity in the first place in concientious folks beyond our local area.

Cholesterol and Social Security

Cholesterol level is mostly related to diet. However, survey of the entire population statistics can be graphed as a bell-shaped curve. A small percentage of people on either end of the spectrum simply defy the odds. Statisticians call them the "outliers". I distinctly remember during my college years hearing on the news something quite contrary to sound nutrition dogma. It was about an 80 year old Georgia farmer who claimed that for years he ate a dozen eggs a day. Are you kidding me? I thought, especially after it was revealed that he was hale and hearty with normal cholesterol. From an egg-lover's standpoint, this gentleman would be seen as experiencing heaven on earth. From a statistical standpoint, he was a rare example of an outlier whose system was extremely efficient at processing fats.

By the same token, there are patients whose cholesterol and triglycerides remain consistently over 300 despite a low-fat vegetarian diet and active lifestyle. This was illustrated when I was asked to participate in judging a science fair at one of our local junior high schools. One student athlete was on six large cholesterol-lowering pills daily. For his project he worked with his family doctor, measuring his cholesterol weekly off his medication. The graph on his poster-board showed a spectacular rise into the 500 range. Later I found out that several of his relatives had suffered heart attacks and strokes at very early ages. Their *familial hypercholesterolemia* was so extreme that they were being studied by a large state university from a different region of the country. Such individuals absolutely require medication to prevent arteriosclerosis from clogging their blood vessels. In fact, it was this kind of historical observation that first suggested the connection between cholesterol and heart disease.

For most of the rest of us, what we eat generally is what we get. With half of all the sickness and death in our country being cholesterol related, every responsible adult should have their test scores on their fingertips. What's you cholesterol? It should be a reflex just like reciting your social security number upon request. You could even rattle it off in your sleep and scarcely remember having done so upon awaking. Is my cholesterol high? Is it normal? Am I one of those fortunate few whose cholesterol stays low regardless? Am I going along with just taking an expensive pill with its own side effects, or have I made a good faith effort to respond with lifestyles changes? Or worse yet, am I on one of those popular weight loss diets deliberately advocating high protein/high fat?

Medical science first documented cholesterol build up during autopsies performed on 18 year-old casualties of the Vietnam War. This is no longer a disease of old people. Start teaching youngsters early about the significance of cholesterol. Every adult should have a *complete lipid profile* by age 21, or earlier if they have a positive family history. The American Heart

Association recommends having this test done every 5 years. Before completing this book, you would do yourself a big favor by having this taken care of.

Here's why: Lipid profile breaks down total cholesterol into High Density Lipoprotein, HDL (I think of it as H for *healthy*), Low-Density Lipoprotein, LDL (L for *lousy*) and triglycerides (they really *try* your health). HDL are the good guys because they *carry cholesterol away* from the blood vessels to the liver where it is eliminated. That's healthy/good. HDL *prevents* the build up of deadly atherosclerotic plaque in the artery walls. LDL on the other hand, carry cholesterol from the liver to the rest of the body. When there is too much LDL in the blood, cholesterol is being *deposited* on the walls of the coronary arteries. That is lousy/bad because it eventually results in narrowing and blockage. This is the basic cause of poor circulation, heart attacks and strokes.

- Total cholesterol: The goal is to keep it below 200 mg/dl. A level closer to 150 is even better.

- HDL (High density lipoprotein) cholesterol: 35 to 100 mg/dl. Higher is better in protecting against heart disease.

- Keep total Chol: HDL ratio less than 5:1. Find out how to enhance that in *Balanced Nutrition* in Chapter 13.

- An LDL greater than 100 increases ones risk for early heart disease.

- Triglycerides (150 to 200 mg/dl) used to assess heart disease risk. Triglycerides increase significantly when blood sugar is out of control. That is why diabetes is such a risk factor.

Medical Causes of Obesity

As you recall, we started off this book with Jessica's struggle with weight. She tells of one of her friends who had tried every known commercial diet. By age 40, her weight was contributing to back problems and swollen, painful knees. She was getting short of breath and had been diagnosed with early heart failure. Her family physician referred her to an endocrinologist at a leading university center a couple hours away. The expert ran a battery of expensive tests. On her return visit he reviewed her results for cholesterol, thyroid functions, hormone levels and glucose tolerance. He told her all her tests were perfectly normal. "I guess you're just fat," he concluded. He gave her a pat on the back - and discharged her!

This poor woman was in tears as she recounted her ordeal. "I know I have a serious weight problem. All I wanted was some help. I didn't go all the way there for a doctor to tell me I'm fat!" The truth of the matter is that ours is more a disease care system than a healthcare system. Physicians are much better paid to perform procedures and quickly prescribe pills than to patiently promote good health. Just because the tests were negative did not mean that nothing could be done from a medical standpoint about the weight problem. Rather than simply scanning the numbers printed out from a computerized test, a little sensitivity and understanding of her lifestyle made a world of difference.

Having said that, the medical consensus is that hypothyroidism (under-active thyroid), accounts for no more than about 10 pounds. This is mainly due to accumulation of fluid. It slows down the metabolic rate. Imagine you trying to accelerate but you forgot to disengage the parking brake. The vehicle is revving up, but barely crawling. The way certain patients

> *When you blame others, you give up your power to change*
>
> Dr. Robert Anthony

describe their meager results for all their weight loss efforts suggests that we may be dealing with some such problem.

Hypothyroidism, however, occurs in only two percent of the population, though it is 10 times more common in women than men. A frequent cause for under active thyroid is *Hashimoto's disease.* The body's immune system produces antibodies that attack the thyroid gland. It can also be triggered by childbirth and/or stress. Thyroid hormone secretion is reduced causing symptoms of chronic fatigue, cold intolerance, dry skin or hair, difficulty concentrating and a rather deep monotonous voice. An over-active thyroid on the other hand causes nervousness, bulging eyes, palpitations and weight loss. Cabbage and soy products, otherwise quite healthy foods, have been reported to reduce thyroid function in certain individuals. By how much, it is not clear. Hypothyroidism can be routinely diagnosed with a simple blood test and can easily be treated once properly identified.

There are other more exotic conditions featuring obesity as a major part of their symptom complex. *Cushing's* syndrome for instance, is a hormonal disorder which affects no more than 15 people per million every year. It affects part of the brain called the hypothalamus or adrenal gland above the kidney. Tumors in the pituitary, and adjacent parts of the brain, result in increased *cortisol* levels causing weight gain. There are other rare genetic causes of obesity such as *Froehlich's Syndrome* (FS) in boys, *Laurence-Moon-Biedl Syndrome* (LMBS), and the *Prader-Willi Syndromes* (PWS). Among those, the most common is PWS with a prevalence of 1 in 12,000 to 15,000. The syndrome can result from brain injury from trauma or surgery. These patients never feel full. If food is not locked away, they literally eat non-stop. (Even perfectly normal people feel like that sometimes). *Polycystic ovarian syndrome,* a common hormonal disorder in women, is often linked to obesity. Clearly these occasional medical conditions, even when taken together, come nowhere close to accounting for the explosive obesity rate throughout society today.

Routine Screening Tests

You may have skimmed through much of the book so far thinking to yourself, "Thank God, this or that does not apply to me." Like Phil at the beginning of the chapter, we really should not wait until there is a problem before seeking professional attention. One patient was doing remarkably well on her weight management program but kept losing past her target weight. After ruling out anorexia, we ran a series of tests. We diagnosed a right-sided colon cancer! She did well after surgery and chemotherapy and maintained a healthy weight thereafter. I used a simple PSA blood test to diagnose my father's prostate cancer when he was completely without symptoms. Thanks to my urology and radiation oncology colleagues, his life was extended well beyond several of his peers afflicted by the same condition. If that was the only accomplishment in my medical career, it would be more than worth it. My heart's desire is to afford all my patients and their loved ones this very same protection.

The **Recommended Screening Tests** for Healthy Adults (page 308) can save your life. Copy the form and seek your doctor's input. Sound weight management is central to preventive holistic health, but it is not everything. Let this be your "owner's manual." If available, use the computer to neatly document your surgeries (year, surgeon, hospital, and results). Update prescriptions; (By whom? For what? How long?) Include over-the counter medications and supplements. It may well be that you no longer need certain ones. Fill out your **Medical History Form** (pages 302-305). Fax or email it ahead to new doctors. This saves your valuable time otherwise spent filling out forms in the waiting room and answering the same old questions over and over again.

Consider that for centuries, medical training was based on a secretive apprenticeship system. The senior physician would privately mentor an intern until he thought the young man was sufficiently trained to hang out his own shingle. It was based on who one knew and maintained by exclusive guilds and rigid class relationships. The advent of the medical school system opened doors for women and minorities, but offspring of physicians are still preferred over 'commoners' in the selection process. Skilled nurses were forbidden from independently performing routine medical services even when a rookie doctor had no idea what was going on. It was quite a struggle for nurse-practitioners to earn respect for their training and experience. The popularity of television shows like *General Hospital, Chicago Hope*, *The Learning Channel* and *Grey's Anatomy* has largely demystified medicine. Detailed medical knowledge is now at the fingertips of whosoever is interested. Physicians remain among the hardest-working professionals trusted with life and death issues. They will always be highly valued for their ability to efficiently sort through signs and symptoms, diagnose, reassure and treat promptly. Nevertheless, even though the Internet has blasted open the locks on healthcare plantation, most of the captives still have not ventured out beyond their traditional confines as passive patients.

Those dedicated to Manna*fast* principles are different. They acknowledge that they must be good stewards of that wonderful breath of life bestowed upon them from above. They motivated enough to at least get a handle on the basics: their blood pressure, blood sugar and cholesterol results. They seek out are conscientious physicians who are supportive of the covenant concept of healthcare. Chapter 20 shows reveals the inner workings of a vibrant *Covenant Group* and the huge difference in wellness that results. These people are proactive, on the ball and ahead of the curve. In so doing, they reduce the chances of falling victim to many of today's common ailments, including obesity.

Teach us to number our days and recognize how few they are;

Help us to spend them as we should.

Psalm 90:12

REVIEW

1. Are you an "apple" or a "pear?" How did you decide that?

2. Compare the BMI chart (page 3) to the Target Weight chart (page 301). Which is gives a better assessment of your weight?

3. How does your Body Fat Analysis (BFA) compare to the desired range for you age and gender?

4. When was your most recent lipid profile and how to you rate it?

5. What obstacles stand in your way of medical screening tests recommended for you at this time?

Chapter 8
Eating Disorders

You are a child of the universe,
No less the trees and the stars,
You have a right to be here.

Desiderata

What a cute little pumpkin, Mrs. Johnson thought proudly when she carried Tonya to her crib in her own room. Tucked under her soft, pink flannel blanket, she would sleep ever so sweetly. Back then, Mrs. Johnson obsessively double-checked the whisper-quiet baby monitor, especially after what she had read about Sudden Infant Death Syndrome. Twenty-four years later, Mrs. Johnson was in tears. She was up again checking her daughter's breathing. Tonya had gone out on her own worked for a few years, but came back to mother as her weight got the better of her. Her life was so empty. Tonya just couldn't stop eating, not because she was hungry, but to fill that hole in her soul.

Now, topping 900 pounds and totally bedridden, Tonya was making those grunting, choking sounds. The discomfort must be unimaginable, gasping for air like that, as if drowning in one's own flesh. She still clutched that same pink blankie, now tattered and faded. Mrs. Remington had tried to get help from all kinds of doctors. The weight-loss surgeons told her to come back after she had lost at least four hundred pounds. But nothing had worked. In desperation she had turned to the pulmonologist (lung doctor). After a series of tests he ordered a bulky mask (C-pap machine) triggered to blow oxygen into her when she breathed. It looked like something a test pilot would wear. Tonya found it cumbersome, to say the least, but it did make her sleep better.

Mrs. Johnson fretted that Tonya must have taken off the mask again. But she knew that once she had sucked enough oxygen into her lungs she would doze off, sometimes for as much as an hour. And like in the old

111

days, with her daughter asleep, Mrs. Remington herself could catch some z's. Her sleep was restless too as she tormented herself with questions like, "How could this happen to *my* daughter? Where did I go wrong?

Confusion Reigns

When food really gets a hold of a person, it takes more than a team of horses to pry them loose. Monkey-hunters exploit this principle by placing nuts in an anchored box in such a way that the animals can see them. The monkeys grab the nuts though a hole small enough to admit their slender hands, but not large enough for them to extract their fists full of loot. Their poor little hands will bleed to the bone as they struggle to escape but they just will not let go.

Wall Street with its $40 billion advertising budget accomplishes pretty much the same thing. They portray models and actresses as emaciated, "I-haven't-had-a-meal-in-days" waifs. Next we see these glamorized lean and sexy models happily stuffing themselves with the calorie-laden foods being advertised. The not-so-subliminal message to the viewers: go out and do likewise. Intelligent women, who swallow the bait, hook, line and sinker find themselves wondering why they too cannot have a body like that. Never mind that even these idolized models and Hollywood stars sometimes use body doubles to look picture perfect. The net result is that in comparison, an increasing number of women become painfully stuck with an overwhelming sense of worthlessness.

Signs of eating disorders show up early. Youthful frolicking give way endless candy bars and getting all dolled up like Barbie. By age 16, half are more preoccupied with dieting rather than preparing for academic or vocational achievement. Needy romance novels and sultry soap operas later define success for the modern American female as (1) snagging a man with enough plastic to shop till you drop and (2) having a skinny "trophy" body to show off. The quest for this ideal leaves a trail of dysfunctional dieting, superficiality and trivialization of modern western womanhood.

Out of depression

Have you ever sneaked food? How did it make you feel? We have all been there, to some degree or the other. *Closet eating,* or being ashamed of the amounts or types of food eaten is the first symptom in the slide to eating disorders. This is fuelled by a culture that glories in promoting over-indulgence. In cruel irony, society then turns its collective face from the monster it has created. Many react to fat discrimination by resorting to even more dysfunctional means to get this wicked genie back into the bottle. Experts agree that when full blown, more individuals succumb from eating disorders than any other psychiatric condition.

Every now and then, we feel upset about something that did not go quite the way we thought it should. This is not depression. It is natural to feel down from time to time. Eventually we may shrug our shoulders and say something like, "win some, lose some" or "All things work for the good." Then we move on. On the other hand, depressed persons suffer continuous feelings of sadness, diminished vitality, dejection and hopelessness. They feel "blue," "dragging" and "lack pep." They are unable to derive pleasure from simple joys - a lovingly cooked meal, a comfortable bed or some peace and quiet after a long hectic day. They remain unresponsive to the irrepressible laughter of children, interesting company, great weather, even an unexpected compliment.

Depressed patients suffer from higher rates of disease. They drop out of school, cannot hold on to a job or relationship. Their socioeconomic status falls and they lose their medical insurance (or never had it to begin with). This severely limits their treatment options. One out of seven commits suicide. Do you know seven depressed people? Scary isn't it? Depression is like death in slow motion. Acutely distraught individuals may use guns, while others may overdose on pills, but many unconsciously use tobacco, drugs, promiscuity, alcohol, and in this case food, as a weapon of choice.

It is rather cliché to attribute binges to emotional reactions and impulsive behavior patterns. Binge eaters know that they are out of control. They exhibit passive-aggressive behaviors focused on securing and engulfing food. They take revenge on the food cornered in the refrigerator. They snap at people, spurning attempts to reach out to them. We do our loved ones an enormous disfavor by thinking that it is simply a matter of just finding the right diet. As weight escalates, they suffer further stress and isolation, spiraling out of control.

Before the birth of the Internet, plus-sized women spent extra in time and money, trolling hard-to-find catalogs and far-flung specialty stores. With the obesity population boom, retailers are competing for a slice of the growing market. According to industry figures, the rate of increase in the sale of plus-sized women's apparel is double that of regular sizes. Yet, despite more accepting store policy, callous clerks and cavalier customers somehow let it slip with snide remarks and dirty looks directed at those seeking XXXL sizes.

Such unwelcoming treatment can be rather devastating. Can you think of anything more humiliating than being stuck in an amusement park ride or having a chair break under you in public? Some resorts have begun niche marketing making fat-friendly vacations and specializing in sturdy, plus-sized hospitality. This has spawned a reactionary association of "fat acceptance." It is often a company of the miserable, mad at the skinny world. This reflex protest however, diverts energy from useful solutions to the problem. While providing some aid and comfort now to those suffering from their weight, such a movement soon becomes beguiling quicksand, in effect, mass surrender to permanent victim status.

Abuse and Neglect

A 35 year-old patient had carried a weight of about 250 pounds all her adult life. Then she began steadily losing weight without trying. She did not mind it one bit seeing that she used to quit any program she started within a couple weeks. She had complained of some difficulty swallowing solids then even gagging on ice cream and porridge. It was only when she developed blood clots in her leg, however, did she seek medical attention. The Emergency Room physician promptly requested a surgical consultation. This condition, known as deep vein thrombosis (DVT), was unusual for women otherwise in good health and not on birth control pills.

As the work-up proceeded, a CT scan showed the liver to be chock full with tumors. The lower end of the feeding tube or esophagus was almost completely blocked off. Well there was the answer. And it was not good. Upper endoscopy (EGD) was proposed. This involved "swallowing" a fiberoptic tube in order to obtain a tissue sample from the esophagus. The procedure is normally performed under intravenous "conscious sedation" with the throat numbed using a topical anesthetic. Patients are not generally eager at the prospect, but in her case, she adamantly refused. "If anyone is going to put something down my throat, they'll have to knock me out, Doc. Completely!" It was only on further review of her medical history that she admitted to being molested at age 14. Counselors speculated that the event made it traumatic for her to undergo any professional oral instrumentation. Until that time she was of average body size. Thereafter she put on weight thus making herself less attractive to men. Even as the biological clock ticked away she had been quite content with a childless life.

If Dr. Siegel was right in theorizing that patients often develop cancers in areas where they were traumatized, I could not think of a more classic example. Clearly not every one with an eating disorder was abused. In the 1980's it became fashionable for various celebrities, and others seeking their 15 minutes of fame, to be "outed" on shows like Donahue and Oprah. They attributed their problems to a laundry list of family dysfunctions. Many such patients are prone to Obsessive Compulsive Disorders (OCD) and respond to adverse situations in certain predictable ways. Secondary gain push fuels these attention-seeking behaviors until they grow into Goliaths that eventually dominate their lives. Unless we effectively deal with the psychological obstacles to a healthy weight, issues invariably arise to sabotage any progress made.

The Bingeing-Obesity Connection

One of the first things the medical student learns is that whatever an alcoholic admits to consuming in a day, it is safe to assume that the actual amount is at least twice as much. It is the rare binge-eater who will come right out the first time and confess how much he really eats. Their initial response is usually, "Not much...I swear!" Others (perhaps conveniently) truly have no idea just how much they eat. Some complain that eating is a natural act and they should not have to think of everything going into their mouths. Well, what we are doing here is using the Food and Fitness Diary both as a diagnostic and treatment tool. It is no more unnatural than instructing an infertile couple to monitor body temperature to schedule precisely when to try.

The reason is that the hallmark of binge eating disorder is secrecy. Patients become remarkably efficient as they "Eat it and forget it." Their journal eventually reveals the candid truth about the amount eaten. Most of our patients had fairly average childhoods. Few admit to having been a fat child. And when that happens, we can often identify a parents routinely using food as a reward or bribe. Work history and personal relationships have a significant bearing on what makes a person massively obese. Acute increase in stress or personal loss often marks the start of escaping into the comforting arms of food. In much of the world, unemployment leads to "lean," tough times where folks have to hustle to survive. In America, just the opposite occurs. Absence of physical demands along with needed government assistance translates into having nothing to do and all the time to do it.

Today with the Internet, options are unlimited. When I first met one of my morbidly obese patients on the bariatric unit, he was chatting online with a housewife in Australia. At that time their cricket team was touring the West Indies so I asked him permission to chat with her for a minute. She was quite the sports enthusiast, knowing intimate details of those matches often lasting five days. It was quite the thrill to talk about something that had become worlds removed from my daily routine. As I handed him back the keyboard, her question scrolled across the screen: "Is your doctor tall, dark and handsome?" He winked at me and typed back, "He is tall and dark alright!"

Such bed-confined patients spend untold hours online chatting, gaming and engaging in a variety of pursuits. All the while, only their fingers do the walking. They literally do not have to burn the few calories from fetching their own food from the refrigerator. In some instances, the front door is left unlocked to facilitate fast food delivery all the way to the bedroom! When families grow tired of their manipulations, the state provides home care aides to assist with baths and housework. By the time he was admitted, our patient was at the point where he could only move his arms from the elbows. He could not lift his legs off the bed. It took a dozen of the staff to roll him one way then the other to change the linen under him. Suffice it to say, several nurses hurt their backs in the process; some even requiring emergency room visits!

Many months would pass before this patient finally admitted his true daily intake before coming to the facility: two large pizzas, a loaf of bread, a gallon of milk, and sometimes a whole chicken, *everyday!* Surely, he was making this up. But then again, how else could someone become that large? An extreme example, perhaps sounding more like what the giant in *Jack and the Beanstalk* would put away.

Indeed, when food gets a hold of a person, without the right kind of help, it is so hard to let go. The same way illegal drugs penetrate even maximum security prisons, so too bingeing on contraband food frustrates the best efforts weight loss facilities. Even in their helpless state, residents find ways to continue manipulating family and staff to enable their addiction. Those motivated to do well take advantage of support services and rise like cream to the surface. The rest become perpetual wards of the state with zero liability for their care. They bitterly blame "heartless" caregivers and an unresponsive healthcare system for failing to make them well. Working on the front lines of the war on obesity demands every ounce of professionalism to maintain morale. One has to be constantly reminded that this is just the nature of the disease. You may be the last chance before this individual plummets into the abyss. Your duty is to gently restore their sense of ownership of their predicament while managing their multiple medical conditions. Once this is attained, healing begins.

Can't Help Myself

Then there was Linda. She conscientiously watched her diet during the day. When her family turned in at night, she would raid the kitchen. Weapon of choice: frosted flakes.

"I just can't help myself Dr. Christian," she would sob, hesitantly reaching for yet another tissue. "And these were not your ordinary cereal bowls. These were mixing bowls, Dr. Christian, cake mixing bowls."

"Mixing bowls, you said, right?"

"Oh yes, Dr. Christian, *six of them,* I just couldn't stop myself."

According to the national association for Anorexia Nervosa and Associated Eating Disorders (ANAD), 7 million girls and 1 million boys are known to suffer from eating disorders. It is easy nowadays for patients to find each other on chatrooms where they trade secrets on radical weight loss and clothing tricks hide the evidence. Binge eaters consume unusually large amounts of food until they are uncomfortably full. Unlike bulimia, (discussed later,) individuals who binge do not try to get rid of the food consumed. This is not to be confused with those who take pride in their devouring prowess, like the gentleman signing up for a televised hotdog eating competition. It could be that he needs the money, has some real talent, or just loves the attention of making a pig of himself in public. A bingeing episode, on the other hand, has no such 'redeeming' qualities. It is specifically defined as secretly eating an amount of food that is much more than the average person would eat under similar circumstances. Bingers favor high calorie, high carbohydrate foods that go down easy such as ice cream, donuts, chips, candy, and cookies. When you hear of someone bingeing on vegetables, let me know.

When more delicious food avails itself, the normal person who is already full may tentatively take it (a little) or leave it. Not so for those who binge. They seem to know only one gear and that is - go for it! The mere presence of food is like a toddler with a knife - at high risk of inflicting grievous bodily harm. More than half of the participants in medically supervised eating disorder programs eventually admit to binge eating. They tend to become overweight at a younger age than those without the disorder. According to the *Diagnostic and Statistical Manual of Mental Disorders*, bingers eat when not hungry and generally lack a sense of control. This occurs at least twice a week over an extended period of time. Stretched stomachs predispose to recurrent hunger. Despite multiple attempts at yo-yo dieting, they inevitably become massively overweight.

Bulimia: Best of Both Worlds?

While bingers overeat and feel bad, for bulimics it is more a power thing. They enjoy doing it because they feel so clever at finding ways to "lose it." Purging is more commonly done by putting the finger to the throat to induce vomiting or with abuse of laxatives or diuretics. This grosses out the average person who sees something definitely wrong with this picture. Bulimics on the other hand see themselves as getting away with the best of both worlds. They can sneakily stuff in their favorite foods and still not show it on the scales. You scratch your head wondering why some people just cannot seem to lose weight never realizing that the normal-looking person next to you is infected with such strong denial of their habits. Although troubled with guilt at first, when finally confronted, these patients flat out say they will never quit: they would rather die than get fat again. Tragically, many females addicted to smoking (like Mandy in the Foreword) say exactly the same thing.

The physical ravages of bulimia result from vomiting and diarrhea. The retching rips at the lining of the esophagus (Mallory Weiss tears). Stomach acid erodes the dental enamel leaving a pale, yellow discoloration such as that seen in the tobacco chewer or smoker. The teeth themselves begin to look more elongated from acid-aggravated, receding gum lines. Laxative abuse can stir up hemorrhoids and rebound constipation from a lazy bowel grown accustomed to artificial stimulation. Diuretic abuse can result in critical electrolyte imbalance from loss of minerals like sodium and potassium so vital for heart function. Cheeks become puffy from retching. Instead of looking cuter, the cold law of diminishing returns takes effect. This ratchets up a vicious cycle of desperation as the patients lurches further out of control.

The typical bulimic keeps the scales on edge, fluctauting wildly up and down with their emotions. Anna Nicole was a classic example. Bulimics tend to be in jobs where weight is more of an issue - cheerleaders, dancers, models, gymnasts, actresses. Public behavior becomes more erratic with deepening depression as behind closed doors, they resort to extreme bingeing and purging. Eventual demise usually stems from suicide, drug abuse or medical complications.

Doctors spend many years studying all manner of disease because "the diagnosis you don't make is the diagnosis you don't know." Family physicians and gynecologists should be particularly suspicious of frequent requests for diuretics to treat "bloating," but really intended for weight control. Loved ones, likewise, must cultivate that sense of when something is not quite right. One clue might be frequent trips to the bathroom after meals. Is she having diarrhea or is she just freshening up again? Is that the scent of regurgitation being covered up with air freshener? Checking may be considered snooping or humbling, but what it turns up wrappers for unprescribed laxatives or diuretics? Watch for obsessive exercising without regard to injury, illness, weather, home, school or work obligations. Bulimia is not self-limiting: it does not correct itself. Only concerned interference can interrupt this downward spiral.

Features of Anorexia

Tabloids and gossip magazines revel in outing the latest high society damsels in distress trying to dodge the curse of anorexia. They have made much mileage with the Olsen twins and Princess Diana as she tried to cope with her prince charming. However, it was angel-voiced Karen Carpenter who had the tragic misfortune of being the poster child for this condition.

At age 16, standing 5' 2" and weighing 140 pounds she described herself as a "chubby teenager." Her doctor started her on a quick-fix diet reducing her to 115. Compliments on her appearance went to her head and weight loss soon became an end in itself.

Karen produced a stunning array of platinum, gold and Grammy award winning songs, holding the record for the most top hits in her debut year. Around age 24, her weight hovered around 80 pounds and she collapsed on stage while singing "Top of the World" in Las Vegas. She was stabilized with intensive medical efforts and appeared to do well thereafter. Her entourage looked out for her, but no doubt enabled her as well. She continued to abuse laxatives and brought up whatever little she ate. By February 2, 1984, she was back up to a passable 108 pounds. On that day her mother reportedly discovered her unresponsive in a walk-in closet. Unfortunately, this time, the best medical care in the world could not alter the prolonged ravages of this eating disorder.

Anorexia is characterized by a loss of 15-25 per cent of the usual body weight. It results in a distorted body image fueled by an exaggerated fear of how society treats fat people. Bulimics binge and purge. Anorexics disdain eating and still purge away the little that they consume. The typical anorexic is a white, teenage female coming from a somewhat rigid, upper middle class family with high expectations. Experts are unclear what the precipitating events may be. Girls at risk tend to be smart, sensitive and otherwise fairly disciplined. Away from the watchful parental eyes, new college coeds are most vulnerable.

Partly to assert their independence and to rebel against childhood restrictions, they begin to cultivating their self-image at the expense of what anybody else may think. When some crisis arises, academic, romantic or otherwise, losing a few pounds gives a sense of control. Compliments may have the unintended consequence of unhinging the anorexic to pursuing further weight loss as an end in itself. The anorexic feels personally threatened when friends or family express any concern about their relentlessly dropping weight. Eating like a bird, she counts calories to the extreme. Diet may consist of a few sprigs of salad here, a couple teaspoons of cottage cheese there, sips of diet pop and lots of water. When pressed, she becomes more evasive about her intake and more manic about exercise, purging or laxative abuse. As a survival measure, the body lowers its metabolism to preserve its remaining weight. When the anorexic notices that it is becoming harder to shed pounds, she becomes more fearful and resorts to even more drastic measures than the bulimic.

Herein is the dilemma in professional weight management: How does one generate the enthusiasm for healthy weight loss without tipping those at risk into the wasteland of anorexia? *Stomach conditioning* guards against that by inserting strong accountability to those who care. Because if the insidious nature of the disease, at some point, only committed clinical intervention is lifesaving.

At 5' 5", 100 pounds, Lizzie was a petite person to begin with. A very dependent and needy person, she did not fit the profile of the typical suburban anorexic. Her mother was a habitual offender, often in jail on drug related charges. Lizzie loved her mom dearly and would always provide her a room whenever released. Invariably, it would not be long before she once again got entangled with the seamy side. Even during one short stay, her mother managed to steal Lizzie's TV and sell it to Lizzie's best friend! Such is the power of addiction. With each contact with her mother, be it prison or home visits, Lizzie would experience fits of anorexia. Her weight would plunge 10, 15, 20 pounds. And she still thought she was fat.

Apart from her socio-economic background, Lizzie was the classic anorexic challenge. She would sequester herself in her bedroom with the blinds drawn for so many days on end that she became as pale as a sheet. From time to time, we would have to admit her and feed her directly into her veins through a "central line", a special catheter inserted in her neck or under her collarbone. We performed an exhaustive medical work-up to make sure she was not being consumed by some dreaded disease. But her real treatment was psychological with lots of counseling.

While facilities exist for the well-to-do, few services are available for regular people. We were frequently at odds with hospital discharge planners to justify keeping her. In many ways, it seemed that she was just not worth the trouble. We ended up pretty much adopting her total care anyway. When she kept missing appointments, we did not give up on her. Suddenly she would call wanting to be seen immediately for chest pain. Often we had to call the sheriff, social workers, relatives or neighbors to check on her when we thought she was falling between the cracks.

She eventually married a patient, family-oriented young man. His stabilizing influence helped buffer the emotional bumper-car ride that her life had become. This was one remarkable case where the weight gain of pregnancy turned out to be a godsend. Someone heard about our work with Lizzie and ask our permission for her to be on a talk show in New York. Lizzie consented to an all expenses paid trip, complete with her first airplane ride from the heartland of Ohio. Limousines shuttled her to the hotel and studios in downtown Manhattan. Even today, desperate families touched by Lizzie's brave appearance on that show contact us for advice.

It is quite a disturbing sight to see someone truly malnourished in a land of plenty. Skin and nails become dry and brittle. They develop *lanugo*: thin, furry, baby-like hair. With their skeletal appearance come menstrual irregularities leading to eventual complete loss of cycle (amenorrhea). Patients tend to be frail, prone to infections, dehydrated, dizzy, constipated, and insomniac. They complain of always feeling cold from losing much of the natural layer of fat insulation. To embrace them is like hugging a bag of bones. The starvation is every bit as haunting as that seen in concentration camps or places blighted by famine. Electrolyte and mineral loss results in chest spasms, muscle cramps and deep bone pain. Lizzie dodged the final stage of excessive thirst and urination indicating kidney failure. This would have been an ominous sign. The end actually comes as a relief to the loved ones who have watched with horror as an otherwise wonderful person slowly withers away before their very eyes.

Treatment for Eating Disorders

If truth be told, we all may show occasional flashes of eating disorders from time to time. Fortunately, positive feedback from family and acquaintances offers a reality check. This helps us to rein in the impulses which constitute the engine of the obesity epidemic. Continuing to rely on one-size-fits-all programs or costly surgical/mechanical solutions only result in more of the same. Diagnosis involves patiently identifying the triggers to abnormal eating behaviors and connecting the dots to the inevitable medical consequences. We have found that a *team approach* in a structured, nurturing environment is most effective. Mental health professionals may provide cognitive counseling and/or antidepressant therapy (such as Zoloft) enabling the patient to focus on their issues and follow a treatment protocol. The goal is to attain the capacity to turn away from that oral compulsion in response to those life problems which we must all face in some way, shape or form.

Social workers play an essential role in mitigating the contributing factors in the home environment. They also provide that critical link connecting patients to support services, such as may exist. Finally, nutritionists must carefully adjust dietary needs and treats based on rate of recovery. These fragile patients gradually begin to see a balanced diet as "the gift of God, for the people of God." Gently and prayerfully, we teach our loved ones how to let go of that food obsession and open their eyes to the wonderful experiences of life that await those who overcome.

One cannot underestimate the pivotal role that family and friends play in resolving this problem. The lucky ones realize that eating disorders never go away on their own. These conditions are rooted in denial and the best thing you can say is, "I will go with you to your appointment." When Tonya was brought to us on a flatbed truck, she could not get out of bed and was dependent on supplemental oxygen to survive. At the time of publication, with medical supervision she has lost well over half her excess weight. She applied her faith to learn how to let go. She still treasures her precious pink blankie, but now walks without oxygen sleeps without CPAP. She is pursuing college credits. Her self-esteem has blossomed to such an extent that she is even doing some plus-sized modeling, getting back at least some of the life she had missed out on as a young woman. Our loved ones eating disorders can be overcome. Mrs. Johnson proved that. She never stopped praying for her daughter, never grew tired of those deceptive self-defeating tendencies and never gave up in getting the best help available.

Expect trouble as an inevitable part of life and repeat the most comforting words of all: "This too, shall pass."

Ann Landers

REVIEW

1. Compare any case of anorexia you may have heard about in the media with issues in your own life.

2. What are the two main purposes of food and how does this relate to eating disorders.

3. What is the difference between Binge eating and Bulimia?

4. What forms can purging take? Do you personally know of anyone who has done that?

5. What is the best way to help someone with an eating disorder?

Chapter 9

Surgical Options

You are substituting one disease with another.
Regular life-long monitoring is critical
to avoid serious complications.

Bariatric surgery Patient Information Brochure

Controversy surrounded the way Prosecutor Star Jones was let go from the ABC's top-rated morning program, *The View.* Some argue that the show lost class with her departure. Others contend she hurt ratings by misrepresenting how she actually shed as much as 150 pounds.

The fact is everybody's doing it! Or so it seems. NBC weatherman Al Roker, Beach Boys daughter, Carnie Wilson, and American Idol panelist Randy Jackson and others have joined the growing list of celebrity poster children for gastric bypass surgery. Roker's fellow reporters put together several gushing prime-time specials on his giant step. For Jackson it meant not only critiquing contestants on their vocal talents, but on their physical presentation as well. After multiple subsequent plastic surgeries, once camera-shy Ms. Wilson even posed for Playboy! Anxiety over a loved one resorting to the surgery has been replaced by an excited "Why not me too?" It is now regarded as the final solution to their struggles, a fairy tale ending to their nightmare of obesity. Indeed, while safer and more accepted than before, the mainstream media is falling dangerously short in sharing with the public a balanced view of the real concerns involved.

Making it Happen

Something just did not seem to fit. He was a portly, distinguished looking gentleman. His starched white coat was draped over too-tight, red-splattered, green scrubs. We gave each other that manly nod as he strode into the elevator. He peered imperiously at me through eyelids puffy from long hours in the operating room. His stubby finger incessantly jabbed the already-lit button for the 4th floor to which I was heading. As we quietly looked up at the changing numbers, out of the corner of my eye I noticed a peculiar metallic object affixed to his earlobe.

Going through that compulsory period of professional hazing, interns were daily reminded that in the pecking order they were "lower than whale (*sediment*) at the bottom of the deepest ocean." It was unthinkable not to accord the utmost respect to senior attending physicians who controlled their destinies. I therefore reserved judgment on his ear piercing... But then again, it couldn't be! In those days, men in his position simply were not into that kind of fashion statement. I knew it was not polite to stare, but the more I looked, the more familiar the object appeared. Suddenly I realized what it was - a surgical staple! Somewhat stouter and shinier than the average office version, this titanium device did not appear to be holding together an incision or serving any obvious clinical purpose.

"Excuse me sir," I quipped in a burst of bravado, "But I think someone just stapled your earlobe."

Well, who told me to say that?! He glanced down at my name tag, his eyes flashing. I instantly felt like looking for a rock to crawl under.

"That's alright, uh...Sam." He smiled awkwardly. "I know." Now he seemed to be reveling in my incredulous look. "I put it there. Every time somebody asks me about it, I'm reminded that I have to lose weight."

Hmmm...I thought. Whatever!

Unlike the precision of ear acupuncture, this was an earnest, though rather exhibitionistic reminder of his promise to himself. The encounter confirmed this basic principle. Obesity is the result of eating more than the body can burn up. The solution is *portion control imposed by some external mechanical means, or the fruit of personal discipline we develop ourselves*. Unwanted weight causes considerable physiological and emotional distress. Each person responds by choosing his own path, some more desperate than others.

> *Equanimity under duress!*
>
> LaSalle Lefall, Jr.,
> First African-American President of
> the American College of Surgeons.

Take Connie for example, head nurse on the surgical ward at one of the hospitals where I trained. She was efficient, vivacious, attractive and carrying about 90 pounds more than desired. Our surgical team frequently admitted *party animals* with broken jaws from bar room brawls or boys just behaving badly. We would evaluate these trauma patients for internal injury and sew up their lacerations. Next, the Internal Medicine consultants

9. Surgical Options

would manage their DT's (delirium tremens: alcohol withdrawal symptoms) and related clinical problems. Finally, the Oral Surgery residents were summoned to wire their teeth together. This fixation was an "internal cast" for healing of the mandibular fracture. Side effects included damage to gums, teeth, and the temporo-mandibular joint (TMJ). As one could imagine, jaw wiring is anything but comfortable. With the tongue locked away for weeks, the patient could only scrub the outside of their teeth. One shudders to think of how they handle getting nauseated!

So imagine my dismay when I greeted Connie one morning and she answered through clenched teeth. I saw the wires and my heart jumped ...Connie had become a *metal-mouth* too! Surely, her fashion-model features could not have required any cosmetic jaw surgery. Was she assaulted or was it domestic violence? I was confused, afraid to ask. "Don't worry, Dr. Sam." She giggled. "I decided to get it wired. I've got to lose this weight. I'm getting married this summer!"

I was so relieved and happy for her. She explained that she could only "eat" through a straw. Jaw-wiring patients limited to a liquid diet indeed lose significant amounts of weight. And so it was with Connie. She had already lost 5 pounds in the previous week and went on to shed another 53. She looked simply stunning for her wedding and lived happily ever after. Except that within months of being unwired, she was large and in charge again!

The Rise of Obesity Surgery

Father of abdominal surgery, German-born Dr. Theodor Billroth, performed the first formal stomach operation in 1885. From that time, surgeons have known that patients having part of their stomachs removed as treatment for cancer or ulcer disease would suffer from "failure to thrive." This was a medical way of saying this individual would stay thin despite best efforts to "put some meat on his bones." Their appearance would be reminiscent of Shakespeare's description of Cassius as having that "lean and hungry look." Back then, such weight loss was considered an undesirable side effect of stomach surgery.

As widespread obesity began to rear its ugly head in the 1970's, some clever surgeons said "Hey! Why don't we do that ulcer surgery on these heavy folks?!" A variety of modifications were made to the original procedure. These are major operations that seal off most of the stomach to decrease the amount of food eaten. Later on, surgeons began to rearrange the small bowel to reduce the calories absorbed. In a way, it is comparable to rails used in bowling for kids having difficulty keeping the ball from rolling off into the gutter. Surgery is viewed as a magic wand guaranteeing a lucky strike every time. However, patients still failing to do the real work of recommended *lifestyle changes* end up unconsciously finding ways to undermine this major operation. Such behaviors included indulging in frequent snacking (grazing) or sipping endlessly on milk shakes. The result is inevitable weight regain even without anything being technically wrong with the operation itself.

Coincidence perhaps, but at that very time effective medical treatment was rapidly making routine ulcer surgery a thing of the past. During my training, it was common to admit at least a couple people each day with bleeding ulcers. These peptic ulcers were generally thought to result from:

(1) Non-Steroidal Anti-Inflammatory Drugs, (NSAIDS)
    pain medicines like Motrin, Aspirin and Narprosyn

(2) Stress.

This seemed to make sense. An array of high-pressured personalities suffered from peptic ulcers including General Stonewall Jackson, Ayatollah Khomeini of Iran, Mrs. Imelda Marcos of the Philippines, President George Bush Senior, and Pope John Paul II. This was more than just an academic interest because my own mother suffered terribly from ulcers. I remember how she could hardly take medicine for her arthritis out of fear that it would further tear up her stomach.

I knew the score when I too, developed the symptoms. I was diagnosed with a special x-ray that involved drinking that chalky 'milk shake.' (Upper G.I. Series). Nothing on television tormented me more than those slow motion ads for healthy, golden-yellow, Florida orange juice. Every few months or so, I would break down and try some only to pay a severe price within hours of the first sip. I dared not leave home without antacid tablets and supply of Tagamet, Zantac or Pepcid. Surgeons being generally Type A, highly stressed individuals certainly were not immune to the final stage of perforated ulcers. Like watching a cop being arrested or a judge on trial, it was a haunting irony seeing a fellow surgeon slumped on the gurney being rushed into the operating room. I was resigned to the fact that any day I would be next to be struck down.

Then, out of the blue, this upstart theory surfaced. Gastroenterologist Dr. Barry Marshall and pathologist Dr. Robin Warren from the Royal Perth Hospital in Australia began asserting that peptic ulcers were mainly caused

9. Surgical Options

by a bacterium named *Helicobacter pylori* and treatable with antibiotics. Needless to say, like everyone else, I was quite skeptical. That was until I had the triple antibiotic therapy myself and was completely healed. I was a new man! Now I can have all the orange juice I ever wanted and not worry about a thing. Both my Mom and I speak with one voice that this is something from the good old days that we do not miss one bit.

The day that news of this revolutionary approach to ulcer treatment first hit the newsstands, stocks for manufacturers of the old antacid drugs tumbled $1 billion. Back then, the average hospital operating room would perform several emergency bleeding ulcer cases each week. As it turned out, with new and improved ulcer medicines (Nexium, Prevacid, Protonix, Aciphex) it is not unusual for months to go by without the average surgeon seeing an ulcer patient. When one showed up it was usually some old recluse who had not been to a doctor in decades. Since the operating room is the major profit center of hospitals, it is easy to see how this change in disease management made quite a dent in revenues. Perhaps in response, like the pioneering Oklahoma Sooner's, hospitals began tripping over each other to establish bariatric surgery programs. After all, this was an operation for which desperate people were willing to take loans of anywhere from $25,000 - $35,000 to pay up front as eagerly as getting the latest model dream car.

Pre-Certification for Surgery

The 1998 National Institutes of Health Consensus Conference and the Milliman and Robertson Guidelines determine which obese patients are candidates for gastric surgery. Basically patients should have a Body Mass Index (BMI) greater than 35, along with co-morbid conditions such as hypertension, diabetes, sleep apnea or significant pain in weigh-bearing joints. Technically, a BMI greater than 40 by itself qualifies a patient for morbid obesity surgery. This often translates to being at least 100 pounds over ideal body weight based on the standard BMI charts in Chapter 1.

Health Insurance companies generally request a detailed listing of weight loss efforts attempted. Beyond the routine commercial Jenny Craig, Weight Watchers and Adkins, many now specifically require HgbA1C (sugar test) above 8, and at least one year of a medically supervised program with professional nutritional counseling a minimum of twice a month. This is an effort to weed out surgery-seekers who try a vanity diet for a couple weeks and then insist that they cannot lose weight. Oftentimes, surgeons are required to submit additional psychological or psychiatric evaluations documenting that the patient does not suffer from glandular or eating disorders, untreated depression, dysfunctional family support, unrealistic expectations, or drug /alcohol abuse. This is in order to evaluate the likelihood of compliance with post-operative instructions, understanding of the risks involved and the need for rigid follow-up, regardless of outcome. Since weight loss surgery is no small ticket item, insurance companies tend to routinely turn down initial requests often by imposing stringent additional criteria not originally outlined in the members' benefits package. Patients have to carry on a several month campaign for approval, sometimes having to resort to the threat of legal action.

Weight Loss Operations

Historically, the first surgery specifically designed for weight loss, *Jejuno-Ileal Bypass*, was based on shortening the small bowel to less than ten percent of its original length. The stomach itself was not reduced meaning that there was no restriction on consumption. Much of the food eaten was not absorbed. This resulted in dramatic weight loss making these pioneers the toast of the town. However, they began developing severe nutritional and metabolic problems. Several patients died before it was eventually concluded that the weight loss did not justify the risk. Jejunal-Ileal bypass is now thoroughly discredited and is mentioned here for historical purposes only. The following are the five main weight loss surgeries being done today:

1. *Gastroplasty*
2. *Bilio-Pancreatic Diversion*
3. *Duodenal Switch*
4. *Gastric Bypass*
5. *Adjustable Gastric Banding*

We will look at what the future holds for each procedure and for other techniques clawing for a piece of the obesity pie.

Gastroplasty

This stomach stapling operation was popular in the 1970's and 80's. The upper stomach was fashioned into a small pouch, which could accommodate a couple tablespoons (30cc) of food. A band of synthetic mesh was used to reinforce the outlet to slow emptying. After the fiasco with the Jejuno-ileal Bypass, we made this procedure *restrictive* meaning that nothing was done to the bowel to reduce absorption of nutrients. Patients had initial promising weight loss. Ironically, although patients would feel full after a few bites, they would seldom feel truly satisfied (satiety). Bingers in particular found ways to overcome the procedure. This resulted in *stretching* the stomach and frequently tearing the staple line. At one time, these patients were convinced that they were on the cutting edge. Within five years, seventy percent regained the weight. Many had to endure re-operation and worse. Gastroplasty is now largely passé.

Bilio-Pancreatic Diversion

The pendulum had swung one way, then the other. Surgeons therefore decided to combine components of both of the previously mentioned procedures. We removed much of the stomach and re-arranged the intestinal tract. Digestive enzymes were diverted away from the food stream for a variable distance based on excess weight. This reduced absorption of fats and starches while allowing near-normal absorption of proteins and sugars. The down side is chronic diarrhea, nutritional deficiencies, brittle nails, bad breath and notoriously foul smelling stools. Despite this, binge eaters tended to favor this surgery because they did not have to change their portion sizes.

Duodenal Switch

The Duodenal Switch is a modification of the Bilio-Pancreatic Diversion procedure (BPD) championed by my colleague Dr. Douglas Hess of Bowling Green, Ohio. Part 1 of the procedure involves cutting the stomach down to the size of a bratwurst. The stomach capacity is 4-5 ounces compared with about an ounce in the standard gastric bypass. It therefore retains better capacity and portion sizes when compared to subsequent procedures while producing superior weight loss.

Unlike the BPD, the Duodenal Switch *keeps the duodenum with its intact pyloric valve in its normal anatomic position*. This major difference retains much of the important gastroenteric feedback neural regulation compromised in the standard gastric bypass. With more of the stomach retained, the Duodenal Switch continues to produce intrinsic factor so valuable to proper nutrition. Iron, calcium, and Vitamin B12 absorption is superior to the BPD. The presence of the duodenum virtually eliminates "channel outlet" ulcers and *dumping syndrome* (nausea, diarrhea, dizziness and palpitations from eating high calorie foods). However, patients are still prone to most of the other problems of its predecessor operation, especially low blood count requiring periodic transfusions, low potassium, protein and albumin which in turn lead to leg swelling.

Interestingly enough, the first part of the operation (limited to the stomach), now called a *vertical gastrectomy,* is increasingly being used as the final procedure for super-morbidly obese patients. Again, this is nothing new. We have known this since 1885. But then, super-morbidly obese patients in those days were as common as hens' teeth.

Gastric Bypass

This is currently considered the "gold standard" of modern obesity surgery. It is the most commonly performed weight loss operation at this time because it has fewer side effects. The stomach is reduced to a small pouch, which holds about 1 ounce of food. The patient actually feels full with just a few bites of toddler-sized portions. The small intestine is cut about 20 inches below the stomach, and is re-arranged so as to bypass much of the stomach while maintaining the flow of digestive juices. There is less interference with normal absorption of food. Patients lose 80-100 percent of excess body weight - *if they adhere to a strict behavioral pro-*

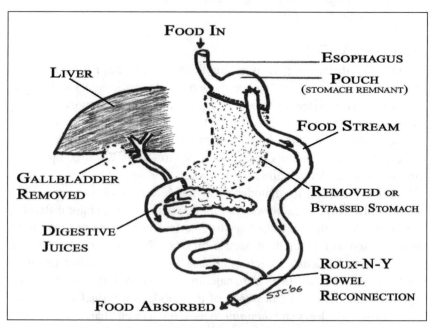

Anatomy of the Bypassed Stomach
(Compare to normal anatomy, page 67)

9. Surgical Options

-gram.

Many surgeons are now performing the procedure laparoscopically, through multiple small incisions. Patients have lower risks of hernia, pain and scarring. Many return to normal activities within 2 weeks. The patient has to be carefully managed for the same problems described above, including gas-bloat syndrome. They are also committed to a lifetime of testing and special supplements. A large part of the stomach is no longer accessible to the endoscope when checking for stomach problems such as bleeding or cancer.

Dr. Mal Fobi, a Cameroon-born surgeon practicing in Los Angeles, made two significant modifications to the gastric bypass procedure. These changes have helped overcome major weaknesses in weight loss surgery. First is the addition of a silastic ring to the outlet of the gastric bypass to minimize stretching. The other was the placement of a gastrostomy site marker providing access to the bypassed stomach for endoscopy, (though that still remains more technically difficult). Touted as the "Surgeon to the Stars," Dr. Fobi has operated on the likes of Gospel singer Andre Crouch, comedienne Roseanne Barr and Randy Jackson mentioned at the beginning of the chapter. Fobi's additional steps are not widely accepted by surgeons because it makes the procedure that much more complex which increases potential risk. The search therefore continues for ways to make the weight loss surgery more natural, durable and safer at the same time.

Adjustable Gastric Banding

Banding meets some of these criteria and is now threatening the popularity of gastric bypass. It involves laparoscopic placement of a silastic band like a noose around the outside of the upper stomach. This deforms the organ into an hourglass-shape forming a small pouch with a narrow passage. The band is inflatable like a blood pressure cuff. This is connected by tubing to a watch-sized port (container) under the skin of the abdominal wall. The surgeon then adjusts the snugness of the band by injecting into or removing saline from the port.

With other obesity operations, the openings to the surgically created stomach pouches can sometimes be *too tight* causing solid food to get stuck. That choking sensation increases saliva production from painful swallowing. Excessive weight loss results in an emaciated and malnourished appearance. On the other hand, if the surgeon errs on making the opening *too loose,* food intake is hardly restricted resulting in minimal weight loss. Since these patients were depending on surgery to limit caloric intake for them, they are quite unhappy after having subjected themselves to such risk and expense. With the adjustable band, the surgeon can get it just right even after surgery.

A major advantage of gastric banding is that it does not open or cut into the gastrointestinal tract. This reduces the risk of infection and virtually eliminates the chance of deadly leak of stomach acid. This has persuaded more people to favor this approach. However, although approved by the FDA, several insurance companies still consider it an investigational procedure and resist coverage. Overall weight loss is generally less than with gastric bypass, though it gives the patient a substantial head start. It is generally reserved for people less than 270 pounds, effectively excluding patients requiring massive weight loss.

The problems associated with gastric banding center around - and here is that word again - *stretching* of the stomach pouch, the part isolated above the band. It balloons out, usually from bingeing, which results in weight regain. Many researchers like Dr. Charles Filipi at Creighton University in Omaha Nebraska, suggest that anatomic stresses such as coughing, gagging or vomiting explain the failure of such procedures. One must bear in mind that any device placed in the body can erode into tissues over time, especially if the organ is a mobile one such as the stomach. Although it is the most "minimally invasive" of all the procedures, lethal threats exist compared to non-surgical massive weight loss.

Gastric pacing is another procedure in its trial stages. Wires are attached to the stomach. The operation is simpler than any of the above because the stomach is not cut or deformed in any way. Surgeons then connect these wires to a battery under the skin much the same way as a cardiac pacemaker. The patient then adjusts the current, inducing a sensation that diminishes hunger. Preliminary results so far are modest. Patients have reduced appetite when their device is turned on though some interpret the unpleasant sensation as nausea. Because they can turn it on or off at will, many feel that it defeats the purpose for stringent mechanical control.

And of course there is *liposuction.* Some patients wish to pass on all the technical stuff by saying, "Just suck it out of me, Doc!" For those who can afford it, liposuction is an accepted part of a menu of "nip and

9. Surgical Options

tuck" services to help limited problem areas. However, this is considered a cosmetic procedure offering little practical help for the truly obese. Liposuction risks include injury to blood vessels and nerves. Fragments of fat can enter the bloodstream (emboli) and block off the lungs with the same lethal consequences as blood clots.

Perhaps the most notorious example was a top druglord south of the border whose girth spread to prosperous proportions on his ill-gotten gains. He underwent extensive liposuction in an effort to elude the Drug Enforcement Agency and Interpol. However his billion-dollar bank account could not shield him from the perils lurking behind the promise of quick weight loss. When he failed to wake up, his ruthless henchmen made sure that his surgeon who would never again perform another operation.

Post-Gastrectomy Diet and Follow-up

Here is the general care plan after surgery:

- Post-Op Day (P.O.D.) #1, the day after surgery: Ice chips, deep breathing exercises, out of bed and walking.

- P.O.D. #2: Sips of water.

- P.O.D. #3: Clear liquids, gelatin.

- P.O.D. #4: If patient shows signs of bowel activity, advance to small amounts of full liquids (custard, soups, etc.)
  Discharge according to clinical pathways protocol.

- 1-2 weeks after surgery: First office check for staple removal. Advance to soft/pureed foods.

- 2-4 weeks after surgery: Second check up. If progressing satisfactorily the patient is advanced to a low fat, healthy meal plan.

Patients begin eating regular foods, but a lot less than before. They are encouraged to chew thoroughly and to avoid drinking fluids at mealtime. Generally speaking, following surgery, there is no turning back. No more bingeing. No more cheating. Like the electric shock in classical conditioning, patients violating these instructions quickly find out that they do so at their own risk. In a sense, the surgery whips them into eating right. Patients freely admit, "If it wasn't for the surgery, I just couldn't stop myself from overeating!"

135

Weight loss surgery therefore can be compared to *Antabuse* (Disulfiram), a drug sometimes used to treat chronic alcoholics. Patients on this medication falling off the wagon and indulging in even small amounts of alcohol suffer a spectrum of unpleasant symptoms that include severe vomiting, throbbing headache, difficulty breathing and chest pain. While an alcoholic can choose to stop taking Antabuse, the surgery patient has permanently traded all choice for lifelong medical monitoring. If all goes well, as is usually the case, weight loss at first can range from 10 to 30 pounds per month depending on starting weight. For persons who have only yo-yo dieted before, this is an intensely exhilarating experience overshadowing any other important considerations mentioned later.

Complications of Surgery

There is always risk with major surgery. These include, but are not limited to anesthesia problems, bleeding, infection, heart attack and death. There are specific additional complications associated with bariatric surgery ranging from early to late.

Leak

Within the first threes days after surgery, staple line breakdown can cause leaking of stomach acid into the abdominal cavity. This is a dreaded early complication showing up as excessive abdominal pain and fever. If the leak is slight, it can be observed for healing over several days while the patient is nourished through the veins or feeding tubes positioned downstream in the bowel. Larger leaks require emergency re-operation to avert septic shock from which it is difficult to recover.

Clots

A small fraction of patients develop *clots* in the deep veins of the legs known as Deep Venous Thrombosis or DVT. Surgeons frequently insert special vena cava filters before surgery via neck or groin veins to prevent potential clots from ascending to the lungs. Clots cause sudden and frequently fatal pulmonary embolus even weeks after apparent normal recovery. Special care is also taken to prevent clot formation by using blood thinners (Heparin, Coumadin, and Lovenox), leg pumps/compression stockings and getting the patient out of bed/walking as soon as possible.

Hernia

Up to a quarter of patients subsequently develop incisional *hernias* from the strain of a large belly. A hernia can be described as a painful, squishy, bulge of bowel protruding between a defect in the abdominal wall under the skin. This can only be fixed surgically. Repair is often delayed after most of the weight is lost, so that the surgeon can also do a non-cosmetic "tummy tuck" by removing unsightly *excess hanging skin*.

For many patients who are financially pressed, this is a factor in deciding whether to have the surgery done the old-fashioned "open" way rather than the slightly riskier, but more elegant laparoscopic method. In other words, patients figure that if they are going to end up with a huge scar anyway, it is to their advantage to have the bariatric surgeon fix the anticipated "hernia" (a covered procedure) a couple years later, rather than having to pay a plastic surgeon out of pocket.

Adhesions

As many as one in five of all abdominal and pelvic operations such as cholecystectomy, appendectomy, hysterectomy, etc. will eventually develop *adhesions*. This is painful scar tissue causing organs to get stuck with each other and to the abdominal wall. The process may take from weeks to decades to become symptomatic. Adhesions often have less to do with the quality of the surgery. It seems more related to the tendency of certain individuals to form exuberant scars. Examples include keloids ("proud flesh") resulting from skin incisions or lacerations.

The first signs of intestinal adhesions are mild and intermittent, but then become chronic and severe. Like a twisted garden hose, it can deteriorate into complete intestinal obstruction. Many products have been devised to minimize or treat adhesions with limited success. Only surgery can restore bowel function and eliminate the pain. However, like a recurring decimal, each re-operation to take down adhesions sows guaranteed seeds for future adhesions, often with increasing frequency.

Nutritional deficiencies

Bariatric surgery interferes with natural digestion. As many as one out of three develop *osteoporosis* and *anemia* because the portions of the gut involved in calcium and iron metabolism has been bypassed. Skin becomes wrinkly. Complexion turns pale and sallow. Even men confess to using make-up to appear normal. Weight loss surgery patients usually require a daily cocktail of vitamin and mineral supplements to help stave off these conditions. Some go on to require repeated blood transfusions.

Women in particular have some extra concerns. *Nails* may become brittle; *hair* may fall out, especially in the first few months (often returning in a coarser texture). Pregnancy during the initial period of rapid weight loss exposes the fetus to nutritional deficiencies. These children may suffer from *low birth weight* and *other developmental problems*. Since physicians can be held liable for diminished performance of children till age 18, many surgeons insist women of childbearing age sign a separate informed consent. This commits them to ironclad birth control measures for at least two years after surgery or until body weight stabilizes.

Cancer?

Researchers have known for some time that cancers arise in areas of chronic irritation. Diverted stomach acid and refluxed bile assaults tissues not normally exposed to these otherwise corrosive substances. We do not yet know all the generational risks of bariatric surgery. But there are anecdotal signs of an increased incidence of stomach cancer. In the long term, it will be interesting to see how does the longevity of weight loss surgery patients compare with those successful at massive, non-surgical Manna*fast* weight loss.

Just the Facts

It was generally accepted that mortality from bariatric surgery was about one in a hundred. That was considered an acceptable risk unless of course, that one was a relative or friend eagerly looking forward to a light and lovable life. However, more recent studies revealed a higher than expected death rate, in some cases up to 13 percent. University of Washington surgeon Dr. David Flum found that up to half of the older patients died within a year of the surgery. (*Journal of the American Medical Association, October 19, 2005*).

> *If God simply granted our every desire, he would be cheating us of our greatest satisfaction – that of accomplishment.*
>
> Anon

With war casualties, for each death there are at least ten who are seriously wounded. The same applies to surgery. One of the main reasons for this undercount is that problem patients often do not announce that they are switching to another surgeon or hospital. After all the initial compliments from family and friends, patients tend to hide their complications. Those who embark on this journey always deserve our prayers and support, but rest assured that any setbacks suffered by celebrity patients are kept under tight wraps for obvious reasons.

9. Surgical Options

I have taken care of a number of patients from other surgeons presenting with a wide spectrum of complications. These range from severe hemorrhoids associated with chronic diarrhea (averaging 4 -12 per day), to chest pain from constant loss of potassium. Some have had to be life-flighted because of bleeding ulcers from the part of the stomach now out of reach. Everyone is aware that bad things can happen with surgery, up to and including not making it. What the average lay person is not in a position to appreciate is the painful social impact such complications have on personal lives.

Laura was perhaps the unhappiest patient ever encountered. Bathroom breaks at work fuelled merciless harassment from immature coworkers who did not take kindly to the fumes. That characteristic malabsorption odor comes from incompletely digested food associated with properly performed weight loss surgery. She also complained bitterly of *new troubling body odor* resistant to frequent showers, fragrant lotions and perfumes. It comes out in the breath and sweat and is almost impossible to mask in face-to-face conversation. She lamented that it ruined intimate relations. Her husband claimed it reminded him of that scent in the room when his mother was dying from cancer. Laura's surgeon dismissed her saying it was all in her mind and suggested counseling. There could not have been a more grateful patient when we provided some measure of relief with a regimen of anti-diarrheal medication and Zinc supplementation.

Orphan Syndrome

It can be extremely challenging to reverse most bariatric procedures gone bad. Re-operative surgery compared to operating on a "virgin abdomen" can be as different as night and day. This is the major reason why surgeons avoid like the plague having to fix another's mistake. No matter how detailed the description of the original operative report, one just cannot know for sure where things are anymore. After all, traditional weight loss surgery is *designed to alter normal anatomy.* Adhesions make dissection more tedious and hazardous. Many surgeons feel they could not be paid enough to risk being drawn into somebody else's malpractice suit. It is to the point that a known AIDS patient having a better chance at getting a new doctor than a problem weight loss surgery patient has finding a new surgeon.

Obesity surgeons are incredibly busy. They are often booked up a year in advance. As such, they tend to have little time for old patients with late complications. Though they might have been previously healthy, these patients now find themselves wondering in a no man's land. They may require multiple additional unplanned procedures and treatments. sinking deeper into a financial hole at a time when they may be earning less regular income. It also affects their ability to switch jobs or relocate because new insurance policies generally *exclude complications from pre-existing conditions or surgeries*.

There is often no negligence on the part of the original surgeon. For instance, forceful vomiting can rip the lining of an intact, normal esophagus and stomach. This is an uncommon condition called *Boerhaave's Syndrome*. The staple line of a bypassed stomach is that much weaker. Throwing up after gastric bypass adds a new dimension of peril. A simple stomach virus can expose a weight loss surgery patient to this rare but significant jeopardy.

Such a step should be entered into solemnly; as a last resort and not on a whim. Unlike surgery for cancer or trauma, the result of this optional operation can be definitely accomplished in a safer, more gradual way. The unsuccessful weight loss surgery patient tends to see himself as the ultimate failure and delays seeking help. I have known of patients to commit suicide not only from regaining weight or depressing recurrent complications, but even from adjustment difficulties to the sudden, massive positive change in body image.

Unexpected major problems can develop at anytime. Furthermore, over a ten-year period, *left to their own devices*, about 90% of patients slowly regain weight. Understandably, how a patient feels about their surgery depends very much on *when* they are asked. During the first couple years when enjoying weight loss without attention to diet and exercise, patients simply rave about it. In the long term, as late complications creep into the picture, a lot fewer patients are inclined to say the same thing. In these cases the stomach may have been worked on, but the eating disorder in their heads remains untreated.

What Were We Thinking?

Most patients do well overall, at least for the first few years. I did the same operation on two sisters a few months apart. Both lost weight nicely. One found it difficult eating meat, the other could no longer stand vegetables and vice versa. Tastes change. Outcomes are not always quite predictable. Many patients say years after the operation, "Best thing I ever did. I don't know why I waited so long. I'd do it again in a heartbeat." Others are not around to speak for themselves. As Forrest Gump said, "Life is like a box of chocolates. You don't know what you're going to get."

As indicated earlier, because of our background in nutrition and surgery, we once offered both dietary weight management for morbid obesity as well as weight loss operations. Patients failing the medically supervised program could then be certified as candidates for surgery. But it was not long before patients would separate into two groups. Those who could not, or would not have surgery, could be motivated to excel. In contrast, patients coming in fixated on having surgery at all costs, tended to do much poorer at losing weight on their own. It was like *Dante's Inferno:* "Abandon every hope, ye who enter here."

Aggressive surgeons actively lure surgery-seekers. Hospitals outsource to sleek marketing agencies for recruitment of the obese. With their expertise in navigating the insurance pre-certification minefield, these business consultants more than pay for themselves by keeping operating rooms humming. Medical, psychological and dietetic consultants are pressured to quickly clear patients for surgery. Those not quite meeting the weight criteria for surgery were "encouraged" with a wink and a nod to come back when they were heavier! That is where I drew the line.

Badge of Bravery

Those opting for surgery generally are the ones having the courage to risk it all for a radical change in life. However, there is another consideration. Throughout history, a fairly constant fraction of every population has suffered from a psychological condition known as *Munchausen's syndrome*. These individuals are not raving lunatics, but clever enough to mimic symptoms and persuade doctors to operate on them. Given equal options, Munchausens' masochistic streak drive them to go under the knife to brag about the adventure or milk more sympathy.

Yet, instead of being selective, fierce competition keeps pushing the envelope with surgeons casting their nets to patients as young as 12 and as old as 75. Frankly, I believe it is wrong to subject a child to a discretionary procedure with the potential for lifelong, even fatal consequences. Once a good faith effort has been made to eliminate medical/genetic causes for obesity, what is left is a child that is purely the product of his environment. Children put through intensive nutritional and activity programs have been able to neutralize the toxic influence of that home. Chapter 17 explains how parents can reverse obesity in children under their watch. When they come of age, these youth can make the awesome decision themselves.

The general public has little idea how wrenching it is caring for someone dying prematurely. During my residency, I remember a very attractive 35 year-old single woman who had weight loss surgery. She enjoyed a couple glamorous fat-free years then developed a late complication of terminal liver failure. Even now I can see her flaming red hair and her ready smile despite her constant pain made worse by eating. All the doctors in the world were helpless to reverse the terrible course of events. I can still hear her voice as if it were yesterday. "If I had only known I that could have ended up like this," she wept, "I would never have done it, never!"

Operations are generally divided into three categories.

1. Emergency: No questions asked. Examples include c-section for fetal distress, immediate angioplasty or coronary bypass for a major heart attack. Another would be lifeflighting the severely injured from the accident scene and zipping them to the rooftop of the trauma center where the operating team is standing by.

2. Elective: The largest category. It can be done tomorrow or next week but hopefully not next month. Examples include an inflamed gallbladder or suspicious breast lump.

3. Optional: Generally non life-threatening operations. There may be a solid medical reasons (breast reduction to reduce back pain) or *cosmetic,* such as Carol Burnett's chin or Michael Jackson's nose.

At different times, obesity surgery may reside somewhere between categories 2 and 3. In my experience, timely professional weight management almost always banishes the need for surgery. It is getting way beyond the point of what society can afford. For a tumor, tonsil or torn spleen, healthcare will do as it must; but the days of unregulated surgery for fat is fast becoming a luxury that premium/tax payers can no longer stomach.

The average hospital CT scan can only bear 450 pounds. This effectively excludes many of our super-morbidly obese patients. On February 15, 2006, The Center for Medicare and Medicaid Services imposed a limitation for coverage of obesity surgery to "centers of excellence." These facilities, (one or two in an average large state), must have the track record of at least 125 cases per year and equipment specially designed to handle such patients. Despite the protests of accomplished surgeons in many major hospitals, this measure is likely to be just the first strike in curbing the exploding costs of weight loss surgery. The net effect of these changes is a operating room traffic jam. Masses of increasingly desperate patients sold on surgery as their only recourse are coming face to face with dwindling numbers of beds and dollars for surgical intervention.

Your choice

An ad for expert financial services features a surgeon in scrubs leaning casually on the nursing station as he calls his patient at home. "Have you disinfected the area? Good. Now make a 3 inch incision between the fourth and fifth abdominal muscles." The troubled patient is seen sitting in a robe, staring at a knife on his kitchen table. His expression is priceless as he mutters, "Shouldn't *you* be doing this?"

The humor in the ad is pungent (Kirshenbaum Bond & Partners for Edward Jones Financial Services). However, there are in fact actual cases of self-surgery. At age 60, Dr. Evan Kane of Kane Community Hospital, Pennsylvania, stunned the medical world in 1921 by removing his own appendix under local anesthesia. In 2004, 40 year-old Ines Perez of Rio Talea, Mexico performed a heroic c-section - *on herself!* Eight hours from the nearest hospital, and having had a stillbirth three years earlier, she decided to take matters into her own hands. Afterward she called the village nurse to sew her up with needle and thread. Mother and baby did fine!

In contrast to such incredible feats, actually doing gastric bypass on oneself is simply impossible. The stomach is located awkwardly under the rib cage, at the very core of our anatomy. Surrounded by critical organs, such operations almost always require general anesthesia and multiple assistants. In contrast, we have proven conclusively that *anyone* can bypass their stomach *nutritionally*. As detailed in Chapter 5, gastric conditioning conducted under proper professional supervision produces at least equivalent weight loss. Like surgery, it is a serious, 'procedure' which must also be carried out in a structured manner with preparatory tests and careful follow-up.

Obesity surgery, on the other hand, has much in common with the stapled ear and the wired jaw: a *physical* intervention that forces the patient to limit total intake of calories. It is a tremendous weapon of last resort to have in our arsenal against the flood of obesity that now threatens to engulf us. Regrettably, it has become idolized and promoted as a panacea when in fact we may be opening Pandora's Box. As a bariatric surgeon, I celebrate the impressive advances that the specialty continues to make, but significant concerns remain. The exponential growth in obesity surgery will no doubt crest in the foreseeable future. Chapter 18, *Corporate Wellness,* details how third party payers are effectively challenging political pressure for unrestricted coverage. Statisticians warn that the surge of Baby Boomers graduating into Medicare will overwhelm the healthcare budget in coming years. Government will have little choice but to further discourage routine weight loss surgery as science points to better, less invasive means of weight management.

Impressive weight loss notwithstanding, the bariatric surgery brochure at the beginning of the chapter clearly concedes it is "substituting one disease for another." Ensuing abnormal bowel function and discomfort can progress at any time to major maladies. On the surface, differences in skin tone and energy levels may appear to be all that separate bypassed patients from Manna*fast* successes. Beyond that, bypassed patients generally do well in our present abundance. But compared to those with normal stomachs, how would they fare in tough times such as a deep recession or some natural disaster interrupting food or medication supply, or even just being lost in the woods? In a turbulent economy with uncertain health insurance, independent health is a precious asset. There many who braved those notoroious "early flights" who eternally regret not having today's improved menu of operations. Indeed, there are many impatiently planning to *permanently* disrupt their digestive tracts, who are now having second thoughts.

Knowing all it involves, guess how many surgeons who themselves qualify for obesity surgery actually choose to undergo it. Odds are most choose to stay in control to the fullest extent possible. Thank God we have options. Non-surgical gastric conditioning is natural and cannot be merchandised in the same way as the scalpel or the pill. It imposes neither hidden cost nor lifetime risk. In light of the above, the question becomes even more pertinent, "Shouldn't *you* be doing this?"

Don't put the keys to your health
in someone else's pocket.

9. Surgical Options

REVIEW

1. How does weight loss surgery compare with Antabuse treatment for alcoholism?

2. What is Munchausen's syndrome? What kind of choices do patients suffering from this disorder make?

3. Discuss experiences with weight loss surgery (yours or someone elses).

4. Compare the benefits and risks of gastric conditioning and weight loss surgery.

5. Should there be any difference in the way premium/taxpayer money is spent for weight loss surgery compared to surgery for cancer or trauma?

I lift up my eyes unto the hills
From where my help comes...

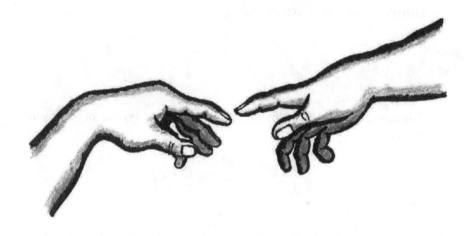

... My help comes from the Lord
Who made heaven and earth.

Psalm 121:1,2.

Chapter 10
Faith and Fitness

We have come this far by faith,
Leaning on the Lord,
Trusting in His Holy Word,
He's never failed us yet!

Albert Goodson, Manna Music, 1963

It was in Antioch that the followers of Jesus were first called by their new name (Acts. 11:26). Society so ridiculed the great lengths these believers would go to imitate their Lord; they began calling them *"little Christs"* or Christians. It was a tough one to live up to, but the name stuck. Despite their many challenges, one cannot imagine these New Testament believers chronically complaining, "I just can't help myself." This is in effect, what the average overweight believer is saying. It is a failure to fully accept the precious gifts bestowed with the New Birth: "Love, joy, peace, patience, kindness, goodness, faithfulness, gentleness and *self-control*," (Galatians 5:19-21).

In Chapter 20, we discuss specific steps that the church, as a local organization in the community, can take in response to the health issues of our day. Notwithstanding this, it is our challenge to first seek divine guidance to inspire the necessary changes within our own hearts. As captains of our souls, we do not have to wait for some religious hierarchy to sanction this season of reflection.

If this chapter tastes like strong medicine, it could be because we are dealing with a serious condition. Purdue University sociologist, Kenneth Ferraro, in a 1998 study confirmed something long suspected. Statistics show that active church members today are more likely to be overweight than the general population. Rev. O. S. Hawkins was even more explicit. From his perspective as CEO of the board responsible for medical and retirement benefits for Southern Baptist pastors, he observed that those in his charge suffered a higher than expected rate of obesity related diseases. In his book *High Calling, High Anxiety,* the Reverend opines that "the secular community is sounding the alarm over the evils of obesity, but Christian churches do not seem to have heard the message."

Doctrinal jingles such as "We don't drink and we don't chew; and we don't go with girls that do," are helpful on shielding us from the harmful practices in this world. However, lifted from the miry clay of traditional vices, experts suggest that we tend to fill the vacuum with eating to excess.

The Forgotten Sin

Ministers know better than to trifle with folks around feeding time. If there is one law that they are still under, it is the 11th commandment: Thou shalt not preach past high noon. The congregation grows increasingly restive with each tick of the clock past 11:30 Sunday morning. Whether the Spirit is moving or not, the preacher overstaying his welcome in the pulpit is likely to witness his audience unceremoniously dribbling out of the pews. In times past people showed some restraint. Today, at the first stomach rumble, they have no compunction excusing themselves for more pressing matters.

Population studies further reveal that Jews, Muslims, Buddhists and certain sects like Adventists, Mormons and Jehovah's Witnesses were less likely to be overweight and healthier than the general population. It is no secret which group surveys deem to be heaviest. Forget creed for a moment. There is no getting around this fact. In spirit, we care deeply for

> *O God our help in ages past,*
> *Our hope for years to come...*
> Isaac Watts, 1624-1748

ministry. We celebrate our missionaries who daily lay their lives on the line carrying the Word to distant lands. Some global neighborhoods still relish ancient atrocities. Stoning, beheading or blowing up civilians on bus or in marketplaces all seem part of the natural landscape. What courage and commitment it takes to bring the Good News of a better way of life! Despite our sacrificial support to missions, it is evident that for many in the church, missing a meal is not very high up on the prayer list. The poor participation in World Vision 30-Hour Famine sponsored by our youth ministry is in stark contrast to the wildly popular potlucks and food related fellowships. To no one's surprise, the more frequent the churchgoer, the greater their weight.

"For *drunkards* and *gluttons* become poor, and drowsiness clothes them in rags," (Proverbs 23:20, 21). How dare the Scripture mention these two vices in the same breath? After all, isn't alcohol use considered a sin? Could our modern churches be revisiting the same excesses that plagued the love feasts of the early church? (Jude: 12). Is obesity undermining the effectiveness of our ministry? In the halls before worship service, much of the talk is about the fad diet of the day. Yet the theology of fitness is practically taboo in most Sunday schools and pulpits. If we fear making our members uncomfortable, how then do we go about making the church part of the solution rather than being part of the problem?

Timeless Truths

Robert Fulghum wrote the best seller, *All I Need to Know about How to Live I Learned in Kindergarten* (Villard Books: New York, 1990). In it he asserts, "Wisdom was not at the top of the university mountain, but there in the sand-pit at kindergarten." Indeed, the brightest minds in the ivory towers of academia, or the clever marketing gurus of Wall Street, have fallen short in delivering us from the clutches of obesity. If runaway weight is indeed a recent development in human history, then perhaps we should reflect on the "kindergarten of civilization" for timeless dietary principles. Wouldn't we be surprised to discover that Scripture provides clear directions for weight control and healthy living? These familiar gems of wisdom will come rushing back to our consciousness the moment we begin reviewing this exciting saga:

Long, long ago, in a culture far, far removed from our own, the tale is told of a band of refugees facing tremendous odds. Having fled an oppressive bondage, they found themselves in a harsh and unforgiving environment. Regrettably, the followers of Moses were troubled that this palace insider had led them out of the frying pan smack into the fire. The 16th chapter of Exodus details what happens next. Here is a compilation of the clearest and most poetic excerpts from the leading translations:

2.   And the whole congregation of the Israelites murmured against Moses and Aaron in the wilderness.

3.   And the Israelites said to them, "If only we had died at the hand of the Lord in the land of Egypt! There *we sat around pots of meats and ate all the food we wanted.* But you have brought us forth into this wilderness *to starve us all to death.*"

4.   Then the Lord said to Moses, "I will rain down bread from heaven for you. The people are to go out each day and *gather enough for that day.* In this way I will test them and see if they will follow my instructions…"

14. And when the dew was gone, behold, thin flakes like frost appeared on the desert floor.

15. And when the Israelites saw it, they asked each other, *"What is this?"* For they were mystified as to how they were being fed. So Moses explained that it was "the nourishment the Lord has given you to eat."

16. Here is what the Lord has commanded: "Each one is to *gather as much as he needs*. Take an omer for each person you have in your tent.

17. The Israelites complied; some gathered more and some less.

18. *He that gathered much did not consume too much*, and he that gathered little still ended up with enough. They gathered each one according to his eating.

19. And Moses said, "Do not leave any of it until the morning".

20. But they did not listen to Moses, but some of them hoarded it until the morning. And it became rotten with maggots, and stank. And Moses got quite upset with them.

31. And the house of Israel called it *Manna*. It was which like coriander seed, and the taste of wafers with honey.

35. ...They ate Manna until they came into the borders of the land of Canaan.

Some dismiss this illustrious episode as "old Jewish fables;" others say, "It's just symbolic." The truth is that this passage is pregnant with meaning. Here are a few insights that have inspired our nutrition practice.

Providence

It is the nourishment the Lord has given you to eat. (vv. 15)

You open the door of your refrigerator. Your stomach propelled you in that direction, but you are not sure exactly what you want. You peer through that fine swirling mist forming as frigid air embraces the humid atmosphere of the kitchen. Frosted meat and fish is stashed compactly in the freezer. Straight ahead sits the chilled milk, juice, punch and half-finished containers of this and that. Your eyes flit from left to right and down to the next shelf in a well-rehearsed unconscious sequence, like reading a book. Do you feel like just fixing a sandwich? ...or these leftovers here saying, "Eat me." Perhaps you are thinking of just grabbing a yogurt or drenching some 2% over your favorite cereal. Fruits and vegetables crisply tucked away are waving their imaginary little arms: *Hey, how about me?!* More choices. What's this on the inside of the door? Pudding? Jam? Over here...eggs, cheese, butter, ketchup and salad dressing, all standing by and looking eagerly at you.

The thought seldom enters your mind, but today you pause to reflect on something you just heard on the news. Those folks in that terrible flood several states away have been out of electricity for weeks. Washed away roads prevent trucks from delivering produce. Without outside help, the prospect of starvation is real. Of course, on paper, such a thing would never happen here. Our military would drop rations from the sky. Red Cross would deliver blankets, tents and medicines. FEMA (Federal Emergency Management Agency) and insurance agents would be on location within days with debit cards and checks to cover the damages.

Yet it takes situations like that to remind us that we did not grow those vegetables, squeeze the juice or catch the fish. Surely, we had to spend our hard-earned cash for those groceries, but disasters have a way of dramatizing our dependence on others. Regardless of how smart and sophisticated, we could be living in a country where food is hard to come by, one perhaps devastated by famine or strife. Therefore, even if our sustenance did not drop down from heaven above, we acknowledge Divine Providence for our daily bread.

Leibe, our Japanese friend from college, comes to mind. She was visiting the States again so we invited her over for dinner. It was clear that she had not changed one bit. Coming from a different philosophical background could not stop her delightful personality from shining through. After the table was set, I thought I would have some fun by asking her to give the blessing.

That sure caught her by surprise! She paused for an awkward moment. One could see the wheels turning. Then she quickly bowed her head and simply said "*Dozo!*"

Okay, I thought, that was nice and to the point. But what did it mean?

"Dig in!" She laughed as she reached for the serving spoon.

Leibe was by no means overweight, but I do believe that "digging in" without pausing to give thanks may have something to do with our total caloric intake. Taking time to center oneself at meals does not neutralize whatever fat, carcinogens, or Salmonella contained therein. However, experts speculate that grace before meals actually facilitates digestion and fosters weight control. Donald Altman, author of *Art of the Inner Meal: Eating as a Spiritual Path* (Harper, San Francisco; 1999), suggests that meal-time should be a spiritual experience, an oasis of calm during your day.

Observe how chickens drink (or most birds for that matter). It is fascinating how they rhythmically crane their necks upward after *each* 'beakful.' It is as if they are saying "Thank you Lord for this water." Likewise, whether we give thanks before each snack or only at sit-down meals, it is harder to abuse food when we are truly appreciative of our Source. Do not allow your family to become like ships passing each other in the night. A weight management program is no excuse for disrupting these precious interpersonal relationships. Even if you choose to just have a cup of tea or nutritional supplement while the teenagers eat three times more than you would ever consider, make that another opportunity to celebrate your self-control. As we check out the well-stocked shelves of grocery stores and the menus of finest restaurants where meals are served on white tablecloths, remember this indeed *is the nourishment the Lord has given you to eat (vv.15)*.

Equivalence
Each one according to his eating. (vv. 18)

Mahatma Gandhi, Liberator of India, put it this way: "The world has enough to provide for everyone's need, but not for everyone's greed." Some perceive this statement as radical interference with one's right to unbridled consumption. Suffice it to say, self-indulgence is at the heart of what ails society today. Some celebrities boast of acquiring so much wealth that even their grandchildren could not spend it all. Yet they strive for more because someone else has a few more homes, a larger yacht, a ritzier jet or is invited to a few more exclusive parties than they are.

While desire for stuff and enlightened self-interest have a reasonable place in the human experience, unchecked it simply becomes greed. Advertisers are schooled in finding precise ways of making us say, "I'll have what he's having." Just the sight someone wolfing down a tempting cheeseburger combo is enough to start one's juices flowing - even if other food choices were being considered! The untrained stomach actually grumbles, "Why can't I have that too?!" Or, "How can she eat that and get away with it?"

Though we would rather not dwell on it more than we have to, we know "life is but a vapor that appears for a little while and then vanishes away" (James 4:14). Whether parent, president, pope, princess, prostitute, pauper, prisoner or pop star, our vital functions will someday be disrupted by disease and cease altogether. The world reacts to this reality by saying "Let us eat drink and be merry, for tomorrow we die." As we move up the *planes of progress,* we rise above this carnal attitude. We cannot take it with us; not our bank account, jewelry, pleasure, fame or food. No matter how tantalizing the aroma or a taste to die for, I must renew my expressed commitment to eat according to my caloric need for each day. In so doing, I acknowledge equivalence among God's children and free up resources to minister to those in need.

Confidence
Let no man leave of it until the morning. (vv. 19)
As teenagers, with all kinds of activities packed into our schedules, a meal was more often than not an "eat and run" affair. We must have appeared to just inhale our servings in a few gulps. Mom would say, "Slow down. The food is not running away!" That would conjure up funny fairy tale images of the gingerbread man. The little pastry person managed to elude a slew of characters, starting with the little old couple. I was really pulling for the guy. He was just on the verge of freedom across the river when he accepted a ride from the sly fox... and the rest was history!

All that "gobbling up" of characters in fairy tales suggests a veiled form of aggression that we dissect in Chapter 8 *Eating Disorders.* With spiritual maturity however, we learn to say "Be still my soul" and tame our ravenous childhood appetites. The art of being able to push back and declare, "I'm done" clearly is not some inherited trait or natural skill. Constantly remind yourself that from a metabolic standpoint, you need to be consuming 10 percent less than 10 years ago just to stay even.

The hamster stores food in its cheeks, the camel stores water in its hump for those long trips across the parched desert. There is no need for us to hoard food within our bodies. This is all that fat is. Let the pantry and refrigerator suffice. Trust God that the food will be there when you need it. In this season of obesity, learn to feel good when you pass on some good stuff today. Your body will thank you tomorrow.

Consequence

And it became rotten and stank. (vv. 20)

Even good food in excess ends up in the wrong places. Be that around your waist, your hips or around your heart…on your gut or on the other side. John Kenneth Galbraith puts it this way, "More die in the United States from too much food than from too little." Whether it is the most sophisticated cuisine from Rachel Ray or Emeril, or the standard fare churned out by the neighborhood diners and fast food joints, surplus food stuffed into the body turns ugly to the eye and detrimental to our health. Moses in his book put it bluntly - excess food stinks!

Independence

They ate manna until they came into the borders of the land of Canaan. (vv. 35)

The Bible mentions "fast" and related words 53 times and "feast" and related words 171 times. This suggests that overall, the good Lord wants more for us to have fun with food than to fast…it doesn't get any better than that! Still, it is like a checkbook. Often when shopping, we would say to the kids, "We can't afford that." Their response would be, "Why don't you just write a check?" Their little brains had no concept that withdrawals from the account were limited by deposits. There are times you have to hold off on some wants in order to splurge in the future on a surprise gift, well-deserved R&R, a really cool outfit or a new car. Ice cream and apple pie is not evil - abuse of it is. This is the Manna*fast* concept. It is not about lo-carb prohibitions against "Our Daily Bread," the staff of life. It is not about funny foods and funny drugs or surgically bypassed stomachs to treat bingeing. It is about balance. It is about celebrating the Creator for every good and perfect gift, while acknowledging a definite place for self-denial in the interest of health.

It is fashionable for worldly folk to be on a diet one day and off the next. But we know better. If our hearts are truly transformed because we are temples of the Holy Spirit, there is never a time when we cease from practicing the totality of these Mosaic principles. Some long for that vision of a heaven with no calories or cholesterol concerns. Yet, even here and now, the yoke is easy and the burden light. Manna*fast* is our calling till we transition to Canaan and cross the Jordan into the Promised Land.

10. Faith and Fitness

A Right Relationship with Food

To a child, Thanksgiving is portrayed in *Disneyfied* images of Pilgrims and Squanto, Pocahantas and John Smith, turkey and stuffing. While the informed adult celebrates the pageantry, he also reflects on a deeper perspective. On October 3, 1863, as the nation struggled to bind the tragic wounds inflicted by the Civil War, President Abraham Lincoln wrote:

> *...We have grown in numbers, wealth and power, as no other nation has ever grown. But we have forgotten God. We have forgotten the gracious Hand which preserved us in peace, and multiplied and enriched and strengthened us; and we have vainly imagined, in the deceitfulness of our hearts, that all these blessings were produced by some superior wisdom and virtue of our own.*
>
> *It has seemed to me fit and proper that God should be solemnly, reverently and gratefully acknowledged, as with one heart and one voice, by the whole American people...invited to set apart and observe the last Thursday of November as a day of Thanksgiving and praise to our beneficent Father who dwelleth in the heavens.*

Some fret themselves that this undermines the Establishment Clause separating church and state. But the President was a man constrained by higher obligations. He confessed, "I have often been drawn to my knees by the conviction that I had no other place to go." Instead of using religion as a guise to further oppress the underclass, Lincoln's faith truly powered public policy. His presidential proclamation was modeled on the Old Testament's call to fasting and atonement. He drew from the ancient virtues of personal stewardship, care for the environment and for those less fortunate. Stirrings within the evangelical community are once again invigorating that link between good doctrine and good works.

Today's Thanksgiving however, still translates into an overeating extravaganza extending through the winter hibernation. Statisticians confirm that the average American gains five pounds over the holidays. Just imagine how much more that translates to for those whose bodies retain cookies! Mannafast provides the formula to not only celebrate and control such weight gain, but also to ultimately reverse it.

To Prevent or Rescue

Bill and Gloria Gaither's *Because He Lives* tells of "How sweet to hold a new born baby. And feel the pride and joy he brings..." For the most part, we begin life so unspoiled, as pure as the driven snow! Do your childhood pictures speak of paradise lost? Life rolls on like a videotape. We choose our own paths. Our DNA begins jam-packed with encrypted instruction to deal with every possible clinical contingency. True, some are born with silver spoons in their mouths while others must scratch for survival from day one. The vast majority of western society however, is well within reach of modern medical science. Yet fast-forward twenty, forty years and most present afflictions, obesity included, we bring upon ourselves.

Godless communism may be on the trash heap of history, but it was built on one sad truth. Karl Marx and other German philosophers such as Kant and Hegel saw the religion of their day as "the opium of the people." Wholesome religion helps us bring our big problems to a God that is bigger than we are. I have witnessed wondrous personal change and evidence God's sovereign intervention on disease processes. I am a believer. Yet I cringe whenever I see the merchandising divine healing.

> *Science can purify religion from error and superstition. Religion can purify science from idolatry and false absolutes.*
>
> Pope John Paul II

There have always been those who distract the poor from pursuing disciplined self-care and do little to improve practical access to affordable treatment. The secular world is not impressed. For all they care, religion as currently practiced is still "the sigh of the oppressed creature, the heart of a heartless world."

We are always called to minister to the infirmed. "Whenever you do that to the least of these my brethren, you do it to me" (Matt. 25:39, 40). Too often, prayer for the sick is like a medical "Mayday!" After years of neglect, we frantically implore God to work some divine magic or send in the medical cavalry to rescue us from some avoidable tragedy. Prayer must first serve as a force-field against disease. Regardless of the cause, ask for strength and compassion not only to comfort others *after the fact,* but also to take meaningful action to help *prevent disease.*

Biblical Fasting

Prohibitions have been imposed in the past on alcohol and cigarettes, but it is impossible to realistically ban food. Eating is the most basic

10. **Faith and Fitness**

characteristic of living organisms. Fattening foods will always confront us as we interact with family and friends in various social situations. Throughout the history of faith, people who were serious about accomplishing something for God or overcoming some besetting sin would commit themselves to a period of self-deprivation.

Review of the great fasts of the Bible, reveals that they were prompted by specific spiritual needs for atonement, intercession, repentance, etc. When King David's love-child was sick unto death, he prayed intensely and did not eat for seven days (II Samuel 12:15-20). We have no precise details in all instances of how stringent were the limitations, whether it was a water fast, or minimal amounts of regular foods. Some were simply restrictive diets like John the Baptist's locusts and wild honey. Modern Christians tend to respond to any occasion with food. At weddings we splurge, at showers we eat. At funerals we eat more.

My first experience with fasting was when Hurricane David slammed into our island late summer of 1979. The weatherman from an Atlanta TV station flew over the apparent total devastation in a Air Force C-130. To quote him, there was "no sign of life" on the island. I was stunned. We always thought that hurricanes were no match for our mountains. Bits of information eventually began trickling to the outside world relayed by Navy ships in Roseau harbor. I was overcome with guilt for not being there to help in Dominica's hour of greatest need. I prayed earnestly for news of my family while listening for hours at the home of a ham radio operator in Rome, Georgia. Driving back to the dorm at about 3:00 a.m., I suddenly became aware that some crazy driver kept coming straight at me. At the last moment, I was swerved unto the gravel shoulder of the road. It was only then I realized that I was driving on the left side - as we do in the former English colony!

To be honest, it was not so much a plan to forego eating for any period of time. Food simply had no appeal. The carefree college life appeared as meaningless as ever. Even as the monster storm accelerated across the Caribbean to the American mainland, many student organizations and churches were spontaneously collecting relief supplies, raising funds and comforting me. I felt so blessed and overwhelmed by the kindness of strangers! Dr. Randall Minor, the college president invited me into his ornate office for encouragement. I can still see his shiny bald head and benign face as he said, "Remember Sam, it's not how hard you fall, it's how high you bounce." On the third day, I finally received a telegram. It read, "House . and . family . are . safe." Words fail me. I was bouncing off the walls in gratitude for God's tender mercies. And food never tasted so good!

Those never having fasted have no idea what they are missing. My hurricane fast was an emergency response. However, the experience served as a preparation for subsequent planned and purposeful fasts. Contrasted to anorexia that arises out a preoccupation with self, a spiritual fast arises out of preoccupation with others - including God. Give up a meal or two and your personal problems begin to pale in comparison. It is amazing how clearly you see the small stuff over which we daily fret. Most of all, it helps redefine one's relationship to food in the grand scheme of things. Obesity comes from overeating. Fasting, and fasting alone empowers you to put food in its place.

This struggle with our appetites allows us to identify with the apostle Paul as he wrestled with himself to do the right thing:

> *When I want to do good, evil is right there with me...*
> *waging war against the law of my mind and making me*
> *a prisoner of the law of sin at work within my members.*
> *What a wretched man I am!* (Romans 7:18-25)

Certain denominations traditionally emphasized times set aside for abstaining from fond foods. Yet, even Lent nowadays often means just taking the option for seafood instead of meat in deference to the passion of Christ. Some may take it further, being vigilant to avoid some pet vice or giving up a personal treat, like chocolate. The underlying theme is the practice of bringing 'wants' under subjection.

Prayer and fasting helped Paul leave a glorious legacy. The legacy of our generation at this point is that of being the fattest the world has ever seen. This coincides with sharply declining percentage of the population attending church. Across Europe it is already in the single digits. News reports show more practicing Muslims there than practicing Christians. With their hollow cathedrals and irrelevant liturgy, European Christianity is already living on borrowed time. The continent itself is becoming a huge mission field. North America is next - unless we fix things now and cease from being tepid, neither hot nor cold. The center of gravity for the Living Church is inexorably shifting to the Third World as the West loses sight of its spiritual bearings. At such a time like this, we ought to temper our appetites and be more fervent in our outreach to a dying world.

Why are Muslims, on average, are leaner than Christians? An obvious answer may be that we have more food. However, could periodic self-denial also have something to do with it? Timed according to the phases of the moon, the month of Ramadan is set aside for fasting. In addition to their compulsory five prayers daily, this is a time to ponder the plight of the poor. The occasion is also used to stir up intense resistance to "crusader" western powers whose actions are portrayed as strategies to steal their natural resources. From dawn's early light, only sips of water are permitted. Restaurants close. The entire community is required to submit to the fast, or else... The month of devotion climaxes in the festivities of *Eid* when restrictions are lifted and feasting abounds.

True Christian fasting has no such ritualistic trappings. It is a deeply personal experience, in private or with like-minded souls freely choosing to covenant with each other. The length and depth of the fast is driven by spiritual need and physical condition. It bestows a fresh sense of balance and keen perspective to one's outlook on life. It is not an external imposition, rather a reasonable sacrifice (Romans 12:1-2), an obedient response to the call to consecration. If we as a culture are to stand strong, we would do well to rediscover this lost art.

Many Christians are intrigued by the Manna*fast* concept and are increasingly interested in applying it to their daily lives. While weight control is a necessary outcome, goal-directed *fasting* is a spiritual adventure! The true giants of the faith all agree that there is no greater tool to empower us to overcome as we strive to do the right thing. Numerous online resources are available for those interested in a deeper understanding of spiritual fasting. Manna*fast*.org is a good place to start.

Move Forward!

Moses had it up to here with his faith-challenged people. As the high drama unfolds in Exodus 14, one gets a sinking feeling that human nature has not changed much. Caught between Pharaoh's rapidly approaching, vengeful army and the 'unmovable' Red Sea, the Israelite reaction was to pout and panic at their predicament. "Was it because there were no graves in Egypt?" They mocked bitterly. "It would have been better for us to serve the Egyptians than to perish in the desert!" Once again, Moses had to complain to God about these would-be losers. Was this what he had traded his privileged upbringing for? Verse 15 conveys the Lord's terse response: "Why are you whining to me? *Tell the people to move forward!*"

So there you have it. Your weight is the Red Sea. Enough excuses! Here's how you move forward. I am about to share with you the *Mannafast Affirmation,* powerful fuel for the soul. Say this affirmation for 30 days and see for yourself how your fitness level increases. Say it first thing in the morning, last thing at night. Declare it with firm conviction, preferably standing in front of the mirror. And once again, with feeling!

This is how it inspires change in your life: Chapter 6, *Move it and Lose It,* dealt with getting your body ready for a day of action and exercise. Affirmations take this a step further. The mind is like a blank slate upon awakening. Your subconscious brain is like a computer waiting to download your orders for the day. Input something positive, something powerful. Do not be surprised at the initial level of resistance you will encounter - mainly from yourself. There is a tendency to dismiss it as simply word games. But does it work? Scripture proclaims that, "Death and life are in the power of the tongue" (Psalms 18:21). Do you believe that?

Get past these doubts and the rest is easy. Banish the negativity that has been a stumbling block in getting the desires of your heart. If you have genuinely experienced a rebirth in your spirit, you cannot help but to condition your stomach for phenomenal weight control.

The Manna*fast* Affirmation

I am at peace and comforted by God's presence.
I believe God's will for me is for abundant life.
I deserve a body, fit, vibrant and full of energy.
I let nothing upset me 'cause I am focused on my goal.
My subconscious spirit makes things happen for me.

I'm understanding the reasons for my weight,
As I develop insight into my relationship with food.
Why I eat, where I eat, when I eat, how I eat.
I know my stomach is getting smaller everyday,
Because I enjoy my food, but less of it.

I have stopped wishing or whining about my body.
I have decided to do something about it. No turning back!
I am part of the multitudes taking charge of our lives.
Others are helping me. There's someone only I can help.
Together, we claim victory!

10. Faith and Fitness

As a surgeon, it struck me how many godly people on worldly diets were ending up frustrated and unfulfilled. People of faith are clearly instructed, "Whether therefore you eat or drink or whatsoever you do, do all to the glory of God" (I Corinthians 10:31). Therefore, incorporate the Manna*fast* Affirmation into your prayers. The secret is to personalize it. Shorten it if necessary; focus on parts that address your specific needs. Repeat it everyday, before each meal, in those stressful and hurtful moments that trigger comfort foods and binge eating.

This *focused attention* and auto-suggestion absorbs spiritual energy, nourishing the tiny mustard seed of faith, growing it to a mighty oak of success. It is not magic. It is mental. Experts agree that we are using only one tenth of the brain's potential. Remember, whatever your God-given mind can conceive and believe it can achieve. It *will* achieve. Studies show that people who actually live their faith through corporate worship and healthy lifestyles are more likely to avoid depression, anxiety, survive disease and enjoy a higher quality of life. Their lifespan averages eighty-three years - at least eight years longer than those with no hope.

Our goal as believers is a "people strong and healthy; full of Godly reverent fear." Ask about our *Church 1000* program. It commits congregations to covenant together to lose a thousand pounds total, (just 50 people losing 20 pounds). If you do not have enough people to lose that much, invite others from the community: an exciting form of win-win, *weight-loss evangelism*. Witness the joy as other others transform themselves from the caterpillar of obesity into the glorious butterfly of the abundant life. That encumbering weight simply melts away, like the parting of the Red Sea. Health is miraculously restored. It is God's way of escape from this modern bondage. *Move forward!* Danish philosopher Soren Kierkegaarde called it "a leap of faith." It has happened for others. Now is your turn. It's your time to shine!

Our prayers can become times
when we reach forward in faith
To take hold of what we will one day become.

James Houston

Manna*fast* Miracle

1. Proverbs 23:20, 21 relate gluttony to what other common vice?

2. What did the children of Israel love most about Egypt and how good was it anyway?

3. According to John Kenneth Galbraith "More die in the United States from" what?

4. What is the most effective tool available to believers for deliverance from bondage to food?

5. Which part of the Manna*fast* Affirmation best addresses your needs at this time and why?

Chapter 11

Wonder Drugs ?

*The desire to take medicine, is perhaps the
greatest feature which distinguishes man.*

Sir William Osler, M.D.
Canadian discoverer of blood platelets.

"Need Fen-Phen." That was exactly what Gertrude's wrote on her intake form when she signed into our office in 1993. Tipping the scales at 132, this 62 year-old office manager stood 5' 3" tall. Her demeanor was of someone accustomed to having things done her own way. I remember well because she was immaculately dressed in formal business attire, which impressed me at first. Then I thought to myself, "Why on earth does this lady feel she needs medication for weight anyway?" Of course, you never know what relationship or self-esteem issues someone may be dealing with.

Nevertheless, the perception of being fat was her reality. She definitely was not interested in the niceties of establishing a patient/doctor relationship or even discussing options. She was paying for her visit and expected to leave with a prescription and that was that. Indeed, those were the days when enterprising physicians were setting up chains of "fat mills." Some of these were in shopping centers or two room offices in association with large commercial diet chains. Patients made it into the examination room just long enough to weigh and perhaps have a quick blood pressure check. Within minutes they would be on their way to the pharmacy. In some cases the drugs were even dispensed right there in the office. And all this was aggressively advertised on billboards and other media.

Gertrude appeared restless as I explained our office protocol on appetite suppression medication. Serious side effects from this particular drug cocktail were already being reported - heart valve disease, pulmonary hypertension, strokes and memory loss. If her obesity was not clinically significant, (BMI over 30) she should not be a candidate for those risks.

I was being even more careful about that time especially after viewing a rather sobering TV news story. It dealt with this 45 year old who felt that if she was ever going to enjoy being nice and skinny again, this was it. She loved to eat and freely admitted that she did not care much for getting all hot and sweaty from exercise. At 5' 7", 225 pounds, or about 85 pounds above acceptable body weight, her doctor had started her on the now illustrious Fen-Phen. The feature went on to describe how her mother, who was in the medical field, tried to share her reservations about those drugs, but it was like talking to a stone wall. That young lady went along her merry way to lose 45 pounds. She remarked how sweet it sounded just telling others that her weight was now "one hundred" and something. Unfortunately, she slowly became weaker and began experiencing chest pain. After a rapid series of tests, the cardiologist referred her to surgery to replace heart valves ruined by Fen-Phen. But the damage was too advanced. It would be her mother who would have the dubious honor of watching her son graduate, get married and have kids of his own.

But Gertrude was in no mood for such sentimentality. "Sorry Doc", she tensely interrupted, "All I want is Phen-Fen. It's the only thing that has worked for me. Can you prescribe it or not?"

I paused, evidently a little too long for her liking. Gertrude abruptly sprang up and stormed out of the office. For one thing, this unprecedented reaction refreshingly suggested that at least one other physician had also laid down the law. All the way, she could be heard hissing something to the effect that she would just go somewhere else. Needless to say, we have no idea how Gertrude did eventually. In medical terminology, we would say she was "lost to follow-up." What we do know is that not long afterwards, lawyers nationwide were in a feeding frenzy with the disastrous complications of Fen-Phen.

Many patients come for professional help with their weight only after exhausting a wide array of weight-loss drugs marketed over-the-counter or online. According to the April 15, 1998 issue of the *Journal of the American Medical Association*, at least 106,000 people die each year from *properly* prescribed medications. That makes it the *fourth leading cause of death* in the United States after heart disease, cancer and stroke. When compared to the 15,000 people who die annually from illegal street drugs, the average person is therefore six times more likely to die from legally prescribed drugs. Let us stop and think for a minute. If that is true, what should be the wise response?

11. Wonder Drugs ?

History of Weight Loss Drugs

Today, we look back at Fen-Phen as a needless tragedy. However, a candid review over centuries brings into sharp focus that human penchant for drug dependence. Old timers made periodic use of mineral oil, castor oil and "natural" plant-based laxatives like Senna to "purge the system." Nowadays laxatives have become a weapon of choice for those desiring to quickly part with the baggage of their overindulgence. Chapter 8, described the wages of laxative abuse.

Our ancestors claimed that concoctions containing vinegar and apple cider were useful in removing toxins from the body, speed up metabolism, and decrease appetite. Today's so-called dieter's teas do nothing for fat, but basically are diuretics that rid the body of excess water weight. Boxers or wrestlers routinely do the same thing, dropping a dozen pounds the day before competition to meet weight criteria. The weight rushes right back the moment they re-hydrate themselves in the ring. These "natural" substances are just the beginning. With weight loss drugs among the most lucrative products, pharmaceutical companies keep churning out a never-ending stream of various chemicals deliberately synthesized or accidentally discovered. In just about *every single case,* adverse side-effects surface sooner or later, oftentimes with deadly results.

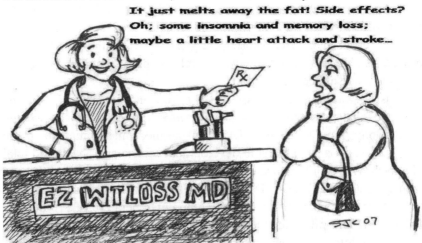

Perhaps nothing dramatizes more the extent to which individuals would go for quick-fix weight loss than the fascination with Dinitrophenol (DNP). This is a chemical long used in the manufacture of photo developers, weed killers, pesticides, wood preservatives and explosives. Early in the last century, that ingredient was a hot commodity as ammunition factories strained to keep up with the spree of international conflicts. Doctors observed that workers in direct contact with DNP developed fever, nausea and vomiting as well as weight loss. Patients got better after a few days off work only to have symptoms promptly recur once back on the job. It was finally determined that the mystery disease was caused when DNP was absorbed through the skin *and sped up the metabolism.*

In 1905, the Czarist military had just suffered a humiliating defeat to the Japanese. On the western front, Russian troops were as good as chopped liver in the face of the vaunted German war machine. Plagued with logistical shortages, these poor fellows were being marched into battle with as few as three bullets! But just as they were able to trip up Napoleon in the past and later Hitler in World War II, the Russians used a scorched earth strategy and "old man winter" as their last resort. They would evacuate entire populations, destroy wells and burn their own towns and villages. Invading armies were thus deprived anticipated shelter and natural resources.

One of Russia's most closely held military secrets was how to keep their soldiers warm internally by giving them DNP tablets. As a result they could endure the frigid Siberian blast, walk over the front lines and simply pry weapons right out of the stone-cold hands of the frozen enemy. Needless to say, after defending the homeland, veterans have long been seen as disposable. What subsequently happened in the United States provides a clue as to why Moscow severely suppressed publication of the long-term side effects of the drug.

Fast forward one generation and Dinitrophenol becomes the darling of American dieters intent on *speeding up their metabolism to lose weight.* Before long, reports began surfacing in the medical literature of severe adverse reactions such as rapid development of cataracts leading to total blindness. One San Francisco newspaper described a doctor from Vienna who took a good dose of DNP for quick weight loss. He was said to have "literally cooked to death" with a body temperature of 110 degrees Fahrenheit! This prompted the FDA in 1934 to assume that Dinitrophenol was in fact doing to humans the same thing it was known to do for weeds and pests. It was pulled off the market three years later. You would think that would have stopped drug-seekers dead in their tracks. But no. Instead they got mad at the government for taking away what they considered their best bet at winning the battle of the bulge.

11. Wonder Drugs ?

Not to be denied, Dinitrophenol raised its ugly head again in 1986, this time as "Mitcal." In no time it began selling like hot cakes. Ironically, the entrepreneur was a Russian-born physician named Nicholas Bachynsky. He established a lucrative chain of weight loss clinics in the Southwest touting his 'unique' product as one that "forces your metabolism to burn thousands more calories." The hook was an offer of 15 pounds weight loss a week "without starving." According to the February 1987 *FDA Consumer*, an estimated 14,000 people paid an average of $1,300 for this treatment. They did so despite signing a consent clearly informing them of the risk of various drastic complications up to and including death.

The state of Texas fined Dr. Bachynsky $86,000 for violating the Food, Drug, and Cosmetic Act by making medical use of a banned substance. Despite all the negative publicity, patients continued to seek out his services. Within three months he was found guilty of contempt of court, charged $100,000, and had his license revoked. Additionally, he was imprisoned for tax evasion. Upon his release, Bachynsky simply moved his Dinitrophenol practice to Mexico and then to Italy. Hordes of customers faithfully followed him every step of the way. In October 2003, Italian newspapers broke the news that Dr. Bachynsky was charged with aggravated manslaughter stemming from the death of four patients.

It simply boggles the imagination just how far people will go for immediate desperate cures when natural options are staring them in the face. The body *always* pays a price in the long run. It may show up as heart failure, cancer or whatever complication, much earlier in life than it might have otherwise occurred, if at all. The intervening years may cloud the connection between that unnatural chemical and the natural consequence. Unlike the search for the Holy Grail or the Rosetta Stone, the not-so-secret answer to obesity lies dormant within each and every one of us. Yet, the frantic search for the magic bullet continues to heat up.

Human Chorionic Gonadotropin (HCG), or *Growth Hormone was* found useful in warding off obesity boys with particular genetic disorders. When it later proved ineffective in fuller-sized adult females, investors turned their interests elsewhere. When research revealed that it could enhance physical performance, they began peddling it to professional athletes. Nowadays, from track and field to Tour de France, there is no shame in using, only regret in getting caught.

Dartmouth College researchers in 1988 demonstrated that *chromium* helps to stabilize sugar levels and weight *in diabetics*. A trace element which the body needs only in tiny amounts, it generally has no effect on the average person who already has normal levels. Excessive amounts, however, have long been known to increase risk of cancer, anemia, or liver and kidney problems. Despite that, chromium picolinate was adopted as the flavor of the day. It began turning up in every conceivable weight loss product. Most hoping for help are still awash in weight.

The deluge of weight loss gadgets and gimmicks include a variety of patches, soaps and thinning thigh creams. Some contain the asthma medicine aminophylline for getting rid of cellulite, although that has never been scientifically proven. The same can be said about the FDA's ban on fraudulent marketing of electric belts. Ads claimed to exercise you into those fabulous six-pack abs while just sitting twitching from self-administered shocks. Regulators also pulled the plug on other pieces of equipment such as those fitted with broad bands placed around the waist promising to vibrate, shake and jiggle away the fat. Regardless how outlandish it seems in retrospect, there will always be enough people willing to try. Instructions typically include staying on 'a sensible diet' and 'that results may vary.' Experts conclude that any transient weight lost resulted from the aforementioned dietary measures and *placebo effect*.

Herbal and Over the Counter Drugs

Some patients proudly announce that they are taking some *natural* or herbal products, convinced that it must be completely safe. Mushrooms are natural, yet we know that people eating the wrong kinds experience similar outcomes as those ingesting arsenic or cyanide. For several years the Chinese herb *Ephedra* was promoted as a "safe natural Phen-fen." Phenylpropanolamine, the active ingredient, was well known to decrease appetite and increase metabolic rate, pulse and blood pressure. For years the FDA had been accumulating data on how Ephedra was causing a higher than expected rate of heart attacks and strokes. Yet, sales persons and gung-ho trainers openly encouraged clients to "stack" or double up on Ephedra products, occasionally with disastrous consequences.

Consequently, the U.S. military banned the sale of Ephedra on its bases after it was implicated in the deaths of over 20 soldiers. While the International Olympic Committee, NCAA, NFL and others may ban offenders for a year or two, Major League Baseball still gives what amounts to a slap on the wrist. It came as no surprise therefore, when in 1999, Steve Bechler of the Baltimore Orioles reportedly took 3 Ephedra pills on an empty stomach before practice. At 6' 2", 239 pounds, he was desperate to get his weight under control to improve his chances on the team. Instead, he complained of dizziness and collapsed, never to recover. It was only after the untimely demise of this 23 year-old expectant father, that the FDA finally took decisive action.

Marketers touted had 'this one little pill' as providing all the benefits of exercise. How could they get away with that? The fact is that the FDA is not mandated to regulate drugs unless they are prescription. Government therefore, limits itself to ensuring these dietary supplements maintain certain sanitary levels and do not make exaggerated claims such as curing cancer or treating heart disease. More people than one would imagine try these supplements, even if many may not finish using it. Naturally, there is a "money back guarantee." But the process of proving that the product was ineffective is so cumbersome, most people simply come to the conclusion that it is not worth their while. It goes without saying that if purchased in some network marketing scheme, prices would be highly inflated and reimbursement would be even more improbable.

The Journal of the American Medical Association published a study by the *Obesity Research Center at the Columbia University College of Medicine* in New York debunking the effectiveness of several popular weight loss aids. Hydroxycitric acid, extracted from the herb *Garcinia cambogia,* is an example of a drug widely marketed as an anti-obesity agent. Another is *Chitin/Chitosan* derived from the shells of crustaceans, such as shrimp and lobster, as well as from yeast and fungi. Studies have failed to demonstrate significant weight loss much beyond that observed with placebo. In the final analysis, neither reams of horror stories nor conclusions of reputable researchers do much to dampen resurgent appetite for these chemical quick fixes.

Fat Blockers and Fake Fat

The modern palate is so accustomed to fat that little else tastes good. Despite the inverted logic of the lo-carb/high fat advocates, dietary fat remains the primary source for heart-hating cholesterol while adding to the excess calories. Knowing this, manufacturers therefore set out to design fake-fat to cater to the fatty tastes of the ballooning population. Proctor & Gamble came out with Olestra, a synthetic fat molecule too large to be absorbed through the intestine. It was marketed as *Olean* and added to popular snacks. The FDA was soon flooded with reports of cramping, bleeding, uncontrolled bowel movements, not to mention a yellow-orange oily discoloration of toilet bowls and underwear.

In a April 16, 2000 letter to the FDA, the *Center for Science in the Public Interest,* cataloged 2,893 complaints attributed to Olestra. It ranged from a woman developing such sudden diarrhea while car-pooling children that she did not even have time to get off the road. A groomsman reportedly threw up and fainted after eating fat-free Pringles chips. Of interest was the fact that the American Medical Association (AMA) allegedly accepted $800,000 from Proctor & Gamble for endorsing Olestra *even before* the product was fully studied. Not only that, it was further alleged that the wife of an AMA vice president received a substantial cut for public relations services in arranging the deal. This just goes to show that we simply cannot take for granted who is supposed to be looking out for us.

Likewise, there is Orlistat, available first by prescription as *Xenical,* then OTC as the popular *Alli*). This is a prescription fat blocker developed for use as part of a low-fat, reduced calorie, weight reduction diet. Since vitamins D, E, K, and beta-carotene are absorbed with fat, patients are instructed to take a multivitamin to replace these nutrients. Like Olean, the main side effect was increased bowel movement urges from undigested fat passing through the system. Patients also were cautioned to expect that orange/brown oily stool and increased gas. When that happens, the patient is blamed for failing eating meals containing higher amounts of fat than recommended. While many patients were prepared to put up with all this in return for measurable weight loss, others were not amused having "accidents" for the first time since day care. As with obesity surgery, instead of risking all this tribulation, would it not make much more sense to gently and systematically train oneself to gradually lower fat intake?

Unintended Weight Gain

Using a careful medication history on the first visit, we can often correlate the onset of obesity with the start of certain medications. The law now requires that pharmacists insert information about drugs with each prescription. Some nervous patients, however, misinterpret that to mean they *will* get every listed side effect. Nevertheless, if weight gain is an issue, scan the package insert to see if references that in the fine print. Your doctor may still insist that this particular medication is the best for the time being. At least you will be prepared to deal with that side effect rather than being shocked that the scale is suddenly being so mean to you.

Here is a brief list of some of the medications known to have weight

11. Wonder Drugs ?

gain side effects:
- Steroids, several depression and high blood pressure medications.
- Insulin and pills to lower blood sugar.
- Central nervous system agents such as lithium.
- Birth control pills.

One of the more common offenders is the long-term, injectable contraceptive. It does wonders for women with heavy, difficult, painful periods and those likely to say "Oops, I forgot to take my pill." Unfortunately, it is almost always associated with significant weight gain from fluid retention and increased appetite.

How Sweet It Is!

There is an interesting story behind the discovery of the first artificial sweetener. Professor Ira Remsen of Johns Hopkins University was working with his graduate student, Constantine Fahlberg, in developing a new drug to kill bacteria. During one evening meal, Fahlberg noticed that something on his finger tasted very sweet. He retraced his steps and discovered that a product concocted during the day was many times sweeter than sugar. Fahlberg and his professor published their discovery together in 1879 calling the drug *Saccharin* (Latin for sugar). Today it is marketed as *Sweet'N Low and Sweetmate.*

Fahlberg then did something considered unethical in academic circles. He jumped ahead and patented Saccharin under his name only, thereby becoming fabulously wealthy. This reportedly formed part of the capital investment for the giant chemical company, Monsanto. Professor Remsen went on to become president of Johns Hopkins University, but reportedly never reconciled his bitterness arising out of the artificial sweetness boom. Saccharin was later found to cause bladder cancer in rats and banned in Canada in 1977. An attempt by the FDA to do the same in the U.S. was overruled by Congress in 1991 after intense industry lobbying.

Another artificial sweetener, *Cyclamate*, was in fact banned in 1969 because of the increased risk of bladder cancer. Yet another *Aspartame*, was discovered back in 1965 by James Schlatter while working on drugs to treat ulcers. Legend has it that he too licked his fingers to pick up a piece of paper – lo and behold, it tasted very sweet! Before being marketed as *NutraSweet* and *Equal,* it had to overcome some very serious concerns. Aspartame barely squeaked through the extended review process thanks to the influence of two very accomplished individuals: then company attorney Clarence Thomas and then chairman of the pharmaceutical company *Searle*, Donald Rumsfeld.

Aspartame is 50% Phenylalanine, an amino acid which at high levels is toxic to the central nervous system. The best evidence for this is a condition called Phenylketonuria (PKU) present in 1 in 10,000 births. These patients inherit a defect in the enzyme that metabolizes Phenylalanine. If fed foods naturally high in Phenylalanine, they develop mental retardation. This is such an important matter that all babies in developed countries are tested for PKU prior to discharge from the nursery. The interesting thing is that 1 in 50 people are carriers for PKU and they too, are affected to a lesser extent to high Phenylalanine levels.

According to a 1984 edition of the *Journal of Applied Nutrition*, Phenylalanine is unstable above 86° F, breaking down into *Methanol* (wood alcohol) *10.9%* by weight. Methanol is known to metabolize into formaldehyde (embalming fluid), formic acid (fire ant venom), and Diketopiperazine (DKP), a known cause of brain cancer. The most notable side effects of these chemicals are vision disturbances and dizziness (especially in pilots). This led the Department of Defense in its May and August 1992 publications *Flying Safety*, to formally warn all its air crews to abstain from consuming diet drinks on duty. Not only that, a wide array of specific complaints have been lodged with Health and Human Services against Aspartame. They range from migraine headaches, to mood swings, chronic fatigue, memory loss, convulsions and even brain tumors.

An increasing wave of perfectly healthy persons now find themselves dependent on additional medicines to treat symptoms likely flowing from the aluminum can. Even the National Soft Drink Association (NSDA) in 1983 fired off a lengthy protest against approval. This was well-documented in the Congressional Review. Once approved however, the NSDA wasted no time in jumping on the profitable bandwagon. Scientists now speculate that the mysterious Gulf War Syndrome may be related to breakdown products from prolonged exposure of diet soda to the desert heat. Check the ingredients on the side of your favorite can of diet soda:

Aspartame per average can (www.nsda.org.) .... 180 mg

Phenylalanine content (50%)... 90 mg
Potential methanol yield per can of diet soda .... 9.81 mg
(90 x 10.9%).

Reference Dose (RfD) for methanol.. 0.5 mg
per kilogram of body weight per day. (www.epa.gov)

RfD for typical 80 kg person (176 lb.) per day ....40 mg

11. Wonder Drugs ?

(Based on studies by Tsang, Wing-Sum, et al, 1985, "Determination of Aspartame and Its Breakdown Products in Soft Drinks by Reverse-Phase Chromatography and UV Detection," *Journal of Agriculture and Food Chemistry,* Vol. 33, 4, pages 734-738 and Determination of Aspartame and Its Major Decomposition Products in Food." Journal of AOAC International, Volume 76, No. 2, 1993.)

The Environmental Protection Agency, an arm of the Federal government, makes this categorical statement: "*At exposures increasingly greater than the RfD, the potential for adverse health effects increases.*" How many cans of diet soda (with about potentially 10 mg of Methanol/ can) would it take to exceed the Reference Dose (40 mg) for this toxic chemical? Next question: Do you know of anyone who regularly consumes more than four cans of diet soda daily?

We often make light of the person who orders a *diet soda* along with a typical high fat, high calorie fast food combo. So powerful is the marketing that they feel entitled to splurging on some candy bars. Actually there is sound scientific explanation for such behavior. Several experts have confirmed that artificial sweeteners affect serotonin levels in the brain, leaving consumers less satisfied. This increases high caloric craving and resulting in *paradoxical weight gain*. It is one thing to control food intake with self-discipline, but it is quite another to fool the body into thinking that it is feasting when there is "just one calorie" to work with. The body reacts by backfiring in different ways. This applies to all the artificial sweeteners, including new ones like *Splenda*.

We would delude ourselves to focus exclusively on diet sodas. Artificial sweeteners can be found in such a vast array of goods that it is almost impossible to avoid. FDA has received complaints for this particular additive in punch mix, ice tea, hot chocolate, breath mints, frozen confections, cereal, even dried fruit, to name a few. Having said that, abusers of diet soda who may be experiencing any of the above symptoms while still gaining weight may be interested in researching the information for themselves. The truth of how aspartame may or may not be affecting you personally resides somewhere between the public relations "harmless" hype and hysterical mixture of urban legends. Good starting points for fair and balanced opposing views are *www.aspertamesafety.com* and *www.aspertame-info.com*.

Current EPA policy is that artificial sweeteners are safe for human consumption at certain minimum levels. In fact we do not hesitate to make limited use of artificial sweeteners especially during the intensive fasting stage of the Mannafast program. However, the best way for heavy users to find out how artificial sweeteners may, or may not be affecting them is by *avoiding it for a couple weeks* and observing for changes. He is wise, who after an honest inquiry into this controversy, makes the necessary adjustment to his consumption of artificial sweeteners.

Promises of Chemical Weight Loss

A number of substances or factors in the body have shown promise in being manipulated to control weight. A fat gene that codes for the Melanocortin 4 receptor protein (MC4R) appears to responsible for early obesity in no more than 5% of the population. In 1994, Professor Jeffrey Friedman of Rockerfeller University identified *Leptin* (from the Greek work for thin) a hormone produced by fat cells that limits appetite. Friedman and others have succeeded in using it to regulate weight in mice, but have been unable to do so in men.

Scientists are also looking at another hormone known as *PYY3-36*. It is secreted by the lining of the intestine after eating and serves as an appetite reducer. Then there is the hunger hormone *Ghrelin,* (from the Hindi word for growth). It reduces food intake by one third in human studies. Researchers at London's Imperial Royal College have also identified a natural stomach hormone, *Oxyntomodulin,* which when injected, limits appetite and raises activity levels. There is speculation that commitment to a structured weight loss program induces natural production of these substances. These intrinsic pathways in turn may be involved in sustaining long-term weight reduction. Could these also be the same substances stimulated by specific acupuncture points?

Several new weight-control medicines are well on their way out of the laboratory. *Rimonabant,* by Sanofi-Synthelab, is designed to regulate intake of food by suppressing a nervous system receptor. *Axokine,* by Regeneron Pharmaceuticals, is an injectable form of a modified natural protein which suppresses appetite by attaching to receptors in the brain. Abbott Laboratories is coming out with a drug that makes the familiar promise to raise metabolic rate; to burn off extra calories instead of storing them as fat. Johnson and Johnson's epilepsy drug *Topomax* has been shown to have some weight loss benefits. Despite the known side effects such as excessive drowsiness, fatigue, as well as difficulty concentrating and impaired coordination, many physicians are using it

11. Wonder Drugs ?

'off label' on perfectly healthy overweight people clamoring for help in pill form.

The appetite suppressant from the rare *Hoodia Gordonii* cactus looms as the wonder drug to beat. South African anthropologists had long observed that the Bushmen of the Kalahari Desert on extended hunting trips would not be hungry or thirsty after chewing on the cactus. Neither did they have that jittery sensation as with Ephedra, caffeine, and many Western diet medications. Hoodia contains a molecule said to be as much as 10,000 times more active as glucose. This messages the brain that the stomach is satisfied even when empty. The British firm, Phytopharm, teamed up with the giant US firm Pfizer to market the drug. Reputed aphrodisiac properties give an added buzz to its sales pitch. With no major side effects yet identified, Hoodia is already being hailed as "the obesity solution of all-time." However, the same reservations apply as with artificial sweeteners. Will it short-circuit the system in our high fat, high sugar, large portion society compared to its effectiveness in the bare desert environment? Should this be the long-awaited, safe, weight-loss wonder drug, then heaven knows we need it. However based on all we have discussed before, one needs to be mindful that late complications can still surface long after formal approval.

Jumpstart

Being spiritual should not be equated to being anti-science. It means that one should be wise and selective. The Manna*fast* approach is to maximize use of the latest technology, but only after it has been proven safer and more effective than traditional approaches.

Medication should not be seen as the solution to food addiction. Just as the effectiveness of pills and patches depends on a smoker's genuine desire to quit, so too appetite suppression medication can play a useful role in weight control. Adipex is one such drug in use for over 20 years that has a well-defined and acceptable safety profile. It provides patients a positive period of weight loss during which time we teach them to analyze their eating patterns. To the extent that they shrink their own stomachs for lasting weight loss, we avoid the use of medication altogether. We use such medication only as an *adjunct to nutrition counseling* as recommended by most State Medical Boards:

- The patient must undergo a thorough history and physical.

175

- Must have a BMI of at least 30 with co-morbid conditions.
- Must be unable to lose weight for at least one month with diet and exercise.
- Must be monitored by the physician every 30 days.
- The course of treatment generally does not exceed 12 weeks.
- Cannot resume such treatment until six months following the present plan of treatment, 'drug holiday.'
- Must have no history of drug or alcohol abuse.

These measures are generally intended to monitor drug reactions and to prevent the build up of *drug tolerance* (the need for more of the drug for the same effect). Our standard practice is to first complete a weight history (Appendix B). We then instruct patients in the use of their *Food and Fitness Workbook,* basic eating plan and tailored exercise program. Approximately three out of four clients do well enough that the issue of appetite suppression medication does not come up. However, many patients who have used appetite suppression in the past will inquire only about medication. After reviewing the pros and cons of appetite suppression, we have the patient sign a witnessed agreement before beginning our plan of treatment. We are also well aware that many patients try to find ways to circumvent these guidelines. In our experience, *many patients who are dependent on medications for weight loss care little for exercise or healthy food choices*. Often, they would cancel or not show for their lifestyle counseling appointment, then telephone the office to try having the medication called into the pharmacy.

A Two-edged Sword

Pharmaceutical companies are wonderful innovators producing miracle medicines to treat dreaded diseases. The vast majority of drugs cause minimal harm and do produce the desired effect touted in their package inserts. It is indeed a blessing to have access to effective medication when desperately needed. Millions of dollars are spent for research and development and millions more for liability coverage. A healthy return on investment is therefore well deserved. Wall Street verifies that drug companies in fact do very, very well. Significant profit is also made by a host of offshore Internet companies. Investigative reports show that online companies frequently sell (knock-off) fake drugs shipped directly to patients not diagnosed or monitored by a physician. If there is a drug reaction, of what help can the impersonal website be? When these patients turn up in the emergency room, no one is quite sure what medications they were on, or how they had been responding.

The advertising mantra today is, "Ask your doctor if (such and such a drug) is right for you." According to the National Institute for Health Care Management report, retail sales of the 50 drugs most directly advertised to patients "accounted for almost one-half of the $20.8 billion *increase* in retail spending on prescriptions from 1999 to 2000." Research proves that despite spending all this money, American health and happiness still lags far behind other developed countries. What should one make of this?

Merck spent $160.8 million on direct advertising of Vioxx to the consumer. Retail sales surge from $329.5 million in 1999 to $1.5 billion in 2000 at the very time that researchers were sounding the alarm of a significant associated increase in heart attacks and strokes. Indeed, any drug can be a two edged sword. Polypharmacy (being on multiple drugs) can create a toxic stew within the body that exponentially increases drug interactions and delayed side effects. At some point, no one pharmacist or physician can keep up and connect the dots between what caused what and when. By the time the FDA intervenes, it is often too late for many.

Most reasonable people would agree that life's goal should therefore be enjoyment of the best of health on the least amount of medication. Right now, only you know for sure how far you are from this ideal. We will have succeeded if this chapter gives even the slightest pause to reflex drug treatment of *lifestyle* diseases for which nutritional intervention may be safer and more effective. Thomas Edison envisioned that "*the doctor of the future will give no medicine but will interest his patients in the care of the human frame for the cause and prevention of disease.*" The obesity crisis will prevail as long as those profiting from the current situation are more clever and more focused than those suffering from it. The health of the nation will be best served when good people quit standing idly by with a "that's-not-my-problem" attitude. Let us motivate each other with inspired gastric conditioning rather waiting to be rescued by some sleek wonder drug posing as a knight in shining armor.

Why do you spend money for that which is not bread?
And your labor for that which does not satisfy?
Isaiah 55:2

REVIEW

1. Discuss a diet drug you have used or one that you are most familiar with.

2. How many cans of diet soda would you consider safe to drink daily?

3. Explain three of the measures employed by State Medical Boards to ensure safety and effectiveness of appetite suppression drugs.

4. Give a couple examples of herbal or over-the-counter diet drugs and comment on their effectiveness.

5. Is it better to limit the amount of fat in our foods or to block it from being absorbed?

Chapter 12
Diet Roller Coaster

*It's not the things we don't know that get us into trouble;
it's the things we do know that ain't so.*

Will Rogers

Hollywood endorsement rather than scientific scrutiny crowns one diet as top dog - for a season. That is until someone has the common sense to see through the emperor's "clothes" and the courage to speak up about it. Case in point: New York's Mayor Bloomberg, a billionaire ex-businessman with a reputation for considerate efficiency, got himself in quite a pickle. Concerned about mounting healthcare expenses, "Hizzoner" took the liberty to chide the caricature of the out-of-shape, donut-munching cop during a January 2004 talk to the city's finest and bravest. And by the way, Bloomberg opined, Dr. Atkins was fat, and his diet may have contributed to his death. Well, who told him to say that?! The press jumped all over him. Besides the fact this was not a nice thing to say, just who gave him the scientific authority to make that call, they railed. Instead of recanting as the Atkins Corporation and others demanded, the Mayor suggested folks lighten up: He invited Mrs. Atkins to a lo-carb steak dinner - no potatoes of course!

As irreverent and improper the Mayor's comments may appear, it did raise a very provocative question. Can diets be harmful? Was this an isolated event? Whatever the cause of Dr. Atkins' heart attack, we may never know for sure. Interestingly enough, the family refused an autopsy. The Medical Examiner was strictly permitted to reveal only basic data: history of heart disease, height of 6' 0," and *weight of 256 pounds*. We are only left to wonder why should this be such a closely guarded secret?

That diet guru was not the first New Yorker to raise eyebrows about the consequences of a deliberate high fat diet. Woody Allen's classic 1973 movie, *Sleeper* was strangely prophetic. The owner of a health food store (played by Allen himself), dies during a routine stomach operation. He is cryogenically preserved and defrosted 200 years later by a team headed by a lady physician. She reports that the revived patient's breakfast request included among other things, wheat germ and organic honey.

"Oh yes," remarks the lead scientist, "These substances some years ago were thought to contain life preserving properties."

"You mean there was no fat? No steak, or cream pie, or hot fudge?"

"Those were thought to be unhealthy. Precisely the opposite of what we now know to be true."

Puzzled, she concludes this dietary discussion with, "Well he wants to know where he is and what's going on."

Overweight patients today are likewise confused and want to know what is really going on. Many of the most popular diets are like science fiction come true. Lo-carb at one point had food companies tripping over each other to portray their wares as *Atkins-friendly.* There news reports that a Utah buffet restaurant had to block a customer from returning to the line for his *12th* serving of roast beef! He strenuously protested, claiming to be on the Atkins diet! Texas cattlemen were in hog heaven enjoying the highest price per pound until Mad Cow crashed the party. Oprah's program challenging the safety of a red meat based diet did nothing to help their stock. Thanks in part to Dr. Phil's astute consultation on jury selection; she narrowly survived a mega-million reprisal lawsuit.

Dieting Through the Ages

From pork rinds to unabashed monster hamburgers, the new millennium presented the weird spectacle of junk food manufacturers on the offensive while producers of breads, cereals, fruit and vegetable juices were scrambling to keep their heads above water. But it was not always so. Unlike what Fred Flintstone would have us believe,

> *Globally, America ranks:*
> *number one in technology,*
> *number one in fatty fast food,*
> *number one in diets,*
> *yet number 16 in longevity.*

our pre-historic ancestors were "hunter-gatherers." The characters in the Book of Beginnings consumed energy chasing after food. They were therefore lean and muscular. Needless to say there was no such thing as "dieting" in those days, neither was there any evidence whatsoever of heart disease. Apart from infections, primitive tribes featured on *National Geographic* indeed conform to this pattern of robust fitness and health.

Any hunter knows that wild meat is lean compared to modern livestock from factory farms, fattened with all kinds of hormones for quick turn over. (This kind of high-protein / high-fat intake is the main culprit for premature puberty with girls developing breast by age 7 and having periods by age 9). Anthropologists estimate that the Stone Age diet was perhaps no more than 20 percent fat. More than half the calories came from *complex carbohydrates* in the form of fruits, nuts, grains legumes and roots – by no means considered lo-carb.

This is not to say that obesity never occurred in those early days. In fact, one dramatic account in Scripture describes the assassination of King Eglon in Judges 3:14-30. It appears that Eglon was a rather hefty fellow who indulged in oppressing the children of Israel. He was eventually stabbed by Ehud, the left-handed Jewish undercover agent. The account very graphically describes how so much belly fat covered the sword to the hilt that it could not be pulled out.

History is replete with those who struggled with the scales though not in vast numbers as today. Britain's King William the Conqueror was Commander-in-Chief at a time when the role involved actually leading his men into battle. As he ballooned in size, his horse slowed to a crawl under the crushing weight, presenting the enemy a target as large as the broad side of a barn. His Majesty realized that unless he got back in shape, he would be toast. William therefore took time out from the manly sport of war to embark on a "liquid" diet (as in ale). The fact that he was eventually able saddle up again is a credit to how seriously he took his responsibilities.

In 1825, French magistrate, Jean Anthelme Brillat-Savarin, published *Physiologie du Gout* (The Physiology of Taste). His theory was that white sugar and white flour were the source of excessive carbohydrates and "fatty congestion." The answer? More fruits and vegetables. In 1862, another Frenchman, physiologist Dr. Claude Bernard began discouraging sugars, milk, breads and pastries while promoting protein. However, dieting as a fad was not introduced into the lexicon until Englishman William Banting, experienced a spectacular stunning health benefits from weight loss.

Middle-age spread for this undertaker to the British upper crust made a mockery of simple activities such as tying his shoelaces. A rupture in his bellybutton added to his woes such that he could only walk down the stairs backward. Weight loss wonder drugs of that era (laxatives, baking soda, Epsom salts, even mini-dose arsenic), proved ineffective. He complained that intense exercise only increased his appetite, further swelling his waistline. By 1862, at the age of 66, 5' 5" William Banting tipped the scales at 202 pounds. Ironically, many of my patients today would give anything for that weight. But that was then and Mr. Banting was beside himself. It was only when he began to lose his hearing that he sought the services of Ear, Nose and Throat (ENT) specialist, Dr. William Harvey.

As fate would have it, Dr. Harvey had just returned from a symposium in Paris where he heard a presentation by the aforementioned Dr. Bernard on combating obesity. While treating the hearing problems, Dr. Harvey applied these concepts to his new patient. What happened thereafter proves that any doctor (or anyone, for that matter) can effectively treat obesity it they take a little more time to point their patients in a more natural direction. Banting dropped 50 pounds and 12 inches off his paunch within one year. His hearing returned to normal and his energy improved. So thrilled was he with his accomplishment that he penned *A Letter on Corpulence Addressed to the Public.* In one passage he gushes:

> *"I am very much better both bodily and mentally and pleased to believe that I hold the reins of health and comfort in my own hands. It is simply miraculous and I am thankful to Almighty Providence for directing me through an extraordinary chance to the care of a man who worked such a change in so short a time."*

That book sparked such a huge craze that in those days anyone losing weight would be described, not as dieting, but as 'Banting.' Variations on the theme were made as the phenomenon spread overseas. Dr. Felix Niemeyer of Stuttgart, Germany, identified protein as the only non-respiratory food. His advice to patients made sense: trim away the fat to get lean protein. By the 1880's, Dr. Helen Densmore had adapted the concepts in *Letter on Corpulence* to achieve significant weight loss in her heavy American patients.

> *There is nothing more frightful than ignorance in action.*
> Goethe

Prosperity Fuels Diet Industry

Fed by resources from the colonies, the wealth of the West multiplied

12. Diet Roller Coaster

dramatically during the 20th century. This drained previously self-sustaining civilizations such that significant segments of the world's population face a clear and present threat of hunger. The World Food Program reports that 25,000 starve to death each day. While $21 can feed a child for a year, Americans spend $40-60 billion a year to shed weight amassed from over-consumption. We are only now beginning to understand how this misuse of earth's resources increases our "carbon footprint" thus contributing to global warming and disastrous climate change.

This concept of food as energy began with Yale University physiologist, Russell Chittenden who was the first to define the calorie as the amount of heat needed to raise one gram of water by one degree Centigrade. In 1917, Dr. Lulu Peters applied the theory to weight control in her 1917 book *Diet and Health with a Key to the Calories*. Thereafter, strong personalities would try tinkering with the ratios of different foods to secure their own cult-like following. A rash of popular diets followed ranging from the sublime to the ridiculous. Dr. William Howard began promoting the *Food-Combining Diet* based on slow chewing and separating fruits, starches and protein in different meals. The *Lamb Chop and Pineapple Diet* was also quite the rage during that period. Dr. Herman Taller published *Calories Don't Count* in 1961. About the same time Dr. Irwin Stillman came out with *The Doctor's Quick Weight Loss Diet*. Both books espoused high fat, high protein and lo-carb. Stillman believed that the breakdown of protein consumes more energy than it generated. His followers were taught to avoid grain, fruits and vegetables – a common thread among lo-carb diets. Dr. Stillman sold over 20 million books and built an empire of followers before succumbing to a heart attack in 1975.

Dr. Herman Tarnower's high protein *Complete Scarsdale Diet* (1978) was a summary of his experiences at his New York cardiology practice. His illustrious career came to a full stop when his mistress, prep school Principal Jean Harris could not take it anymore. About that time period, Philadelphia Osteopathic physician Dr. Robert Linn produced a nutritional supplement comprising of ground-up animal by-products and promoted it in *The Last Chance Diet*. For the 58 of his customers who died of heart attacks, it did turn out to be their last diet before it was banned. Marion White's *"Diet without Despair"* advocated mineral oil laxative. However it resulted in symptoms such as bloating, diarrhea and excessive passing of gas. The *Cambridge Diet* was another upscale lo-carb (320 calories), high protein diet venture. Thirty dieters perished from heart attacks before the FDA and the United States Postal Service put a stop to it.

Has anyone stopped to ask why the more diet books we have, the fatter the population becomes? *The Zone* by Barry Sanders Ph.D., *Protein Power* Drs. Michael and Mary Dan Eads and *South Beach* by Miami cardiologist Dr. Arthur Agatston offer a few more bells and whistles but repackaging the same old platitudes. Glamorous sounding names target certain wealthy niche markets. Dr. Peter D'Adamo's *"Eat Right for Your Blood Type* entices readers to snack as often they like once it goes with their blood type. While these represent the tip of the iceberg of diet books, there are the more mainstream support-oriented programs. In 1948, Milwaukee housewife Esther Manzin founded *T.O.P.S* (Taking Pounds

> *Eating natural, non-processed foods automatically reduces calories and increases nutritive value.*

Off Sensibly) based on reduced calories, food diaries and support group meetings. Jean Nidetch used material from a New York City Department of Health clinic to start *Weight Watchers* in 1963. *Nutri/System* was launched in 1971 followed by *Jenny Craig* in 1983.

A healthier vein of weight-loss books are available such as *Pritikin Principle* in 1979. Later, President Clinton diet adviser Dr. Dean Ornish advocated strict limits on fat consumption in *Eat More, Weigh Less.* He also highlighted meditation and group support. Unlike Atkins, low fat diets have demonstrated actual reversal of coronary heart disease. Unfortunately, Ornish finds it necessary to genuflect as well before the altar of "eat-all-you-want, eat-as-often-as-you-are-hungry." This fails to adequately address the contagious eating disorders of our times. It neither promotes gastric rest nor reduces actual stomach size. Ornish dieters are therefore more vulnerable to that oral compulsion, habitually relapsing into eating tasty, high-fat, high-caloric foods when the opportunity arises. Mannafast, on the other hand, treats overeating rather than quibble obsessively about fat content. Its smaller stomach / reduced volume natural approach goes beyond the Ornish diet and is consistent with today's bariatric surgery principles.

The personal longevity of the typical diet guru pales in comparison with someone like *Jack LaLanne*. He has consistently preached low fat and exercise since the days of black and white television. Even in his 90's, Jack is still physically active, outperforming researchers and reporters half his age! How many of the famous lo-carb/high fat proponents from his age group are still around to challenge him on the relative merits of their approaches?

Why are high protein/high fat diets so deadly? Studies show that this kind of unbalanced, quick weight loss results in formation of ketones in the bloodstream. This causes dizziness and nausea, further decreasing appetite. Ketones results in *halitosis* (bad breath), increased uric acid production and kidney stones. Ketones also stimulate loss of calcium leading to osteoporosis and weakened teeth. Side effects make these diets unsustainable in the long run and rebound weight gain often follows. More importantly high fat/lo-carb diets increase the excretion of potassium and sodium thereby interfering with heart rhythms. The vast majority who have no idea the consequences these popular weigh-loss methods would do well to analyze the causes of death of leading diet doctors and their followers.

Fake Diets

It was Santayana who said that 'Those who do not remember the past are doomed to repeat it.' The biggest drawing card of new diets is the false hope that here comes something you have never seen before. Readers of this chapter are not likely to have the wool pulled over their eyes again. They can now recognize fad diets for short-term success and long-term havoc. Persons struggling with their weight are exquisitely vulnerable to hype and fables. Like the patron of that Utah buffet restaurant, there is always the ultimate temptation of eating to excess and weight loss at the same time. Lookout for any of these *five common features of fad diets*:

- Typically tease by offering "all you can eat."
- You don't have to exercise
- Burns fat during sleep
- Sleek marketing plan
- Tricky money back guarantees

Our worldly nature seduces us into labeling ourselves by the diet of the day. Surely, fad diets are based on some element of science with each offering some good advice. However, a wide range of factors (illnesses, medications, relationships, stresses) influence the best approach for a particular individual. I am therefore troubled when I hear intelligent people and devout folks fervently proclaim themselves to be followers of such and such a diet. The *Three Little Pigs* felt equally secure. They built their houses of different materials, but only when subjected to the huffing and the puffing that we saw the difference. Likewise, this chapter's brief analysis of competing diets teaches us that short-term weight loss is one thing, while long-term health is quite another. In comparison, Gastric conditioning is based on balanced nutrition and balanced living. Progressive, scientific, portion control actually shrinks the stomach in such a way as to make relapse quite unlikely.

As Mayor Bloomberg suggested, diets come and go. The diet roller coaster will continue to lurch one way and then the other. Waiting lines will always be long. But you and I know better than getting on that ride. It just leaves a bad taste finding out that the diet once raved about may actually be undermining the health of many. Weight control really is so simple "even caveman could do it." It is not something that you have to figure out. Just remember that commercial interests run rampant with a constant drumbeat urging wanton consumption the moment we come to the point of saying "That's it! This weight's got to go!" Instead, signal that you are serious about sustainable, "green lean" gastric conditioning. In the moral economy, we have been appointed stewards, not only of our own bodies, but of Mother Earth as well. Manna*fast* is a liberating lifestyle choice of grounded people of faith. It is built upon a Rock, not a fad diet that you go on and off like vagaries of fashion. Your *Mannameter* Lifescore serves as a daily reminder that as long as you keep doing the right thing, pleasing results are sure to follow.

People occasionally stumble over the truth,
but most of them pick themselves up
and hurry off as if nothing had happened.

Sir Winston Churchill

12. Diet Roller Coaster

REVIEW

1. Which was the first major lo-carb diet?

2. What is the worst harm caused by unscientific diets?

3. Which kinds of diets have been shown to reverse heart disease?

4. Which two features of fad diets are you most familiar with?

5. What are the essential features of a responsible eating plan that gives lasting weight control?

21. **Corn**   Source of Southern grits and Mexican tortillas. High in
   _____   lutein. Cardioprotective, helps macular degeneration.

22. **Cucumber** Apply directly to relieve tired swollen eyes. Helps derm-
   _____   atitis and sunburn. in silica, strengthens connective tissue.

23. **Eggplant** in vitamins, minerals and the flavonoid *nasunin*;
   _____   protects from cellular damage. Removes excess iron.

24. **Grapefruit** in sodium, in potassium and in fat burning enzymes.
   _____   Helps weight loss. Reduces cholesterol. Protects heart.

25. **Grapes** Darker more effective. eyesight. Fights cancer. varicose
    veins. heart disease. (Red wine/"French Paradox").

26 **Kiwifruit** (Chinese gooseberry) Effective against respiratory illness.
   _____   meat tenderizer *actinidin*. New Zealand dessert: Pavlova

27. **Lentils** High in protein, fiber, folic acid and trace minerals.
   _____   cholesterol and cancer risks. Controls blood sugar.

28. **Lettuce** Mediterranean origin. Helps sleep. vitamins, choline and
   _____   chromium, water content, "free" diet food.

29. **Mangoes** invitamins and minerals. Regulates thyroid. As effective
   _____   as drug treatment for traveler's diarrhea, *Giardiasis.*

30. **Mushrooms** in iron, Selenium, Vitamin B6 & B12, cholesterol.
    Strengthens bones. Kills bacteria and cancer cells.

+_____% **TOTAL VQ**   (VQ Assessment # 4 on page 234).

Chapter 13
Balanced Nutrition

*For too many people, a balanced meal
means a donut in each hand.*

Anon

The story is told of a missionary trekking through the jungle when he came face-to-face with a pair of hungry-looking lions. "Oh Lord," cried the missionary, "Please grant that these beasts are Christian, vegetarian lions." The rain forest grew strangely silent. As if in a trance, the lions not only appeared to kneel, but even closed their eyes. The missionary breathed a sigh of relief, secure in the belief that the savage predators were suddenly sanctified. Convinced that they had fallen asleep, he tiptoed past them rejoicing. Just then, he thought he heard a low, guttural growl. He turned around. Beneath their furry eyelids, the lions were eying him with keen interest. The sound rumbled into a deep, bone-chilling roar vibrating the vegetation around him. It sounded strangely like "Thank Thee Lord for this food which we are about to receive..."

> *Eggs* *contain vitamins B12 and D, riboflavin, and Folate, and is an excellent source of protein.*

Isaiah 65 prophesies of a time when the lion shall lay down with the lamb. The return of paradise would signal curtains for hunting and being hunted. Not so fast. The National Rifle Association (NRA) would counter that such a scenario conflicts with the Genesis portrayal of Divine favor on Abel's *animal sacrifice* over Cain's offering "from the fruit of the earth." Though theologians may explain this was in essence a precursor to Christ's blood atonement on Calvary, hunters remain unimpressed. In their eyes, this is just the first piece of evidence that a meat-based diet is superior. The two camps have been at loggerheads ever since.

Nutritionists too, wrestle with this controversial issue that so directly impacts obesity and health. Missionary or lion, all living things have to get that *protein*! It forms the building blocks of life. There are only two known sources, plants or animals. "Neither" is not an option. Protein is a major source of iron needed to build rich blood.

It is well established that iron is better absorbed from lean red meat, chicken and sea food. However, adequate amounts can be absorbed from enriched breads, legumes, cereals, prunes and raisins, especially when combined with foods high in vitamin C. Which protein source is better simply for weight loss? Which is better for long-term health? Is high-protein diet the wave of the future or is there such a thing as too much meat? You and I answer this question with every bite we take.

This chapter sets forth to scientifically analyze the human digestive system as compared to other creatures. It will clue us in to what kinds of foods are best suited for human consumption. We will then look into the matter of where dietary fat, milk, eggs and fish fit into the scheme of balanced nutrition. How valid is it to condemn certain foods from a religious or moral standpoint? What scientific proof do we have to back up our particular choices?

Red Meat vs. Green Pastures

Lawsuits were filed on behalf of any vegetarian who ate fries from a leading purveyor of fast food. Although the company purported to use only pure vegetable oil, they continued to add small amounts of beef fat to its fries because their customers seemed to be just loving the flavor. According to a report in the Chicago Tribune the company agreed to a public apology and to pay $10 million to charities that support vegetarianism (not to mention $2.4 million to probably steak-chomping plaintiffs' attorneys). The settlement also included an agreement to form an advisory board to respond to vegetarian dietary concerns.

The debate about meat consumption is not all black and white. Christians come in different stripes, the broad categories being Catholics and Protestants; Jews as Orthodox and Reformed, Muslims as Shiites, Sunnis and Nation of Islam. Vegetarians likewise come in different "sects and denominations." They all generally assert that their diet is more compassionate and in harmony with nature. Strict vegetarians however, will eat absolutely nothing from animal origin. Some go to the extent of not wearing anything involving fur, suede or leather. Others excuse animal materials such as wool and angora that do not require taking of life. *Lacto*-vegetarians are somewhat less dogmatic and do not mind a *milk* mustache. Lacto-*ovo*-vegetarians are even more casual and will have *eggs* to go with that. The vegetarians are fond of saying that they "eat nothing that has a face or a mother." (Poor fathers!) Such confusion had led some to suggest that vegetarian is just an old Native American word for "bad hunter!"

13. Balanced Nutrition

Vegans go all the way. Even animal products like honey and yeast are off limits. Reincarnation doctrine influences them to equate chomping on a drumstick with munching on great grandpa's leg. Historically, their zeal against taking advantage of animals has led to violent campaigns against vivisection in the teaching of practical anatomy. From time to time, activists release tapes showing them "liberating" lab animals and destroying expensive equipment used at research centers. Many cosmetic manufacturers are cowed into posting politically correct labels such as, "No animal experimentation or testing was used in production." Movies nowadays likewise remind us that, "No animals were deliberately hurt or killed during production of this film." All this has fuelled rancorous debate on more humane means of butchering.

*According to research, people with the **fewest heart attacks***

- *Eat lots of fruits and vegetables*
- *Avoid processed meats*
- *Exercise 3 times a week*
- *Do not smoke*
- *Do not abuse alcohol*

Society is successful in shielding the sensitive from how Bambi becomes venison. It is one thing to enjoy a fine steak. It is quite another to appreciate what really happened to Bessie. Anyway you cut it, that warm creature with those soft, gentle eyes is transformed to protein on your plate. Artistic genius Vincent Van Gogh stopped eating meat after a visit to a Paris slaughterhouse turned his stomach. Undercover video documents cases of wanton animal cruelty even at our most advanced livestock facilities. One included workers viciously stomping birds to death then processing them for a major finger-licking chicken franchise.

As we become more civilized, two culinary practices are coming under scrutiny. Crustaceans have become *cause célèbre* with protests against dunking live lobsters in boiling water. Activists are targeting certain advanced Pacific countries for the practice of tossing *screaming shrimp* on the "barbie" (barbeque). This is done table-side, much to the delight of the diners dedicated to guaranteed-fresh meals. The city of Chicago recently banned *foie grois*, the French delicacy of fatty liver produced by pushing a tube down the throat of ducks and geese to force-feed them into obesity. It was behavior like this that fired up Irish dramatist George Bernard Shaw to offer meat-eaters a stinging rebuke: "While we ourselves are *the living graves of murdered beasts*, how can we expect any ideal conditions on this earth?" Fighting words!

For many red meat lovers, vegetarians have long been suspect. That debate has raged ever since the first cavemen fantasized about the refrigerator and grunted, "What's for dinner?" There are those who look down their collective noses with a superiority complex at what other folks eat. They denounce certain foods as unclean, junk, or plain nasty. Everyone seems to be yelling something different. Orientals view Westerners as inhumane for eating holy cow. Pet lovers are repulsed by what they see ending up on the menu in certain Asian cultures. Some AIDS researchers blame eating African "bush meat" for the spread of the virus to mankind. People for the Ethical Treatment of Animals (PETA) wrap their naked bodies in cellophane packets as a form of protest in front of grocery stores. They go as far as erecting billboards with the Blessed Virgin cradling a dead chicken in her arms. Environmentalists badger indigenous tribes for feeding on of endangered species, while Muslims and Jews, embrace each other in reviling everyone else for eating swine. Enough already!

Gut Check

Imagine we were to back off a bit; we could just get along enough for anatomy to provide some insights. In the same way that bedroom slippers may not be appropriate for the gym, work or reception, so too the digestive organs of different life forms are uniquely configured to the foods best suited for healthy living. Consider how vegetarian/herbivore teeth are primarily incisors designed for chewing grass. In contrast, the Creator endowed carnivores have big mouths and sharp teeth for biting and devouring prey. The more civilized Homo sapiens have a small mouth-to-head ratio compared to classic carnivores. Think back: Tyrannosaurus Rex - big mouth, meat-eater. Brontosaurus - small mouth, plant eater.

Over here, observe closely: Primates (human/monkey family) have 32 teeth: 12 molars, 8 bicuspids, 8 incisors and 4 canines. Though we would rather disown them, biologists tell us that there is scarcely a 1 percent difference in our DNA make up. Theater audiences cringed in their seats as sharp-fanged King Kong lumbered up that New York skyscraper after the fair maiden... except the producer forgot to tell us that this ferocious looking mountain gorilla actually lives almost exclusively on fruits. Which raises the question, if our closest relatives in the animal kingdom hardly eat meat, then why should we?

But there is more to that story. The carnivore stomach is a simple sack and does not contain ruggae like that of the human. Herbivores on

13. Balanced Nutrition

the other hand have rather complex stomachs. As a matter of fact, they have anywhere from three to seven distinct compartments. Additionally, they are endowed with the enzyme *cellulase* specifically designed for the breakdown of coarse vegetable matter. As we saw in the anatomy and physiology section of Chapter 5, humans do not produce cellulase. Neither do we possess multiple stomachs, (though the way some eat, makes one wonder!) Ours is more complex, transitioning into the distinct *sections*: antrum, body and pylorus (page 67). However, unlike herbivores that tend to bring up their food to chew the cud, once our food hits the spot, we would rather not have anything further to do with it, thank you. As long as it keeps heading south, that works for *most* people - except for those afflicted with particular eating disorders. All this is to say that the structure and function of the human stomach is rather intermediate between that of a true carnivore or herbivore.

The bowel of humans, primates and herbivores in general is about 10 times the length of the trunk. This permits longer times to complete digestion of fruits and vegetables. The shorter bowel of carnivores (only 3 times trunk length) means a shorter transit time and less exposure to the more toxic by-products from the breakdown of meat. As every surgeon knows, intestinal obstruction causes accumulation of harmful metabolites and bacterial proliferation. This helps us understand why meat-eaters have smellier stools and higher rates of colon cancer.

A study done at England's University of Newcastle found that people who eat high amounts of red meat and processed meat were five times more likely to suffer intestinal problems such as ulcerative colitis.

Let us back up to the earlier and less offensive aspects of digestion. It is interesting to note that production of hydrochloric acid (HCL) is the unique feature of the carnivore. This is not found in herbivores. Here then, comes the million-dollar question: Does the human stomach produce acid? Naturally, today, we all know the answer to this question. But that was not always common knowledge, at least, not before we travel back in time to a place Ohioans call "that state up north." In fact, this discovery is by far one of the most colorful in the history of medicine.

Dr. William Beaumont in 1822 was serving as the Army surgeon stationed at Fort Mackinac, Michigan. He was called urgently to treat Alexis St. Martin, a Canadian hunter who was shot in the abdomen when

193

a musket accidentally discharged. St. Martin's wound healed in such a way as to create a permanent *gastrostomy* or window into his stomach. Dr. Beaumont was able to drop various food substances directly through this opening and actually watch the digestion process. For example, he tied a piece of meat on a string, lowered it through the opening and documented how the stomach rumbled as its gastric juices worked on the food. When he published his fascinating *Experiments and Observations on the Gastric Juice and Physiology of Digestion,* it was hailed as a landmark study in the annals of science.

Of course, humans produce HCL. Anyone who has suffered from acid reflux or heartburn can testify to that. Furthermore, biologists point out other important comparisons. Both herbivores and humans get vitamin C from their diets, whereas carnivores produce their own internally. Herbivores and humans perspire; carnivores get rid of excess heat by panting. Humans have teeth like primate fruitarians, gastrointestinal tracts more or less in between those of herbivores and carnivores, and they produce stomach acid like carnivores. All that should help answer the New Age question, "If vegetarians eat vegetables, what do humanitarians eat?" Seriously though, a 1999 article in the journal, *The Ecologist,* concluded that human "physiology definitely indicates a *mixed feeder.*"

> *According to the 40 year long Framingham Study, no deaths has been reported from heart disease with a cholesterol under 150.*
> *-Am. Journal of Cardiology '98*

The conclusion of the matter, therefore, is this: humans were created not to be typical carnivores or herbivores but *omnivores,* (eaters of a wide variety of foods: fruits, vegetables, grain and meat). Dumbo, the flying elephant, could get quite obese on his herbivore diet. Canadian geese migrating south for winter stop to rest and feed from place to place. Occasionally, some birds feasting excessively on grain grow too fat to fly. This all comes back to the basic Mannafast principle that it is not so much the type of diet but the *amount* of whatever is eaten which results in obesity. Armed with these facts, how then do we make wise nutritional choices for effective weight control and optimal health?

13. Balanced Nutrition

Balance

Traditional Eskimos subsist during the long winters on the fatty meat of whale, seal and caribou. They eat hardly any fruit and vegetables. Traditionally, they do not suffer from the kind of obesity and heart disease seen today in their native cousins on the reservations. Once they adopt the standard high fat, high volume American diet combined with little exercise, disease and death rates shoot up to the levels discussed in Chapter 4. It would appear that geographic eating patterns have to balance total lifestyle in order to produce good health and longevity.

The modern term "flexitarian" describes one who strives for the right balance of fresh fruit and vegetables while resisting high meat consumption. This is the intelligent approach in the post-Atkins era. It recognizes that organisms in nature generally subsist on living food; (except for vultures, buzzards and saprophytic fungi which live on dead food). Humans putting themselves in that category do not do well. Processing kills food in order to preserve it. In a sense, this removes it from the viable food chain and natural order. Of course, raw meat and fish do not appeal to most people. Doing so would vastly increase the risk of Salmonella, hepatitis, and mad cow disease.

> *A study of 88,000 women found that those eating the most animal fat were nearly twice as likely to develop colon cancer as those eating less animal fat.*

Raw vegetables and fruits, however, are very much 'alive.' They are loaded with enzymes and vital nutrients. No manufactured pill or capsule can ever contain the incredible balance of vitamins and nutrients found in the natural state. It takes more than just knocking back a daily handful of unproven herbal supplements to make one healthy. While these manufactured products may have certain benefits, we need to be reminded that they can in no way match the real thing.

Fewer than 9 percent of Americans eat the recommended five daily servings of fruits and vegetables. Incredibly, some of the most popular diets today seek to steer adherents even further away from whole foods. Why then should we be surprised at the outcome? NASA's nutrition is packaged for highly mobile life. But rest assured that the focus is on harnessing the natural goodness and preserving that balance. It is interesting that many patients when stricken with cancer plunge into holistic ways to fight the disease. They invariably start 'eating healthier' coming up with a "macrobiotic," more vegetable-based diet. More often than not, it is too late. Balanced nutrition and healthy lifestyle *prevents* cancer. That should be the emphasis rather than just a narrow focus on weight loss.

No matter how suspicious one may be of "Big Government," the time has come to put confidence in the updated nutritional guidelines and responsibly apply them directly to our daily meals. The masses are led by their taste buds and tradition into predictable pitfalls. Just a little changes here and there yields amazing results. It is not unusual for us to see a roughly 50 point drop in cholesterol, *without medication*, after just three months on Manna*fast*. Many of our patients had been on the high-fat Atkins diet. They had been jubilant about losing weight in the short-term, but had no idea what effect it was having on their cholesterol levels and long-term health.

> So this patient with a weakness for juicy steaks says, "If animals aren't supposed to be eaten, then why are they made out of meat?!"

Every minute in the United States, two people die from heart disease making it by far the leading cause of death. All responsible medical authorities advocate reduction in cholesterol levels to improve heart health by *shifting to a diet that is more plant based.* Interestingly, a researcher by the name of E. L. Alderman found that Coronary Artery Bypass surgery does not "cure" the underlying condition in the truest sense. Writing in the journal, *Circulation*, November 1990, Alderman described a ten year follow up of Survival and Myocardial Infarction. He found that surgery improves *chest pain* and function, but does not really increase *long-term* survival as much as cardiac rehab.

As an intern, I had to draw blood on a patient in preparation for blocked up blood vessels in his legs. My job was to make sure all his results were on the chart and that he was good to go first thing in the morning. Well, the gentleman had just decided to have one more splurge on a hamburger combo with milkshake and fries. The lab technician showed me the unusually thick, greasy layer that separated out after spinning his blood down in the centrifuge. This was when I saw for myself how food choices directly influence health.

When you think of it, that makes a lot of sense. What exactly is

13. Balanced Nutrition

OBSOLETE FOOD PYRAMID

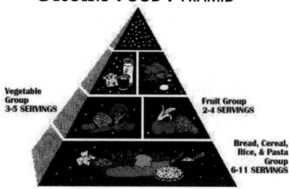

NEW USDA APPROVED FOOD PYRAMID

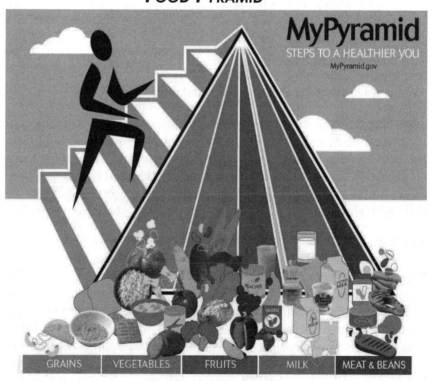

cardiac rehab anyway? It is basically a structured program of exercise and balanced nutrition. I was fascinated to observe that within a month or two of diagnosis, the typical heart attack victims would report, "I have never felt better."

Surely, appropriate medication and surgical intervention is crucial. However, it is only after a close call with the grim reaper that a good percentage of patients become motivated enough to make dramatic lifestyles changes. They finally are forced by their families to quit smoking, lower their fat and salt intake and do some regular exercise. Before their heart attack they ignored those recommendations or at best, only paid lip service. Those, like my patient, who continue eating as before, soon compromise again the improved coronary blood flow provided by angioplasty or bypass.

> *The preponderance of evidence over decades suggests that a more vegetarian diet is far healthier. Few reputable nutritionists would dispute that.*

Tropical rain forests are being cleared at an alarming rate for supplying meat beyond our natural requirements. Studies show that meat production consumes 15 times more energy and more than 25 times more water that vegetables. Reduction in meat consumption therefore decreases greenhouse gases and climate change.

Saturated Fats

We all know that fat plays an important role in making food taste delicious. Saturated fats are found mostly in meat, whole-milk dairy products (cheese, milk, and ice cream), poultry skin, and egg yolks. They raise total cholesterol, but those from plants such as coconut and palm oil are healthier in that they also raise the "good" HDL cholesterol as well.

Trans Fats

The real culprit today is trans fatty acids. This is produced when liquid vegetable oil is heated in the presence of hydrogen. It makes oils harder at room temperature to produce margarine. Some of us can probably remember a time when *lard* was used generously as a staple in baking. While growing up we used it to grease the pans for holidays and birthday cakes. As a reward, the helper would get the first taste, piping hot from the oven. What the Foreman Grill ingenuously gets rid of, in times past we would skim off to use again. Even so, people were a lot more active and "pigging out" was nowhere as socially acceptable as it is today. Anyway, when we discovered that too much lard and butter was bad for the heart, the new margarine seemed like the perfect substitute. But in truth, this is a synthetic substance that almost never gets rancid or even attracts insects! Somehow, these little bugs instinctively knew what it took us decades of research to find out. It was a mistake though it made sense at the time.

CATEGORIES OF FAT

Type of Fat	Main Source	State at Room Temperature	Effect on Cholesterol Levels
Monounsaturated	Olives; olive oil, canola oil, peanut oil; cashews, almonds, peanuts, and most other nuts; avocados	Liquid	Lowers LDL; raises HDL
Polyunsaturated	Corn, soybean, safflower, and cottonseed oils; fish	Liquid	Lowers LDL; raises HDL
Saturated	Whole milk, butter, cheese, and ice cream; red meat; chocolate; coconut and palm oil	Solid	Raises both LDL and HDL
Trans	Most margarines; vegetable shortening; partially hydrogenated vegetable oil; deep-fried chips; many fast foods; most commercial baked goods	Solid or semi-solid	Raises LDL

Trans fats have the worst effect of all. They not only raise LDL (bad) cholesterol, but also lower HDL (good) cholesterol. Trans fats add flakiness to pastries. They are found mostly in processed snacks and fast foods such as French fries and onion rings, commercially prepared baked goods such as cakes, cookies, donuts, and muffins. They are not poisons in the short term or in limited amounts. But what we gain with convenience and taste from packaged foods and vending machines, we often lose in terms of nutrition. Once again, the rule of thumb is that the more altered the foodstuff, the more harmful to our systems. The state has taken the initiative in outlawing the use trans fat use by restaurants and food companies. A significant drop in heart disease is sure to follow.

Healthy Oils and Fats

From a purely weight loss standpoint, all oils are equally fattening. Each tablespoon yields 120 calories. However, they have different effects on cholesterol levels. Unsaturated fats come mostly from *plant sources*, such as vegetable oils, nuts, seeds and fish. They are divided into two main categories: *monounsaturated* fats (which are found in high concentrations in canola, peanut, and olive oils) and *polyunsaturated* fats (sunflower, corn, soybean and fish oils). These good fats decrease bad cholesterol (LDL) and increase healthy cholesterol (HDL) levels. Mono-unsaturated fats are more effective in this respect. However, the polyunsaturateds include those essential fatty acids (omega 3 and omega 6) discussed later in the chapter.

Give a Man a Fish...

...the saying goes, and you feed him for a day. Teach him to fish, and you feed him for a lifetime - or maybe you just created another part-time widow. Depending on where you are, fishing ranks right up there with football and golf in snatching husbands away for the better part of the weekend.

If this be a vice, however, it is a splendid one! Few things compare to fishing when it comes to relaxing and bonding with kids, especially fathers with sons. I remember when we took our little ones to the festival. Satisfied folks seemed to be skipping along with large, cuddly, stuffed animals. Lady luck was not smiling on me. *What kind of man was I that I could not even win something for my kids?* I felt miserable. Then I paid 50 cents for one of those "always a winner" games. The kids were instructed to stick their little "fishing poles" into a hole in the booth. The charming attendant behind the partition then attached a cheapie plastic toy to the end of the line. Their eyes twinkled with glee at having "caught" something! Together with some wild rides and cotton candy, that let me off the hook. My love for fishing only doubled as I taught them fishing for real at the neighborhood pond. The excitement of the first nibble, the frustration when the bait was gobbled and gone, then finally - "Gotcha!" I can think of no other activity in which they shared in more enthusiastically: preparing our catch and serving it to Mom.

13. Balanced Nutrition

Fishing is an integral part of the commerce and culture for islanders. I therefore found it fascinating the different prevailing attitudes to fish consumption across the continental United States. On the East and West coasts, people have a particular spring in their step seeking out the choice catch at the wharves or fresh fish markets. Compare that to the central and mountain states. Just talk of *eating* fish and some folks look at you like, "What planet are you from?" In these parts, fish jokes are about as risqué as they get. Many a Midwestern housewife would gladly get down on her hands and knees to do bathroom chores rather than be asked to prepare fish. Should she deign accompany her husband on a fishing trip, far be it from a "lady" to bait her own hook. And God forbid she feels some action on the other

> *Whatsoever hath fins, and scales in the water, in the seas and in the rivers, them shall you eat.*
> Leviticus 11:19

end; she quickly surrenders the pole for him to haul it in. The very thought of a flopping fish is as scary as a mouse let loose in a classroom of girls. Out yonder, the manly art of recreational fishing reigns supreme with its own celebrities and television channel.

Frequent public service announcements warn about local fish contaminated with carcinogens such as mercury and polychlorinated biphenyls (PCB's). This, no doubt, deepens the general taboo that eating fish is bad. Meanwhile, a robust sporting goods industry promotes big bucks competitions for specially tagged fish. After hours at the waters edge or on specially designed boats with the beverage of choice, fishermen return with tall tales about "the one that got away."

In the context of history and global cultures, the humane-sounding practice of 'catch n' release' is not only unusual, but actually quite traumatic to fish. An emergency room physician treating a patient unfortunate enough to be accidentally snagged does not rip out the hook but rather carefully advances, cuts and removes it to avoid further injury. Not so with fish. Having no front paws, they use their mouths for so many functions other creatures take for granted. Furthermore, the protective coating over their scales is disrupted by handling. Released fish are thereby exposed to an array of bacteria, viruses and toxins. Not surprisingly, reports indicate that as many as 30 percent with hook-damaged mouths soon perish when thrown back into their natural habitats. Fish are part of the circle of life. If they could talk, perhaps they would be gulping, "You caught me, OK Let's get on with it! Please don't play games and let me suffer like this!"

Sacred history and science converge to highlight the importance of fish in the life of the faithful. The Gospels are generously sprinkled with stories and parables featuring fish and fishermen. In His glorified body, what did Christ eat? Broiled fish! The Greek spelling for fish, ICHTHUS is an acrostic for **I**esous (Jesus) **CH**ristos (Christ) **TH**eou (God's) **U**iou (Son) **S**oter (Savior). The early believers lived in such constant fear of persecutors that on meeting a stranger they would tentatively scratch a semi-circle on the ground with their feet or using a stick. If the 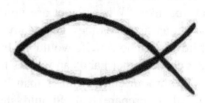 other person was like-minded, he would make a complementary semi-circle to form that well-known fish symbol. Before cathedrals, Bible tracts, or televangelists, that brave and simple act was a sermon in itself.

The awkward irony today is that places where the gospel flourishes, fish consumption flounders. This, at a time when scientists are more emphatically endorsing of omega-3 fatty acids. Found primarily in such fish as salmon, tuna, mackerel, lake trout and sardines, these nutrients block the formation of leukotriene B4 and prostaglandins responsible for inflammatory response. Fish-eaters therefore suffer less joint pain, migraine headaches, lupus, asthma and obesity. Omega-3's also thin the blood shielding the artery walls from accumulating that gooey cholesterol. It reduces irregular heartbeats and arteriosclerosis that contribute to the mortality of heart disease. Cardiologists now recommend fish at least once or twice a week as part of a low fat diet. Avoid breading and deep-frying as with most fast-food fish sandwiches. That simply defeats the purpose.

Newer medical research is pointing to a definite link between mental health and omega-3 fatty acids. Because they are highly concentrated in the brain, these substances are believed to have a mood-stabilizing effect. People with depression have been found to have abnormally low levels of these fatty acids. Depressed people become more sedentary and more obese. It all adds up.

Most of the fish caught in America goes into pet food. Pets, (or *Animal Americans* as they are now called), are therefore often healthier than patients. Surely, they would wish their owners would likewise benefit. That much-maligned fish odor during preparation is easily neutralized with a little lemon. For those particularly sensitive to being called 'sardine breath,' a simple after-dinner mint keeps everyone sociable. Most will agree that a fish meal sits lighter on the stomach than steak and is less likely to cause reflux. Those still not persuaded should consider omega-3 fatty acids or fish oil supplements to cover any gaps in good nutrition. Isn't it ironic that today it takes science to persuade us that faith without fish is a moral contradiction? The time has come therefore, for us to restore the profound nutritive benefits of fishing above its cherished recreational attributes.

Easy To Eat Right

Thousands of articles and books have been written on the topics we touched on in this chapter. We did not attempt to resolve controversy, only to show the relevant logic of food science. Research confirms that obesity is a direct result of not only how much, but also what exactly we have been eating lately. Today's Standard American Diet (SAD) is 33 percent heavier in dairy products, 50 percent more in beef and 280 percent more in poultry than a century ago. For the most part, we take little advantage from having access to a wider array of healthy foods than did our parents. Pledging *at least couple meatless days a week* would therefore be an excellent start to our nutrition makeover. It is easier than one would think once we have the foresight required to modify our traditional menus.

In times past we were not fully aware how years of unbalanced "meat and potatoes" processed food consumption gave rise to obesity and disease. Our generation has witnessed the complications from attempting to quickly undo the consequences using glamorous diets, drugs and surgery. The message in the missionary's heart at the beginning of the chapter must therefore be translated into ways of eating that lead to improved health and weight control. Proverbs 4:23 exhorts us to "Guard your *heart* with all diligence for out of it come the issues of life." In like manner, Manna*fast* guards our *stomachs* with all wisdom, for out of it comes the issues of health.

Your choice of diet can influence your long-term health
prospects more than any other action you might take.

C. Everett Koop, M.D., Former Surgeon General

203

Review

1. Is the human digestive system designed to consume meat?

2. Was Jesus vegetarian?

3. What are the health risks of excessive meat consumption?

3. What is the advantage of eating fish?

5. What is the difference in effectiveness between nutrition supplements and fresh fruits and vegetables?

Chapter 14
Health Freedom Ring

While I have been fighting,
Rome has grown mad and corpulent and diseased.
I did this. And now I shall make it right.

Marcus - The movie *Gladiator*

"Struck by the poverty...in rich America." So said Archbishop Paul Cordes, Vatican envoy touring New Orleans and surrounding areas devastated by Hurricane Katrina. Was he reacting to reports of the wealthy fleeing harm's way in private jets while arranging for their pets to be whisked away in air-conditioned tour buses? Or was he as horrified as the rest of the world watching helplessly while the killer storm tore into the neglected masses? Rather than a place of refuge, the Superdome quickly descended into a living hell. Surging floodwaters washed away any veneer of civility to become emblematic of the widening gulf between the classes in modern USA.

Congress quickly confirmed what many suspected. Federal, State and Municipal leaders fell woefully short in planning for a crisis looming for decades. With much of the "Big Easy" below sea level, the populace had to trudge to overpasses and other higher ground for safety. Politics and patronage poisoned disaster management. In large measure, the poor, the elderly and the incapacitated initially were left to fend for themselves.

July 10, 1893: Dr. Daniel Hale Williams performs the world's first successful heart surgery at Provident, Chicago's only integrated hospital at the time. The patient goes on to live another 20 years.

Healthcare workers were forced to make unthinkable decisions. The morbidly obese featured disproportionately among those left behind. Helicopters had to pluck stranded residents from rooftops. These powerful aircraft designed to haul heavy military payloads could be seen straining to lift the corpulent - one at a time. It took a disaster of this magnitude to dramatize how chronic poverty is compounded by overweight.

Keep these searing images in mind as we challenge specific taboos in this chapter. In a culture priding itself on rugged individualism, personal weight is often seen as a private matter between an individual and his doctor. The fact is that overall fitness also profoundly impacts the fate of groups in society. How can each of us help to bring greater health equity throughout the entire population? From my visit to New Orleans, working with Native Americans or migrant workers and other under-served populations, I am deeply troubled by persistent trends in minority health. Why are activity levels so low in certain neighborhoods? What kind of social and legislative initiatives can we promote to make things right?

Nourishment or Noose?

Sharlo's Strange Bargain by West Indian author Ralph Prince (1968) presents interesting parallels to the Charlie Daniels Band 1979 hit, *The Devil Went Down to Georgia.* It tells an intriguing story of the sweetest fife player in the village having an encounter with a tall, mysterious, ageless man with white flowing hair. In exchange for his beloved musical instrument, the man made Sharlo an offer he could not refuse. It was a magic *calabash* (a bowl made from a tropical gourd) overflowing with all kinds of delicious food on demand. Neither the story of the Grimm Brothers' gingerbread house nor the Biblical feast of Belshazzar made my mouth water more. Imagine, all one had to do was recite this goofy rhyme requesting your favorite dish - and there it was!

Anyway, Sharlo struck a deal pledging never to disclose his source - otherwise bad things would happen. *"Sharlo no longer worked, and even in hard times people wondered where Sharlo was getting his food from."* The story went on to describe how he grew *"so fat that he could scarcely open his eyes...His belly sagged over his belt like that of a pig hanging down."* (While I would never approve of anyone being described in such fashion, fiction writers were not constrained by political correctness when Mr. Prince spun his tale). Unlike the Charlie Daniels' ballad, however, the Devil did get his due. Prince wrapped up his yarn with Sharlo breaking his end of the bargain. He spilled the beans to a persistently curious friend whereupon he disappeared without a trace.

As Archbishop Cordes discovered, malnutrition is rampant in America. Sociologists described growing *food deserts* in barren, poor urban communities where healthy food in well-stocked supermarkets can only be found more than an hour away by foot or bus. By default, a proliferation of convenience and liquor shops supply low quality fattening foods. The result is a paradoxical combination of growing pockets of real hunger in the midst of endemic obesity. Still, as with the Devil's calabash in Caribbean folklore, to what extent are we ourselves to blame for the bad things happening in minority health these days? Sharlo's sedentary lifestyle and compulsive eating habits were directly linked to his destiny. How hard are we fighting to *prevent* disease? How can other nations are healthier than the US while using less medications and surgery. Slavery, segregation and racial profiling no doubt play a major role in our present predicament, but until we face up to obesity as the very root of this new insidious form of bondage, we cannot truly set our people free.

The Diversion

The prophet came to the stark realization that "My people are destroyed for lack of knowledge," (Hosea 4:6). The ostrich buries its head in the sand to hide from surrounding threats. Similarly, by totally immersing ourselves in sports and entertainment, we think everything is cool. Is it? Knowledge of our own historic accomplishments leaves much to be desired. Instead we are easily dazzled by those who have made it. The Oprahs, the Lebrons and P. Diddys of the minority community tend to divert attention from how much worse the masses are doing.

> *All families have the right to quality healthcare and the responsibility to practice good health preserving habits such as proper diet, exercise and emotional well-being.*
>
> Rose Sanders, Esq.
> Selma Alabama Voting Rights Museum, Declaration of Family Bill of Rights and Responsibility

When we take a good hard look at where we are heading to, we observe that the African-American high school graduation rate at 83.7 percent, still trails the 91.8 percent for whites. Who is responsible? An astonishing 70 percent of African-American babies are born out-of-wedlock, compared to 27 percent for Whites. Who is responsible? 53 percent of African-American households are headed by single females, the majority falling below the poverty line. Who is responsible? The average income for African-Americans is 61 percent of whites. Incarceration rates for males in their 20's: Whites:1.7%, Hispanics: 3.6%, African-Americans: 12.6%. Equal justice?

The sad state of affairs is further reflected in the comparative diabetes rate: Whites: 12 percent, Hispanics: 16 percent, African-Americans: 26 percent! Since diabetes is a major cause of kidney failure as we saw in Chapter 4, a visit to any dialysis facility in the country reveals that the majority of the patients are minorities. *Miami Heat's* Alonzo "Zo" Mourning battled back after his kidney transplant to earn his NBA championship ring. This truly remarkable achievement still does not negate the fact that patients with kidney failure generally continue to have greatly increased risks from *associated cardiovascular disease.*

Historical analysis reveals that one side prevailed in the Civil War, the other side prevailed throughout Reconstruction. There result was a time when minorities had no access to quality health care. So oppressive was the Jim Crow culture that it engendered enduring myths in the African-American community. Dr. Charles Drew, Chairman of the Department of Surgery at Howard University, is credited with inventing blood transfusion. This medical breakthrough immediately saved countless American lives in World War II. In 1950, at age 46, Dr. Drew

> *I've always believed that if you put in the work, the results will come. I don't do things half-heartedly. Because I know if I do, then I can expect half-hearted results.*
> Michael Jordan

was involved in a tragic motor vehicle accident near Haw River, North Carolina. Despite official denials, many still believe the cruel irony in reports that he was turned away from a segregated hospital and the chance for a life-saving blood transfusion.

Today, access to healthcare remains a major issue; though not nearly as blatant as it was back then. Yet, in the year that Dr. Drew left us, the overall cancer mortality rate for African-American males was only 178.9 per 100,000 – actually *better* that the 210 for white males. Today, according to the Centers for Disease Control and Prevention, the cancer death rate for African-American males has shot up to 330.9, far worse than the 239.2 for white males. What happened? The expected lifespan as of the middle of the first decade of the 21st century:

Caucasian: 80.5 (female) 75.4 (male)
African-American 76.1 (female) *69.2* (male)

Sports Addiction

How could it be that we were healthier back then with less health care? One reason is that we remain too enamored with the belief in our physical prowess. The annals of sports provide some clues to the best strategies for raising healthy activity levels in the minority community.

Way back in 1908, Jack Johnson had to go all the way to Australia to become the first African-American boxer to seize the world heavyweight championship. Only then did reigning American champion Jim Jeffries, who had earlier refused to fight Johnson, attempted to snatch back the title. When Johnson prevailed in Las Vegas in 1910 Jeffries incensed fans terrorized black neighborhoods. Government had to ban showing the film in order limit the body count.

In Yankee Stadium, 1936, Germany's Max Schmeling stunned the world of pugilism by knocking out Joe Louis, the promising *Brown Bomber*. Schmeling, a reluctant Nazi icon, was transported in glory on the Hindenburg airship for dinner with Hitler. As they looked at the video together, *The Fuhrer* was described as dancing with joy each time his man landed a telling blow. In a super-hyped rematch two years later, Louis returned the favor. Before the largest worldwide radio audience up to that time, he decked Schmeling in one round to become undisputed world boxing champion. Like Jesse Owens, Louis contributed immeasurably in debunking Hitler's notion of Aryan supremacy. Before that fight, he was invited to the White House for a pep talk by FDR. Despite his ethnicity, this time films of the match were widely used in propaganda against the enemy. After serving his purpose, Louis was promptly impoverished in his native land. He succumbed to drugs, barely surviving to collect Social Security. Frank Sinatra paid for his heart surgery and his magnanimous German opponent paid for his funeral. Schmeling, meanwhile, went on to run a profitable Coca Cola franchise and living to the ripe, old age of 99.

Imus' spectacular meltdown following his characterization of the Rutgers University women's basketball team was not unique. Before him, CBS had to fire sports announcer Jimmy 'The Greek' Snyder for attributing Black so-called natural giftedness to "breeding in slavery." Referring to the ascendant Tiger Woods as "that little boy," professional golf veteran Fuzzy Zoeller urged him "not to serve fried chicken or collard greens" for the PGA Champions Dinner. In his brief foray as a sports commentator, one leading radio talk show host chose to *diss* Eagles' Donovan McNabb (son of the lovable Chunky Chicken Soup lady). He argued that Donovan was overrated and that the media just wanted a Black quarterback to succeed. Ex-General Manager for the Los Angeles Dodgers, Al Campinis, proclaimed that Blacks could never coach because they lacked the necessary thinking and managerial skills. How do such tortured souls handle seeing two African-American coaches, Indianapolis' Tony Dungy and Chicago's Lovie Smith, in the SuperBowl?

The point is not to recite a litany of verbal abuse. It is no secret that legends like Muhammad Ali, Jackie Joyner-Kersey, Arthur Ashe, Walter Peyton, Venus and Serena Williams, Reggie White and Kirby Puckett have all had to overcome various forms of demeaning prejudice before being showered with accolades. In a perverse way, it is that very triumph in the face of such adversity which has so endeared the African-American athlete to his struggling community. Yet, the resultant excessive reverence may be turning out to be more of a curse than a blessing.

The persistent belief that we may run faster and jump higher certainly is not translating into health and longevity. As the Romans would say, *Quam cito transit gloria mundi!* How quickly passes the glory of the world! The health of these powerful role models often plummets to the bottom of the scorecard soon after retirement from a sparkling sports career. Families are often left behind with little more than fading trophies and fragile records.

A painful disconnect exists between *valuing* of athletic ability and the *actual involvement* in a regular athletic/exercise activity. The *Journal of the American Medical Association* reports that African-American men who are obese at age 20 will die 20 years before their peers, which is by age 50. Take a look at the 100-meter dash in any national or international

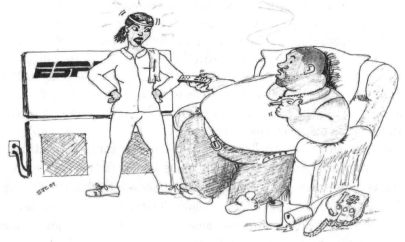

track & field games - almost uniformly black; the 100 meter dash for centenarians (100 year-olds, *they actually run!*) - uniformly white. Could it be that a 'senior tour' of the NBA today would look as lily-white as the college teams of the 1950's?

14. Health Freedom Ring

There is no greater place to show some love, man-to-man, than at the barber shop. The bonding and banter is boisterous. You better be able to hold your point or face being verbally beaten into bemused submission. Yet, barber-shop talk proves that few other groups anywhere come close in paying more adulation at the altar of celebrity athletes. After graduation, African-American exercise activity drops so dramatically that many of these same vocal fans could scarcely walk a mile even if their lives depended on it. Right there must be the epicenter of our health initiative.

Hair Today - Gone Tomorrow

The root causes of obesity in the African-American community are far from obvious. However zeroing in on a rather mundane physician office encounter may shed some insight into solutions for this chronic problem:

"Apply a small amount of antibiotic ointment daily to the incision and keep it dry for the next three days," I instructed Melissa, who is White, after excising a cyst from her scalp. Fairly routine post-op instructions, I thought as I focused on charting her visit.

"THREE DAYS?!" She protested, "Gosh! What about washing my hair?"

"Come on now, not washing your hair for a few days isn't going to kill you," I glibly replied. As the receptionist scheduled her follow-up appointment, Melissa said nothing - just looked at me funny.

That got me thinking. I began to wonder whether rather trivial differences in racial attitudes toward hair-care could actually be impacting health more profoundly than all these

> *Bring your best to the moment. Then, whether it fails or succeeds, at least you know you gave all you had. We need to live the best that's in us."*
> Angela Bassett

hallowed government programs. This prompted me to seek the opinions of experienced hairdressers, beauticians and barbers on the matter. What I discovered (and this was by no means a scientific poll,) was that many African-Americans felt Caucasian "straight" hair somehow gets greasier faster, thus requiring frequent washing. Conversely, "curly" hair is thought to produce less grease and therefore does not need to be washed and styled as often. After spending big bucks and long hours on a precious perm, our women hardly have any appetite for getting their "do's" ruined in a drizzle or even a little perspiration. They baby their hairstyles with a passion as moisture of any kind makes for a bad hair day. On the other hand, Caucasians were reflexly aghast at the notion of going days, or even weeks without shampooing.

Some may see these findings as shedding some light on the relationship between hair-care and fitness. Others may respond, "Don't even go there!" Nevertheless, it does raise some provocative questions. Do African-American women avoid swimming, and outdoor ventures because of their hair? Does this inactivity extend to the bedroom where annoyance at messing up the hair puts a cramp on intimacy?

Let's face it, feeling good about ones hair has a lot to do with a woman's sense of comparative beauty. My medical school classmate, Dr. Cheryl Burgess, now a prominent Washington DC dermatologist, proposes a more complex interplay of social factors affecting the relationship between weight and hair care. Yet there seems to be an unnecessary contradiction between having pretty hair and being pretty *and* fit. In the African-American community, eating disorders such as anorexia are considered weird and are practically unheard of. Plus-sized stars like Aretha Franklyn, Nel Carter, Queen Latifa and Monique are not only well-accepted but celebrated without reservation. It is a source of pride to be perceived as "big and beautiful," "big-boned," or "a whole lot of woman." Black males, the more successful ones in particular, though very vocal in their praise of their dreamgirl *Nubian* queen, often select "trophy mates" from other races. Is this the result of lingering inferiority complex or could it in some way be related to activity levels? Many African-Americans express aversion to exercise because "It looks too much like work." As they say, *if Mom ain't exercising, ain't nobody exercising!* Reversing childhood obesity is going to take a little more than just telling kids to go outside to play.

Before the Civil Rights era, hot combs and harsh chemicals were routinely used to make African-American hair "more manageable." Trend-setters like Angela Davis and Jimmy Hendricks led the charge by sporting huge afros and using more Black identity hair-care products. But with *Superfly*, hair-straightening returned with a vengeance. *Icky* Geri-curls not only consumed much time, but also left oily signatures on dance partners and pillows. Fortunately, we are re-learning that "nappy is happy." Braids or locks are gradually being rediscovered as being lower maintenance. It used to be that society considered such hairstyles unkempt, immoral and associated with a back-to-nature *Rasta* subculture. Whoopi Goldberg is among the many celebrities to demonstrate that such hairstyles are no longer seen as an impediment to upward mobility. Mainstream ads (such as United Colors of Benetton) now portray sophisticated consumers of all races as gravitating to more natural and functional styles.

14. Health Freedom Ring

Life, Liberty and...

A quick glance at Black Entertainment Television is enough to convince anyone that African-Americans excel in rhythm, comedy and how to party. Without a doubt, when it comes to that kind of *pursuit of happiness*, we have that nailed down. The *life* part too. We have survived in the context of history where less hardy species have been utterly wiped out from the face of the earth. The *liberty* part, however, is still somewhat in question.

The economic empowerment acquired by recently arrived ethnic groups continues to elude us. The Irish, Hispanics, Asians, Indians, Eastern Europeans fleeing communism, even Arabs and Jews fleeing Middle East madness all rightly point to the discrimination they too had to endure. Theirs is in no way comparable to the harsh dehumanizing experience of slavery. Nevertheless, they have organized their close-knit families and worked diligently together to quickly leap ahead into the mainstream. While our unique melanin content makes it more difficult to blend in, we still have to give an account for not taking better advantage of the available opportunities. We need to redirect envy at the successful foreign-born and begin by celebrating our own accomplishments and potential. How can we get any respect if we persist in demeaning ourselves by using the N-word then turning around and castigating others for doing the very same?

Self-inflicted maladies continue to sap our collective energy relegating us to the bottom rungs of the socio-economic ladder. At the same time, the deteriorating state of healthcare in the African-American community may well be no accident. Today, policies of the Department of Health and Human Services generally appear above board. However, there is sufficient reason to question whether the manner in which these are currently applied actually contribute to perpetuating inequities.

In 1879, America's first African-American professional nurse, Mary Eliza Mahoney graduated from the New England Hospital for Women and Children Training School. Her career was marked by accolades for calm, efficient and tender care of the sick. Her service to community was in stark contrast to that of Eunice Rivers, the head nurse for most of the bizarre Tuskegee Syphilis Experiment. Conducted secretly from 1932 until 1972, it was a giant stain on the records of a succession of Surgeon Generals, both Democratic and Republican. In this program, 399 African-American males in one of the poorest counties in Alabama were deliberately *infected* with syphilis. Furthermore, they were systematically deceived into believing that they were receiving free medical treatment, all in the interest of so-called medical science. Heartless government physicians simply continued with business as usual documenting the ravages of the disease.

That was not too long ago. Many of us physicians in practice today were well along in our schooling when a voice crying in the wilderness blew the whistle on this crime. No one was ever convicted. As woman at that time, Nurse Rivers' was both a victim and co-conspirator, claiming that she was trained not to question doctors and was *just follow orders.*

Looking at these events in the historical perspective provides a reliable guide for effective action. Following World War II, Mahatma Gandhi, taught the modern world what could be accomplished with fasting. His single-minded resistance brought the British Empire to its knees. Dr. Martin Luther King traveled to the subcontinent to adopt Gandhi's tactics of self-sacrifice. His approach of redemptive suffering and noble African-American leadership bore much fruit during the civil rights era. That was a time when people of

> *No, people don't expect govern-ment to solve all their problems. But they sense, that with just a slight change in priorities, we can make sure that every child in America has a decent shot at life.*
> Barack Obama

conscience from all races placed their bodies on the line for causes they believed in. Today, such self-denial is passé. Our people who have made it just do not seem to care. They do not want to be inconvenienced. Pie-in-the-sky churches preach unearned blessings and magical cures rather than prayerfully organizing to deliver those held captive by preventable diseases. Sadly, the majority of our own health care professionals are carrying on with business as usual. The Tuskegee mindset still rules: implementing directives from above, more committed to turning a dollar rather than interceding for the most needy.

Active Public Policy

Fast food giants serve as the kitchens for the poor. Profits, not nutrition, are their primary focus. They typically respond to negative press rather than social conscience. Wendy's stock fell following the heart attack of its founder Dave Thomas in 1996. Thereafter they began pushing healthier choices in a bid to keep up with Subway which had overtaken its second place position in the fast-food race. McDonalds CEO Jim Cantalupo also succumbed to a heart attack at age 60 in 2004. Concerned about its role in the obesity epidemic, the company afterward became more proactive by promoting adult Happy Meals featuring salad, bottled water and a pedometer. Government is finally pressuring the restaurant industry to stop peddling trans fats to the unsuspecting public.

Once again, comparison to nicotine addiction is instructive. Within a year of New York City imposing tobacco control strategy (involving taxation, workplace smoking ban, and smoking cessation assistance,) prevalence of smoking decreased sharply by 11 percent. At first there was a whole lot of whining and complaining, but in the end, the 140,000 ex-smokers were appreciative that the city had taken bold action to help them quit. It is indeed heartening to see an increasing number of municipalities and states standing up and making that bold move.

Massive weight control is a personal triumph for the individual. Studies show this reduces patients' overall medication costs by over 90 percent which translates into substantial cost savings for third party payers, health plans and society as a whole. More importantly, patients transition from dependence and heavy healthcare utilization to being productive members of society. Resources invested in changing

> *The ultimate measure of a man, is not where he stands in moments of comfort and convenience, but where he stands at times of challenge and controversy.*
> Rev. Dr. Martin Luther King

behavior therefore saves a whole lot more than our preoccupation with expensive medicines and grand hospitals filled with high-tech equipment. Government must consider using proactive fiscal policies to discourage high-calorie, low-nutrient fattening foods and use the proceeds to subsidize the cost of health-promoting fruits and vegetables

Specific Goals

The Old Testament describes Zechariah's vision of a valley of dry bones coming to life. Nehemiah had to organize the people to build up the defensive walls of Jerusalem. I see modern day versions of this renaissance with role models like Ohio's Health Director, Dr. Alvin Jackson. While at Fremont's Community Health Services, he was featured in publications like *USA Today* as being in the forefront of advancing health initiatives for migrant workers and its mobile clinic response to Hurricane Katrina. State funds were obtained for faith-based minority health programs. Al and his wife Gail invest their time and treasure leading at-risk youth on college tours. I can think of attorneys who are not just interested in holding their troubled minority clients ransom for their fees. Instead they take the time to encourage these youth to read a good book or steer them to some program whereby they can better themselves. Such mentorship provides examples to all of us who are committed to reversing these disturbing trends.

Minorities are disappointed when popular vanity diets do not work for them. With names like "South Beach," and "Scarsdale," (Chapter 12) what else should one expect? These diet do not cater to people who make do with chitlins instead of caviar or tamales instead of tofu. We must instead build on our faith traditions to fuel our resolve to be strong and fit through disciplined exercise and eating more *itals:* naturally nutritious foods.

Let us now step outside our comfort zone and examine some very basic goals for the next 5 years. We can do this:

1. Reduce Obesity rate by 10 percent. Weigh everyone in every class, in every church, every year. Protect their confidentiality. Calculate the average and use it to monitor and compete with peer groups. Recognize parent fitness awards at basketball games

> *I would unite with anybody to do right and with nobody to do wrong.*
>
> Frederick Douglass
>
> Abolitionist

2. Increase high school and college graduation rate by 10 percent.

3. Reduce dialysis rate by 10 percent.

4. Foster a culture of self-respect and hard work.

5. Before the Internet, mobile libraries made an impact in helping combat illiteracy. Based on Montel Williams successful bus distribution, *Partnership for Prescription Assistance,* let us do the same thing for fruits and vegetables. We must think outside the box and come up with creative strategies to get healthier foods into isolated in urban food deserts. The goal is preventive. A healthier population will have less need for drugs.

Let this be the ministry of churches, organizations and individuals who have been blessed. According to an Arab proverb, "If the mountain will not come to Mohammed, Mohammed must come to the mountain."

14. Health Freedom Ring

If the people are not coming for their health checks, let us bring health checks to the people. We must seize control of our health as a powerful instrument of economic liberation and empowerment in a pluralistic society. The civil rights agenda must now move from equal access to the voting booth to equal access to treatment plans, health clubs and walking trails. Each of us has a job to do, beginning with ourselves. The time has come to reject the historic role thrust upon us by society; that of merely being sports performers and court jesters, a group always pleading for government assistance, the bottom of the totem pole, the caboose in the train of human development.

The next Tuskegee Experiment or Katrina Disaster is likely to be more insidious and widespread. We stand on the shoulders of giants before us like the Frederick Douglass, Harriet Tubman, Sojourner Truth, Malcolm X and Martin Luther King. Their blood, sweat, tears and Mosaic sacrifices have granted us the position as Joshuas to bring the dream to full fruition. Past struggles were against historical prejudices, powers and principalities. Today's struggle is primarily against our own social disintegration and self-care complacency. If our health indices continue to deteriorate on my watch, in areas under my sphere of influence, let it never be said that it was because I did not speak up or mobilize. Wouldn't it break Dr. King's heart to see how African-Americans have turned the opportunities of the 'promised land' into being *among the fattest people in the world?*

Perhaps you have wondered what role you would have played in historic crises like the persecution of the early church, slavery, the Salem Witch Hunt Trials, the Holocaust, the Civil Rights and African famine. While the obesity epidemic may not be as dramatic, it makes similar demands on all our consciences, regardless of race. As you complete your *Mannameter Lifescore* today, think of ways in which we can move from the politics of protest to the power of pride and example.

Women need to communicate to their hard-working, sports-possessed men they ain't that tough if they do not stick around to enjoy the fruits of retirement. Men need to assure women that they are loved more for their charm and vitality rather than for glamorously inconvenient hairstyles. Our country's best years are ahead. Indeed, it is only as pull ourselves up by out own bootstraps that we can truly join in that lofty chorus:

America! America! God shed His grace on thee,
And crown thy good with brotherhood, from sea to shining sea!

217

REVIEW

1   How is obesity related to socioeconomic class in America?

2. Describe the relationship between hair care and fitness.

3. How can lessons from smoking cessation efforts be applied to the battle against obesity?

4. Why is obesity considered a new form of bondage?

5. What steps can population groups take to secure their own health freedom?

Chapter 15

Keeping It Real

*God-centered thinking does not deny the reality of our
present situation, but it does put our troubles into perspective.*
Richard Exley

D ashing through the wintry mix seemed enough of a work-out
for Phyllis. Chased by the biting cold and out of breath, she
trailed Jessica across the health club parking lot. That handicap
spot was looking even better now. After all, which challenged individual
would want to be out in such weather?

Freeze that scene for a second. It is moments like these that
flutter the fragile flame of motivation. All the government statistical
reports and lofty recommendations of talking-head scientific experts
do little to energize it. Close observation of the nitty-gritty of daily life
reveals that grim fanaticism in the end fuels bad outcomes. It takes a
charming joie-de-vive to somehow overcome and delivers personal
triumphs. Just watch:

The friends pulled at the stiff door and stomped off the slush
unto the mats. The warm indoor atmosphere embraced them. For one
woman, the whiff of chlorine blended with that fragrance of fresh linen,
furnished images of fun and fitness. For the other, it conjured odors of
sticky sweat and senselessly sore muscles. They were "best buds," but
on some things they were miles apart. A couple of those "fitness freaks"
held the inner door for them. Everyday folks they were, in all shapes and
sizes, enthusiastically wishing them a good work out. They must have
come in before dawn. Already they were heading off to their appointed
tasks with that purposeful and energized look on their faces.

"Are you kidding?!" Phyllis mumbled beneath her breath,
wishing she could be snug-as-a-bug under her comforter. "They must

be on something..." There was no way she could look that awake so early in the morning unless she was on her second cup of cappuccino. After losing only 55 pounds following gastric bypass, Phyllis had started regaining. Others had such great results. If anything had to go wrong, she lamented, sure enough, it would have to be me.

Working it out

At one time Phyllis felt like the cat's meow, the fortunate recipient of the latest and best technology medical science had to offer. Reflecting on the process, she felt that once her insurance was approved, she was rushed to the operating room before having a chance to think things over. Mad at the world, she found herself snapping at everyone - including that so-called friend Jessica, dragging her out here on a day like this. She finally had to admit to herself that this was perhaps the major motivation to consider surgery: She did not want people to ever badger her again about exercising. Now here she was, right back to where she started - almost.

"Good to see you again Jess!" Chirped the receptionist as Jessica swiped her membership card into the registration console. "And the name of your guest is..."

"That's Phyllis, Phyllis Farrington," she responded, visibly shivering as she signed in on the clipboard. The receptionist presented two sets of fluffy towels from the warmer, crowning them with keys to the women's locker room.

"Cold out, huh?"

"Tell me about it." Phyllis mumbled, still tightly clutching her coat around her. Jessica offered to take her gloves and clasped her friend's hands tenderly between the toasty towels. That felt so good! Eyes gently shut; Phyllis smiled blissfully as she cradled the warm linen between her neck and shoulder.

Her reverie was way too short. As the automatic doors ushered them into the main corridor of the airy gym, Phyllis was regretting her decision even more. She hated crowds. At least, she was relieved by how much the initial buzz of activity seemed to have so quickly subsided. Maybe she would not have to deal with all those people staring at her cellulite after all. Well aware of her friend's mood, Jessica tried keeping up a lively chatter by proudly pointing out the various amenities added in recent months.

But they did not quite have the locker room all to themselves. As they changed, a svelte specimen of humanity sashayed from the shower.

15. **Keeping It Real**

Seemingly oblivious of their presence, the woman strutted across the room and alighted on the mats in front of the full-length mirror. Like some mythical nymph, she admired herself in different poses. She seemed to be about their age, yet everything looked so firm, so toned. Tossing her head, she mopped the rivulets cascading from her hair. The two friends just stared at each other. Jessica just knew what Phyllis would be thinking. Think fast, say something clever, she thought.

"I guess she never had to deal with this." Phyllis teased, grabbing her own love handles for effect. She was not sure that came out right. In any case, the hair-dryer seemed to offer some kind of cover as she made faces in the direction of the *hard body* preening over there.

No luck.

"I-don't-think-so!" Phyllis shot back, emphasizing her point by doing that little head thing. She peered self-consciously from behind the locker door then repeatedly poked her friend in the chest with a stiff index finger. "That's-why-I-hate-these-places!" She hissed.

"Can't compare yourself with her," Jessica argued. "Come on now, I bet she never had kids."

"So?!...She's a natural, but she doesn't have to flaunt it like that."

"Flaunt it?" Whispered Jessica, "She was so into herself, I don't think she even noticed us."

"She did too. Didn't you see her wave - as you were grabbing yourself?"

"Nooo!" Jess covered her mouth in dismay. "Gosh! I'm so embarrassed."

"Chill girl," cooed Phyllis, "I bet half of the people come in here just to show off; y'know, the meat market thing…"

Now Jessica too, was having second thoughts about the morning. This chick was giving her a complex. Yet she took solace in the fact that her friend seemed to be loosening up some, even though at her expense. She also knew that behind the grumpiness was a wild streak a mile wide just waiting to come out. Given half a chance, Phyllis would find some way to have her laughing her head off in a heartbeat.

They ventured uneasily into the heart of the gym. Jessica took a businesslike sip from her water bottle and set it down along with the towel next to the exercise bike. "I had this trainer…"

"What trainer?"

"He told me five minutes of warm-ups every time." Jessica continued, pushing against the wall, stretching out those calf muscles.

221

"Is that the Leon you were talking about?" Her friend's face lit up as she mirrored some basic stretches before also hopping onto the stationary bike. "Is he going to be here today?"

"I don't know. He sometimes comes around to offer some advice and maybe sign up private clients."

"You said he was ripped, right?"

"Did I say that? Well anyway, it's time for *us* to get ripped."

CNN's *Robin & Company* was on the television facing the array of exercise equipment. The news anchor was interviewing some young Hollywood hunk.

"I think she's hitting on him! Can you believe that?!" Phyllis remarked as they pedaled away.

"Oh, she is just being herself. The guys love it. They just can't seem to get over her electric smile."

"Yeah, I remember when they used to say I had an electric smile. Those were the days, my friend."

"Actually, I remember overhearing the guys in college describing it as dazzling. Phyllis was always the girl with the dazzling smile." Her friend blushed. "And you still got it, girl!" Jessica added.

"Hey, I'm trying. But look at me now."

Things were warming up, alright. Jessica checked to see whether her pulse was in the target zone before moving on with her circuit training routine. She heaved a 20-pound weight onto the leg-curls machine. Jessica gracefully mounted the bench on her tummy and shimmied into position so that the padded bars were situated just above the back of her ankles. Gripping the handles, she pressed her pelvis down as she hoisted the weights with her muscular legs. It felt good that she still had a lot of power from her days of high school volleyball. Between deep breaths she mentioned to Phyllis that she was concentrating on her hamstrings in this session.

"Hamstrings? Y'know, that word, it makes me think of different kind of cuts, like tenderloins, rump roast, fillet mignon…how about you?"

"Oh, you silly goose! Focus, girl. How about your upper body? Why don't you start there?"

"Okay, slave-driver; I should use the butterfly machine for that, right?"

"Yup. Go for it!"

Phyllis sat upright on the bench, her arms horizontal, bent upward at the elbow. She pushed inwards on the padded armrests as the weights on the pulley drew them apart. Jessica was observing her, offering a suggestion here and there. She did look a little klutzy getting started, but once she got accustomed to the equipment, it did not seem that bad. Actually, Phyllis seemed to be whispering some little rhyme under her breath. Nice, Jessica thought, she's getting into it. She paused and listened intently to pick up the lyrics.

"I must, I must - I must increase my bust." Phyllis sang in rhythm with the machine, her forearms ending up in front of her face.

"Girl, I haven't heard that song since high school!"

"Ha! How could anybody forget! You know I need all the help I can get."

"Yeah, didn't you say you were going to get one of those silicone jobbies?"

"Don't remind me, Jes. The only time I had anything there was when I was pregnant. But my husband won't even hear of it."

"I have to agree with Fred on that one. I wish I could transplant some of mine to you. You know, guys never look me in the face first. All that is for them is eye candy. They don't care how much it hurts my back and how the straps cut into my shoulders. Believe me, Fifi, You're okay. You just have to get toned."

"You know what? You may have a point. I can feel it in my pecs!"

"Actually that's a real good exercise for exactly what you guys're talking about." Boomed a deep, rich voice. For the second time that morning, the ladies were caught off guard. It was Leon – and he almost seemed embarrassed at his own comment. He quickly excused himself, apologizing for interrupting the girl-talk. Phyllis eagerly started asking about some training tips, but succeeded only in fumbling her words. By the time she had dabbed the sweat from her face, the door had shut behind him.

"Girl, you should see yourself!" Jessica giggled, "You reminded me of when the kids first laid eyes on Micky for real at Disney World."

"Hmm, hmm, hmm! He looked fine, let me tell you! You've been holding out on me, girlfriend!"

"Me?! Holding out? Look, Leon's real nice to everybody; a little bit of a charmer if you ask me."

"Well, you know what they say – looking at the menu, doesn't mean you have to place an order!"

They erupted in convulsions of mischievous laughter.

"So what lucky client you think he's meeting with now?"

"*Mrs.* Farrington!" Jessica interrupted in mock exasperation. "Come on now. Let's get back to the basics for today…"

Manna*fast* Miracle

Breakthrough

Phyllis' routine after running the kids to school was to whip up a couple of scrambled eggs. She would have that with a pop tart or waffles and linger with some hot chocolate. But today she found herself settling for whole grain cereal in soy milk, a slice of cantaloupe and a tall glass of orange juice. Refreshed after her shower, she reclined in the La-Z-Boy, rehearsing in her mind how interesting and different the morning had turned out. Before tackling her chores, her thoughts fast-forwarded to the afternoon when Fred would return from work. He would head straight for this same chair. Grabbing a beer, he would switch to the sports channel and settle in till dinner. During that time he'd ask her to fetch him a couple more cold ones. He knew her standard answer, "Pour you own poison." He would grumble, but she drew the line. If anything came up with the kids during that time, his final answer was always, "Go ask your mother."

She loved teasing Jessica, letting her think that Leon was the main attraction. She was always committed to her family and now really committed to her health. A month had passed and Phyllis was feeling better than she had in years. Ten times better, it seemed, than those giddy months following her surgery when the pounds seemed to just fall away without effort. For the first time, she was being honest with herself about exactly what she ate. Later, they agreed to meet with a group of like-minded people committed to taking their health in their own hands. That, more than anything else, seemed to confirm her new attitude. Now, even Fred seemed to appreciate that.

> *When the pain of change is less than the pain of remaining the same, then change will come.*
>
> Anon

Mastery over Food

This is a character trait which favors no race, gender or IQ. My own appreciation of that fact evolved during my years of surgery training program at St. Barnabas Medical Center in New Jersey. We were fortunate to have a Chief of Surgery who had spent some of his best years in leadership at Charity Hospital in New Orleans. As a special "Fat Tuesday" treat, Dr. Nance would fly in the choicest Cajun cuisine for his Residents. Gumbo, Jambalaya, crawfish - the works! We even heard of the legend of how these were once lobsters that followed the French

15. Keeping It Real

Acadians (Cajuns) forced out of Nova Scotia by the British. Following the crustacean's long walk overland, they shrunk in size and were celebrated as crawfish on their arrival to the Bayou on the Gulf coast.

No other young docs were lavished such attention. It is important to understand the context. We would frequently a meal or two during emergencies or when tied up on long cases in the operating room. Having to eat hospital food for days on end somehow stirred deep craving for pizza or Chinese food. So when pharmaceutical sales 'reps' showed up to 'sponsor' our 4 PM Chiefs rounds, residents were ravenous. Once we had our fill, the rep would pitch their goods. Like icing on the cake, they would leave generous amounts of free stuff such as pens, golf balls, post-it note pads, Broadway tickets and designer confections, all sporting the drug name or company logo.

That is why Trent impressed me so much. A bearded, plain-spoken guy from rural Pennsylvania, few would confuse with some heartthrob from the silver screen. The dude never cared much to indulge in the feeding frenzy. He would partake at the end, maybe. While the rep had the rest of us literally eating out of his hands, Trent would sit confidently on a desk at the back and unleash a barrage of difficult questions. What were the side effects of this medication? How valid was the research to back up its claims? What were the cheaper alternatives?

Anyone of us could have raised these issues if we were not otherwise engaged. Some perhaps thought him a tad rude for boldly challenging our guests or just plain stupid for not digging in before it was all gone. Or maybe he was just trying to be different. Throughout those grueling years, Trent set a towering example of dignity and self-control which few have matched. Way back in Genesis 25:29-34, Esau traded his birthright for a pot of stew. Regardless of station in life, history is replete with the stories of people habitually swapping their well-being for the dictates of their bellies.

Studies show that up to 90 percent of traditional dieters regain it all within 2 years, and then some. These numbers can be discouraging. However, studies of the ten percent who do maintain reveal some very consistent characteristics. After reaching their desired weight those who adopt a Mannafast lifestyle seldom allow it to fluctuate more than ten pounds in any given year. They simply refuse to let it happen. They track their monthly progress on the Weight Maintenance graph (page 231) and

Manna*fast* Miracle

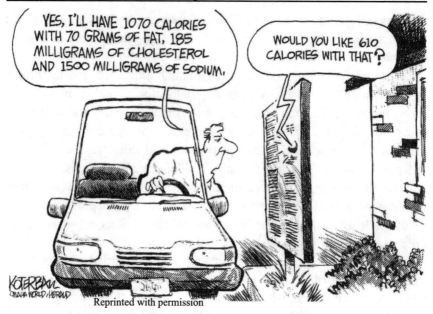

Reprinted with permission

we are really on a roll. We are all subject to the common snare of food addictions even after making a spectacular start with our gastric conditioning? Dough, distraction, disagreement, disease and disaster are *the five D's* just waiting to trip us up into relapsing. We are all vulnerable in some way, shape or form. It is only as we acknowledge that can we take the necessary precautions to finish strong!

Dough

Money is a factor in any human activity - even for the air we breathe. Technically, it is free. Yet we know that the respiratory systems of many susceptible people are daily pummeled by pollen and pollution. They would benefit from special filters or moving to an environment with cleaner air. Unfortunately, large swaths of the population do not have the funds or the skills to relocate, even if they wanted to.

Fitness is likewise *affected* by finances, but not dictated by it. How often do you hear folks excuse their weight on not being able to afford a health club membership, fancy home exercise equipment, nutritional supplements, a diet counselor, fitness trainer, even surgery? Properly utilized, these can all make a difference. However, none are essential. The minute you find yourself blaming finances, stop. We can improvise. We can substitute. Where there is a will, there is always a way. What matters is

226

desire, the willingness to make the effort. Either you have it in you or you do not. Mannafast is all about how to acquire that desire, how to nurture and maintain it indefinitely. Associate with believers who value their bodies as *temples* of the living God. If you cannot find a Covenant Group (Chapter 20) in your area, start one!

Distraction

There is no debate about the anguish and confusion resulting from the loss of a loved one or the loss of a job. But positive events can also throw us off track just as thoroughly as negative ones. The common denominator is that the predictable routine of life is turned upside down. From the championships, (whether high school, college or professional) to the final episode of the top-rated sitcom, there are times when it seems that everyone is caught up in that one monster television event. Austrian psychologist Dr. Hans Seyle's research on this topic earned him the title of "Father of Stress." While weddings, vacations, hosting the holiday dinner are by no means bad things, they can certainly be disruptive. Georgia's "Runaway Bride" was a rather dramatic illustration.

Then, consider Marcia. She did not make national headlines, but her experience equally exemplifies the obligations which all of us must one day face in life. Marcia had lost a remarkable sixty pounds on the Mannafast program and had truly turned her life around. At that point her mother took ill and was transferred to the intensive care unit at the Medical University of Ohio in Toledo. Marcia's father had passed a couple years before. Her three brothers visited only occasionally and contributed little support, if any. As her mother got weaker, Marcia would pack the kids off to school and dutifully rush off on the ninety minute trip to the hospital. She would hurry back to pick the kids up from school. Exercise? Forget it! She reverted to being a fast food junkie during that hectic schedule as her mother agonizingly lingered another three months.

There were all the arrangements and estate matters that fell on her shoulders. When we saw Marcia about seven months later she looked like she had been through the wringer. She appeared withdrawn and bloated. The verdict rendered by the scale was that she had in fact regained most of the weight. Having comforted others, Marcia was receptive to consolation and encouragement. She ploughed right back into the program losing seventy-five pounds. This was about her long term goal to begin with. *Eight years* later, Marcia, continues to defy statistics. Distraction in the form of heartfelt grief had come mightily against her. Yet, like an increasing number of others, she continues to faithfully persevere. It amazes me to this day how well she continues to do.

> *Now faith is the substance of things hoped for, the evidence of things not seen.*
>
> Hebrews 11:1

Disagreement

Greg's mounting DUI's had not only sunk his marriage but even earned him a couple stays in the slammer. Through AA, he finally cleaned up his act and had been sober for a commendable seven years. One day his boss, in his words, began "riding" him for no apparent reason. He really needed the job and dared not talk back. On his way from work he passed the drinking establishment where he used to "split hell right open." He hesitated. Just one little drink, he told himself, just a little pick-me-up. He went in. It was not long before he was on that proverbial slippery slope back into his old ways. His father had died of cirrhosis of the liver, a condition with jaundice as one of its late symptoms. It was not until a co-worker told Greg that his eyes looked yellow that he panicked enough to make an urgent office appointment.

Addictive behavior to alcohol has striking similarities to eating disorders. For some people, all it takes is being upset by something which may seem trivial to others. After losing thirty pounds, this young housewife was on a roll. She kept her office appointments secret because of her husband's complaints that she was just wasting money. This time he noticed something different. Brenda was getting compliments from both men and women. Whatever was going on was a threat to his sedentary lifestyle. With tears in her eyes, Brenda reported how he started bringing home a dozen donuts and just placing the box on the kitchen counter. This was sabotage - on a

> *Be confident of this one thing, that He who has begun a good work in you will carry it on to completion.*
>
> Phil 1:6

grand scale! She resented that, but out of love for her husband, she quietly submitted to sharing in his donut attack. Many are too ashamed to get help. This is the kind of disagreement about priorities in a family which does not show up in raw statistics of "diet failures." Multiplied boxes later, there she was in my office, an emotional wreck. She eventually did well after strengthening her with specific coping strategies.

It is evident that people do not begin regaining weight because they somehow forget basic weight management principles. They regain weight because they lose focus. When something goes wrong they regress into the "oh-what-the-hell mode." Even the most tranquil of homes or workplaces will have its disagreements. Be vigilant not to allow a falling out with anyone become an opening for the pounds to pile back on.

Disease

Just as the fitness program is shifting into high gear, an old ankle sprain can start acting up again. Now, even climbing stairs is a chore. Your joints can predict changes in the weather before the meteorologist forecast. Illness is enough to throw many dieters off track. Hospitalization, unexpected health challenges like the passing flu or an occasional tumble tends to disrupt our fitness plans. Setbacks precipitate fatigue and frustration. Even after we recover physically, our fleshly nature still seeks pampering with a "poor me" attitude. Be mindful of what tripped you up in the past. After a reasonable period of rest and recuperation, get ready to rumble back into your wellness program.

Disaster

Do you remember where you were when the news broke? My first operation for the day had been postponed. The patient was not ready for surgery even though we had gone over the preparations over and over. Now the entire schedule had to be adjusted, a sour note that threatened to color my whole day. After tying up a few odds and ends at home, I was finally about to leave for the office. My hand was on the door to the garage when the phone rang. Should I answer it? After all, if it was anything important they would know how to reach me.

I walked back and glanced at the caller ID. It was my office. "Doctor. Put on the TV!" My receptionist blurted out. What's up with that, I thought; no greeting or anything. I was just short of irritated.

"Quick!" She added, "The TV. Just put it on!" I sensed mounting tension in her voice. I rested the phone on the counter and trudged over to the remote control. Though striving to maintain a surgeon's calm in a crisis, my attitude was more like, "This better be good. This day just is not going well."

The screen flickered to life. The image that flashed before my eyes appeared like twin chimney stacks of some giant ocean liner at full steam - except the background was that unmistakable skyline. No question, those were the twin towers! June and I had taken the kids to the observation deck of the World Trade Center just five years before - almost to the day! I listened with horror to the estimated number of people trapped above where the planes hit. What kind of day were they having? Just then, June rushed in from taking the kids to school, She too was shaken by what she was hearing on the radio.

I had completely forgotten to hang up the receiver. My receptionist had to page me asking if they could go home to get a television. Sure. June and I remained glued to the screen. Breaking news was coming in that a jet had crashed into the Pentagon. Then it was reported (wrongly) that the State Department may have also been hit and another might have gone down in Pennsylvania. Skyscrapers and large government offices across the nation were being evacuated. Multitudes were fleeing Manhattan. Giant clouds of smoke engulfed Gotham City like some surreal grade B Godzilla movie. Phones were jammed. I could not reach my siblings working in New York City or Washington DC. We were clearly under attack. As rumors swirled about a plane heading for the White House, I scrambled into my Army Reserve uniform and called my Combat Support Hospital unit.

The days that followed blurred into each other. The entire nation emerged from the gloom of collective grief and erupted into a frenzy of fervent patriotism. Apart from the disruptions reverberating throughout the economy, everyone not directly involved in rescue or relief seemed to be moving slower, unsure of the changes to come. That was a catastrophe like none other in our lifetime. Unless shaken out of the funk, news addicts like me could listen for updates on the half-hour on various radio stations, TV channels and websites along with binges of reading every newspaper and magazine editorial within reach. Naturally, other aspects of life suffer. As it turns out, spectacular events can be used as an excuse, a cop out.

This is not limited to so-called acts of God such as a hurricane, earthquake, tsunami, forest fire or a man-made holocaust like September 11th. Each family is guaranteed its own private disaster or loss. Accidents, sudden illness or a relative in a pickle can wrench us away from cherished plans and carefully scripted timetables. Man proposes, it is said, and God disposes. Faith strengthens us emotionally to deal with the insidious depression devolving from disaster. *When duty calls or danger, be never be never lacking there.* Personal transformation plans like weight control can quickly get lost in the shuffle. More often, even positive things such

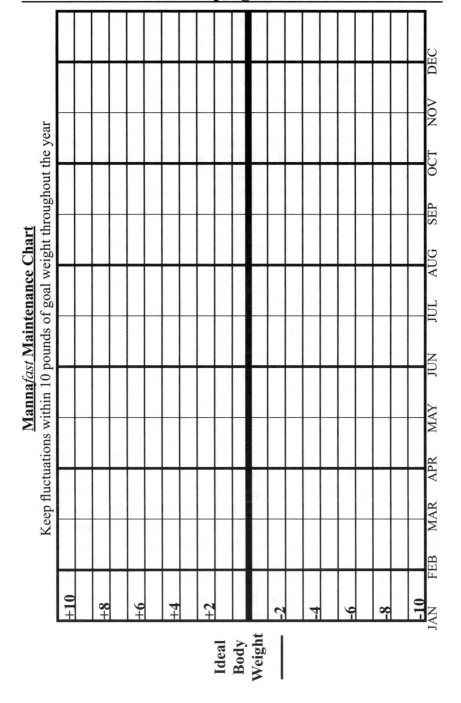

Manna*fast* **Maintenance Chart**

Keep fluctuations within 10 pounds of goal weight throughout the year

as returning from vacation to find a backlog of "to do's" that finally derails our sincerest resolutions. We must make the commitment that come what may, we will make time to fulfill our duty to ourselves and others. It is only by sealing the deal *beforehand* can we insulate ourselves from falling victim to inevitable circumstances beyond our control.

Ironclad Maintenance

The story is told of a devout believer trapped in a tree by rising flood waters. Her neighbors rowed by in a rubber dinghy offering to take her to dry ground. She refused. That boat looked too insecure. A Coast Guard rescuer descended from a helicopter, but she fended him off. No way was she going up in that noisy, shaky thing. God would save her. But the waters rose and washed her away.

At the Pearly Gates, she complained to St. Peter, why did God not save her? "God tried to rescue you by boat, but you refused," replied St. Peter. "The Good Lord tried to rescue you by air, but you turned that down too. There is only so much God can do."

In hindsight, Phyllis' original weight problem stemmed largely from real disagreements with her husband. She was not unhappy enough to abandon her marriage, but neither was the situation one conducive to thriving. Confused and devoid of direction, she pouted and pined, growing plumper and plumper. However, God sent Jessica into her life. Once she latched on to that lifeline, she was able to draw on her friend's strength to overcome. When in a downward spiral, be on the lookout for help outside of yourself. God always provides a way of escape (I Corinthians 10:13).

There is absolutely no valid reason why the average non-pregnant, otherwise healthy adult cannot maintain their healthy weight well within 10 pounds during any given year. Start charting your monthly weight changes on the preceding page. If it even looks like it getting out of line - *"Ding, ding, ding!"* That's a sure signal to bring out the big guns loaded in Chapters 5 and 10. Heed this early warning system and you will never have to consider obesity surgery, I can guarantee you that. Anytime one loses his way, it always because of one of the broad categories discussed above. Respect yourself. Seize this opportunity. Deal promptly with any of those Five D's threatening your success and you'll have it made!

Forget the former things; do not dwell on the past.

See, I am doing a new thing! I will give you a new heart.

Isaiah 43:18,19

15. **Keeping It Real**

REVIEW

1. Describe the positive or negative feelings individuals experience in a health club setting.

2. What is the maximum weight fluctuation that a healthy, non-pregnant adult should allow during the course of a year?

3. Describe a particular episode or time in your life when you showed the most mastery over food.

4. In your experience, is weight gain more gradual and steady or is it more often a slippery slope involving giving up?

5. Which of the 5 D's has been more of a problem in your efforts to stay healthy?

VQ Assessment #4

31. **Nuts**   Rich in vitamins, controls diabetes. Lowers cholesterol.
_____   Cardioprotective, adds 3 years to lifespan.

32. **Oats**   Great breakfast source of complex carbohydrates. Fights
_____   cholesterol, cancer and constipation. Smoothes skin.

33. **Okra**   Common in Southern and Caribbean cooking. High in
Calc. B6, and folic acid ~ neural tube defects in fetuses.

34. **Parsley**   Diuretic as a tea. Rubbed on skin for mosquito bites.
_____   Prevent pregnancy? Can cause oxalate kidney stones.

35. **Passion fruit** High in fiber and vitamins. Relieves headaches,
_____   muscle tension, hypertension, anxiety and insomnia.

36. **Peas**   High in protein, iron, and vitamins. Regulates bowels.
_____   cholesterol. Balances blood sugar. Reduces cancer risk.

37. **Peaches**   High in lycopene, lutein, potassium and flavonoids.
_____   heart disease, strokes macular degeneration and cancer.

38. **Pineapple**   Rich in *bromelain*. Effective for carpal tunnel,
_____   inflammation, warts and bronchitis. Anti-cancer.

39. **Pumpkin**   More than just for pies. Promotes youthful, healthy skin.
_____   Pumpkin seeds lowers prostate & lung cancer risk.

40. **Prunes**   vitamins, potassium and copper. Treats constipation.
_____   Relieves diabetes, heart disease, arthritis & colon cancer.

+ _____ % **TOTAL VQ**   (Final VQ on page 250)

Chapter 16

Fluid and Figure

If you look at what you have in life, you'll always have more.
If you look at what you don't have in life, you'll never have enough.

Oprah

Her husband was finally discharged from the hospital. The cardiologist made it very clear: no intimate relations for at least two weeks. Such activity could risk a second and possibly fatal heart attack. Not wanting to take any chances, he decided to sleep downstairs on the couch. However, after nearly a week, he could stand it no longer. Waking from a restless sleep and throwing caution to the winds, he marched upstairs towards the bedroom. He almost jumped out of his skin as he bumped into someone creeping down the stairs.

"Where are you going?!" She exclaimed, trying to regain her composure, "You forgot the doctor's orders?"

"Well Hon'," he replied defiantly, "I've decided that if I'm going to die, I'm going to die happy…"

"Oh man!" She beamed. "Don't we think alike or what…I couldn't help myself either. I was just coming downstairs to *kill* you!"

Size and Sexuality

The gentler sex has special biological attributes. This chapter examines the importance of self-esteem and love in a woman's health. And that is not only in the romantic sense. There seems to be a greater need to give her heart to someone or something, not only to a guy, but also a galpal, pet, plant, pastime, career, even sacred vows. Those gender differences sometimes hamper weight control efforts, but not if we focus on how they can help.

In an age of blasé openness about sexuality, women of faith struggle to find the balance between purity and passion. While having made great strides in all fields of endeavor; certain constant themes contribute to that feminine mystique. Many women feel they were at the back of

235

the line when the good Lord was bestowing attractiveness. Nature may appear cruel at times, but do not despair. Mona Lisa's exquisite looks and Beyonce's fabulous "bod" is by no means the be all and end all.

If the tabloids tell us anything, it is that the fame and fortune immunizes no one from the trials of life. Diana may have been the fairytale princess, but as the details of her life began to surface, a lot fewer women were eager to trade places with her. No matter how hard it is to accept, at the basic level, the world's sexiest women can experience only as much joy as the girl next door. To fully digest that is to learn to cherish the love in one's life. In fact, *true contentment depends much more on what one does with what they were given.* Regardless of appearance, constantly remind yourself that you are special, you are unique and you deserve to be just as happy as the next person.

But I'm Fat

Spiritual maturity empowers us to make the tough choices that create our own destiny. The 31st chapter of the *Book of Proverbs* extols the industrious characteristics of the virtuous woman. But as the specter of the obesity epidemic sweeps the land, millions of women find their good stuff stifled under increasingly thicker layers of insulation. How often have we heard, "She's not bad-looking, but she sure is a big girl!"

> *His banner the over me is love.*
> *Strengthen me with raisins,*
> *Refresh me with apples,*
> *for I am faint with love.*
> *His left arm is under my head,*
> *His right arm embraces me...*
>
> Song of Solomon 2: 4-6

The Proverbs' woman excels in social skills, exhibiting admirable nesting instincts and domestic management. This woman of faith is a hard worker. Without her, the average church today simply could not function. *Song of Solomon* expresses in no uncertain terms that it is okay to enjoy the finer things of life, paying attention to one's figure, and savoring the physical delights in the proper context. By extension, it validates that feminine yearning for flowers, candlelight dinners and having doors open for her.

John Gray puts it this way, *Men are from Mars, Women are from Venus.* It speaks to the fact that females tend to be more relational, verbal and sensitive; men, more direct and action-oriented. And these differences begin to show up in puberty with girls showing more pronounced bodily changes than boys. This is associated with a higher incidence of eating disorders. Females are challenged with weight in a way that males never will. Pre-menstrual fluid retention, hormonal changes from birth control, pregnancy, possible hysterectomy, and eventual menopause can all be associated with unintended weight gain.

When we look at weight in the historical and global perspective, we observe that during the Renaissance period, the classical artists depicted the most desirable women as full-figured and voluptuous. Twiggy, the 95-pound British model, broke unto the international stage in the 1960's. It was not until then that it began to be "in" to be thin. But on the other side of the world, in areas yet beyond the reach of total western cultural penetration, the heavier-set woman still rules. In those environments, having a frail Alle McBeal type frame could scare locals into thinking

> *Switzerland has the highest consumption of chocolate in the world: 26 lb 6 oz per person year*

famine was around the corner. Instead, leading ladies in these matriarchal societies are the ones endowed with powerful hips and full curves. Such features are suggestive of a robust lioness, capable of fending for her household.

While parents in the West are preoccupied with their daughters' further education, girls surviving gendercide in these cultures are made to double, even triple their weight to secure early marriage. No professor or doctor gives them the formula on how to get fat. They are simply sent off to special "academies" where they are force-fed huge amounts of *high fat foods* and *forbidden from engaging in physical exertion.* As young as age eight, they are fattened like geese. They are compelled to guzzle scarce gallons of whole milk, never mind some even suffocate in the process.

Compared to others on the planet, the modern Western woman does not fully appreciate how lucky she is. While she obsesses till the last moment about taking in on her wedding dress, brides of the Hima tribe, for example, are fattened up for the big day. This particular custom has nothing to do with being strong and invincible. Instead, being barely able to waddle "down the aisle" is considered the height of attractiveness. These brides spend their honeymoons eating and sleeping. "Busting out all over" projects irresistible sex appeal to the men of her village.

In the final analysis, in areas where the threat of hunger is an ever present issue, the plus-sized lady connotes privilege, power and connections to the food supply. In contrast, obesity in the wealthiest countries disproportionately stalks the boonies and reservations, the ghettos and barrios where poverty and crime create obstacles to exercise.

Puffy Periods

In utero, boys and girls are anatomically quite similar. In fact, all human embryos are essentially female. At some point, the Y chromosome begins to differentiate or change the groin into distinct male genitalia. Experienced obstetricians and radiologists can often pick out the outline on ultrasound by the second trimester. While growing up, it is not abnormal for some girls to have tomboy attributes. An earlier growth spurt can make them somewhat more precocious, even dominant little missies. By the early teens, girls are often taller than boys of the same age. They break their classmates' hearts with older dates. But then testosterone kicks in. It melts boys baby fat, dismissing their mothers' features, chiseling more hard-edged, angular bodies. By age 15, males surge ahead in size and physical strength, but not necessarily in emotional maturity.

Girls meanwhile begin accumulating more subcutaneous adipose tissue (fat) which translates into feminine curves in all the right places. Breast buds bloom under the first blast of estrogen, transforming maidens into the softer, gentler, more nurturing repositories of future generations. The lining of the uterus sheds after each monthly preparation to receive the fertilized egg. Periods are therefore reminders that women are God's chosen vessels of the greatest creative act in nature.

Females have about 500 lifetime chances to conceive. Some have done so over twenty times. Others have completely passed on the opportunity for a variety of personal and clinical reasons. But all have had to deal

> ***Evening Primrose***
> *(Oenothera biennis) is rich in gamma linolenic acid (GLA) useful for breast pain, premenstrual syndrome, and mood problems.*

with the challenge. Historically, menses has been associated with being "ill-disposed" and "unclean," (Old Testament). Even today, the rare girl having the misfortune of not being adequately prepared reacts with horror at this mysterious bleeding condition: *menarche* (the first period). Most girls quickly learn one way or the other, how to physically manage those monthly duties. However, from an emotional standpoint, many today still have to grope for meaning.

Though pursuits of the heart traditionally sprout amidst such settings

16. Fluid and Figure

as sunsets, socials and scenic drives, the same can also blossom between burettes, beakers or Bunsen burners. When June invited me to her lab, I watched with amazement the way she delicately handled her tiny biological subjects who volunteered their little kidneys for the cause of science. My fascination grew as she attached their fragile ureters to fine capillary tubes to figure urine output. Being a medical student at the time, I eagerly offered to assist in the microsurgical aspects of her research. Needless to say, she had quite the time keeping me focused.

Notwithstanding, June and I did learn something about fluid retention. In our practice we subsequently observed how premenstrual syndrome is associated with bloating, sluggishness and discomfort from tighter rings and shoes. Young women then tend to become more sensitive, introspective and insecure. Unless we challenge this cyclic feeling of fatness, eating disorders can develop as this notion morphs into reality.

Salt reduction and eating more fruits and vegetables often help. In extreme cases, a mild diuretic may be prescribed. Furthermore, some unfortunate women inherit really difficult periods, enduring more than two weeks a month of cramping, clots, back pain and irritability. Modern sanitary techniques and hormonal manipulation often relegate periods to mild inconveniences. The new drug, *Seasonale*, promises to sharply reduce periods to one every three months. Long-term consequences are unknown at this point so believers in holistic health are hedging their bets.

However, even among the most educated men, the topic is still taboo. Their reactions range from "gross" to "let's not even go there." They joke crudely among themselves about the nuisance of their partners "PMS-ing" or being "on the rag." Many sex education classes fall short in sensitizing males to these periodic female changes? It is only when eager to start a family that a missed period is greeted with anxious excitement until joyfully confirmed by the pregnancy test.

Religion and culture heavily influence what a woman will or will not do on their period. Men need to be respectful when women opt out of swimming or other physical activities during that time of the month. Yet, an enlightened, healthy woman does not allow a normal period to disrupt her personal exercise program. Some cutting back may be necessary but staying active results in lighter, easier flows anyway. As a matter of fact, athletes with significantly reduced body fat percentage may go for months without a period, (amenorrhea).

Problems with periods are a frequent issue in weight management. Remember Sarah in the *Plan* section of Chapter 3? She was the one who bought all those weight loss nutritional supplements and still gained weight. Well she had reached that point in life when it suddenly dawned on her that her biological clock was ticking away. If she was going to have a family, she had to take decisive action. Her heart was in the right place but her planning was too impulsive.

As I reviewed her medical history, I observed that she had been on an injectable hormonal therapy for *endometriosis* (growths on the uterus causing very painful and heavy periods). This is one of several drugs known to be associated with a significant degree of weight gain. We discussed the matter with her gynecologist. Surgical removal of her *fibroids* relieved her of those horrible periods. Thereafter, we were then able to structure a program in which she went on to loss 107 pounds.

Pregnancy Weight Gain

It was the sixth month and Muriel was having those cravings again. "Honey, could you go downtown and get me a couple of them candied apples?"

Farmer Brown rolled over and rubbed his eyes. He had not heard the roosters crowing so he knew it was nowhere close to daybreak.

"What time yer think it is?"

"Two o'clock."

"Woman, you're crazy?! Y'know harvest starts at dawn. I do declare. I'm gonna get me some sleep even if it means I have to carry yer out to the barn myself!"

Fast-forward one hundred years: It was the sixth month and Myra was getting those cravings again. "Honey, could you go downtown and get me an extra large milk shake… and make it chocolate this time."

"Yes dear."

Women will remember every favor bestowed with astonishing detail: which friend brought them what, or who rubbed their feet - especially during that first pregnancy. Each mother also has fond memories of what exactly she craved, from Kit-Kats to pickles and everything in between. Usual foods may become unpalatable. Morning sickness may last throughout, with only a few things staying down. It is mostly unpredictable; a metabolic response in much the same way that tastes change in cancer patients. Cravings are rooted in an innate drive to fill any nutritional gaps in the maternal factory's frantic search for baby building blocks. Before grandma's generation, when malnutrition was a very present danger, that impulse was vital to producing viable offspring. However, the average expectant mother today is more likely to be overfed.

On one level, it is all quite cute actually. Indulge the mom-to-be; after all, she's the one doing all the work. However, it really becomes a problem when cravings are calorie-dense. Weight skyrockets and sugar is detected in the urine (gestational diabetes). This is occurring at a time of reduced overall physical activity. As her due date nears, she is shocked at her weight and complains that she "feels like a cow." It then dawns on her that "eating for two" is no excuse for eating twice as much, all in the name of that poor, innocent little baby.

How the Stars Do It

Celebrities can afford to take a year off for maternity leave. Several months after the must-see cute baby pictures are splashed over the tabloids, she is back to work seemingly just where she left off.

"Look at her! Why, it's just not fair," some might say. "If I had that kind of time and money, I'd look that way too." Yes, they may have personal trainers, private chefs and liposuction. But the main reason these stars regain their youthful figure is that they are *highly motivated* to do so. A whole entourage of agents, financial planners, advertising consultants and film companies feed at her gravy train. Their livelihood is tied to her continued good looks.

The average mother gains about 30 pounds with pregnancy. Half of that, the *water weight* of pregnancy washes out fairly rapidly. While celebrity moms routinely bounce back to portfolio-perfect physiques others are lulled into thinking that the remaining weight will respectfully excuse itself in due course. Not so. More than half of the added poundage still clings by the time baby #2 comes along. As the process repeats, the average mother of two is 30 - 40 pounds heavier than her pre-pregnant weight. Babies demand attention and in an increasing number of instances, father is absent or extended family may not be close enough to make a difference. So as the new mother busies herself with the tighter domestic schedule, she is able to devote less and less time to herself. The weight then quietly creeps up until she is *weighing more than she did when she was most pregnant*. The temptation is to feel resigned to that traditional "matronly" appearance. But she has to make a conscious decision not to just " let herself go." A year later, no one should not be able to tell that she delivered simply by looking at her waistline.

The average young mother contents herself with statements like, "He says he loves me just the way I am." As sweet as that sounds, the reality is that her mate is subjected to an increasingly materialistic and seductive marketplace. Technology brings the claws of the competition within closer striking distance than ever before. In comparison to computer-enhanced pictures of silicone fantasies, his partner begins to look increasingly plain and uninteresting. Somewhere in the murky depths of the typical male psyche, a voice whispers hoarsely, "That sure ain't the deal that you bargained for when you went to the altar."

Granted, weight control should be for the individual's own health and self esteem. In theory, the vows are "until death do us part." But even religion, as currently practiced, is hard-pressed to prevent half of *all* marriages from falling by the

> *When women are depressed, they either eat or go shopping. Men invade another country. It's a whole different way of thinking.*
>
> Elaine Boosler

wayside. So as mom flips again through those wonderful wedding pictures, she should be asking, "Why tempt fate?" It takes energy and commitment to keep oneself presentable for one's mate - something that, by the way, goes both ways.

Nature's Best

Some have compared breast to toys made for kids, but which dads get to play with most of the time. Granted, this is not a popular topic, but one which we must tackle in any comprehensive review of weight loss. How breastfeeding impacts obesity in children is discussed in the next chapter. This section reviews the important role of the breast in weight management for new moms. Is nursing simply a matter of personal preference like chocolate, vanilla or strawberry, or are there deeper emotional and personal health benefits?

The World health Organization sets forth that breastfeeding should be "a global goal for optimal *maternal* and child health and nutrition." According to the UN, "All women should be enabled to practice exclusive breastfeeding and all infants should be fed exclusively on breast milk from birth to four to six months of age." How close would you say we are to this ideal? Especially in developed societies, most mothers enter the hospital having already decided to bottle feed. Motivated by profit, formula companies nail down their customers early.

16. Fluid and Figure

Cigarette companies were free to use the same strategy until the 1970's. Attractive sales reps at street corners handed out cigarettes samples to young future smokers of America. They exploited human psychology in its crudest form. *Free stuff!* Of course, 'carding' was unheard of back then. Even kids and committed non-smokers would therefore come around again to get more for their relatives and friends. When a mother on assistance is hooked with free formula *before* birth, what chance is there of persuading her *after* delivery that nursing is better? As doctors in training starting a family, we were offered an unlimited supply of formula. Is it any surprise that hardly a peep was heard from this generation of health care professionals regarding the advantages of breast milk?

How is the maternal bond formed? First, it arises during those nine months from appreciating the miracle of developing a new life within the mother's very being. Feeling that baby kick is priceless! Still, this part is somewhat invisible. Secondly, and more importantly, the maternal bond is nurtured with breastfeeding. This part you can definitely see. Forensic psychologists link the upsurge in infanticides to greater physical detachment on the part of mothers. This is associated with an unfortunate increase in child abuse. Some of these mothers are very religious and even claiming that "God told them" to commit those horrendous acts. Studies show that mothers who nurse are at a significantly reduced risk of developing that dangerous degree of post-partum depression.

> *I have no hesitation in saying that (of) the American woman ... nowhere does she enjoy a higher station. And if anyone asks me what I think the chief cause of the extraordinary prosperity and growing power of this nation, I should answer that it is due to the superiority of their women.*
>
> Alexis De Tocqueville

Consider Michelangelo's *Pieta* unveiled way back in the year 1500. It still ranks as one of the most renowned sculptures in history. Look again at how the Blessed Virgin tenderly draws to her bosom the limp body of her beloved Son. Nothing better illustrates genuine maternal bonding as a natural outcome of nursing. It is almost impossible to detach emotionally while breastfeeding.

To be fair, modern formula is a wonderful advance in food science. It has the highest of guarantees to be nutritious and hygienic. In many,

many instances, it is literally a godsend. Mothers who bottle feed need not feel guilty or worry about forming nurturing bonds with their babies. It is just that chances are better with the breast. Bottle-feeding is perfectly justified and especially understandable when one just has to get back on the job as soon as possible because bills have to be paid. At the same time, pumping and breast-milk banks are also effective options.

Have you ever seen a skin-and-bones person and think, I wish I could give her some of my fat? A nursing mother is the only one who can actually do that! She passes those calories directly to her baby. Not only that, bust-challenged ladies are simply tickled by the fullness of their lactating bosoms. Ah! Now not only do they lose weight, they organically enhance cup size as well. Furthermore, nursing hastens the uterus' return to pre-pregnancy size. It then hormonally suppresses ovulation and menstruation resulting in natural birth control.

Shunning use the breast for its intended purpose has inherent consequences. Scientists confirm that *nursing reduces breast cancer risk by up to 50%.* Yet, the first reaction of communities alarmed at a spike in breast cancer rates is to try pinning it on other offenders like pesticides in the water and pollutants in the air. You have perhaps seen mothers awash in tears because inverted nipples, inflammation, or weak suckling by their babies deny them the privilege of breastfeeding. Meanwhile, there are those who can, and do not. The facts are there. Resources on websites like www.lalecheleague.org make that choice so easy. Regardless of your family's past experience with breastfeeding, here are a few quick points to consider:

Breastfeeding Tips
1. Breastfeeding is an inalienable right which must be accommodated.
2. Do not "diet" while breastfeeding. Save the nutrients for baby.
3. Breastfeeding greatly reduces cancers.
4. Breastfeeding enhances sensation
5. Breastfeeding is the most intimate form of human bonding.

Love Handles and Thunder Thighs

Certain body areas tend to be more troublesome than others. There are those in the performing arts and others whose self worth is tightly coupled with meeting society's beauty standards. For them, liposuction and plastic surgery are business propositions. However, such artificial measures do not generally make people truly happier. Because of the risk of scarring and numbness, it can be a trade off between "look good" for "feel good." Such patients tend to be somewhat annoyed when their new figure is not noticed and admired. A study by the Canadian Public Health Agency recently found that women undergoing certain cosmetic procedures were 73 percent more likely to commit suicide

Bat wings (flabby underarms), love handles, thunder thighs, *all respond to targeted exercise routines.* Granted, some women have to work much harder at it than others. At least their self esteem does not plunge with complications such as painful scars and the need for touch ups when the fat comes back. Even that resistant "roll" that often develops over a c-section or hysterectomy incision responds regular sit-ups and crunches. I never cease to be amazed how the fat disappears when clients work at it consistently with professional guidance. It is true. Give it your best; the body will do the rest.

Menopause Challenges

Interesting changes occur at menopause that place women metabolically closer to men, but not quite. The ovaries involute, meaning they shrink, and greatly reduce estrogen production. For some, the cessation of periods represents a disturbing finality to the ability to

> *Black Cohosh*
> *(Cimicifuga racemosa) studies have shown this to be as effective as estrogen therapy in reducing the symptoms of menopause.*

conceive. For others, it is a celebration. A gravity-challenged bosom and decreased pubic secretion accompany the tendency for more fat accumulation above the waist. For a number of years until quite recently, society tried turning back the clock with liberal estrogen replacement therapy (ERT). This was touted as the fountain of youth for menopausal women. Once again we discovered that it was not wise to fool Mother Nature. We reaped a whirlwind of increased cancers and clots. The current recommendation is to go with the flow of power surges (hot flashes,) treating them with soy products and natural estrogen-like nutrients. Medications like Premarin are now generally reserved for *disabling symptoms* that interfere with sleep and normal social functioning. Only the lowest effective doses are recommended. Caring relationships provide a balm for mood changes associated with the change of life. As with postpartum depression, one must be sensitive enough to gauge when support is adequate or when medical treatment is necessary.

Making Men Do It

According to National Institutes of Health statistics, an average of 12 percent of men do not have an annual medical check-up compared to 6 percent of women. Does that mean that men require less healthcare or just that they are more resistant to seeking help? What we do know is that across the board, the male lifespan is about six years shorter than females. In fact, they seldom darken the door of a doctor's office until they are dragged in when they are too sick to work or play. They tend to feel bulletproof and invincible. You see it in drinking to excess, speeding or otherwise living beyond the limits and not expecting consequences. That testosterone surge searing an indelible macho image onto the adolescent male consciousness is also responsible for self-neglect later in life.

> **Dong Quai:**
> *(Angelica sinensis) a Chinese herb useful in the treatment of menstrual cramps, infertility and menopause.*

By virtue of that portion of their lives given to childbearing, women are more accustomed to the notion of periodic medical check-ups, sick or not. Women learn early to "lose their dignity" the first time they are positioned in the stirrups on the examining table. Men should overcome their coyness and agree to schedule their counterpart prostate exam around the time his partner has her mammogram or Pap smear. The evidence is clear. A man with a woman in his life lives longer. By the time retirement/ assisted living rolls around, women out-number men four to one. The woman therefore has little choice but to strive keeping her man healthy if she desires companionship into the golden years.

Women of all ages know that it takes more than just suggesting and nagging. Sometimes, even making appointments for their husbands, fathers, sons or significant others may not be enough. They have to go with them to make sure it happens. In any case, having the couple in the office gives a fuller picture of a medical condition. It can be pretty amusing actually, listening to some high-powered executive or supervisor stumble on the sequence of his symptoms or timing of his medication. The wife may say something like, "No honey, that was a catheterization you had in 1999, your bypass was in 2001," or "It's the blue pill you take twice a day and the white one you're supposed to take only in the morning."

At no other time in history has it been more of a challenge to maintain reasonable body weight. Figure and fat percentage are distinctly important markers of personal health. Women are the gatekeepers of health for the family. They make the grocery decisions. They take the kids for their shots. They see to the medical needs of the men in their lives. Especially for those committed to the purpose driven life, the female experience seems often wrapped up in child-care and man-care in different phases of life. This is not to say that it should only be the woman's responsibility. The facts simply show that when mothers are health-assertive, childhood obesity is reduced and fathers enjoy longer, fuller lives. Society becomes more serene and communal health rises as a result. Women are breaking through the marble ceiling into higher positions of church, corporate and political authority. From my medical office vantage point, I have no doubt that the nation's health security will fare far better when that responsibility lies squarely in the lap of the woman.

God grant me the serenity
To accept the things I cannot change;
The courage to change the things I can;
And wisdom to know the difference.

Serenity prayer

REVIEW

1. How do periods influence self-esteem and obesity?

2. What are the benefits of breastfeeding?

3. Describe the weight gain pattern with each pregnancy.

4. What are the key steps in mothers retaining a romantic allure?

5. Males or females, who are stronger?

fearfully

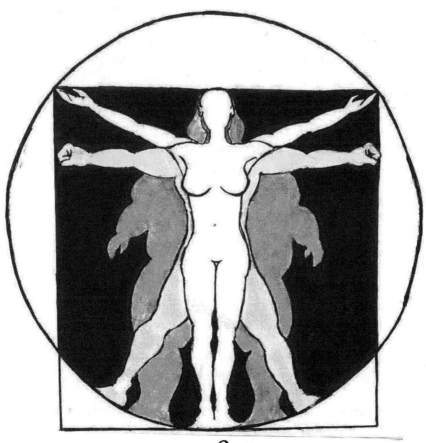

&
wonderfully made

psalm 139:14

Vege-Qoutient: Assessment #5

<u>Scores:</u>   More than once a week---10; About weekly---9 Monthly---5 to 8.
Few times a year---3 to 4;   Never or few times in your life--- 0 to 2

41. **Radishes** ↑ in fiber, vitamins and minerals such as copper and
_____   magnesium. Choleretic: improves gallbladder and liver.

42. **Spinach**   Nutritious Source of strength for *Popeye*. First cultivated
_____   in Iran. ↑ in oxalate, can cause gout & kidney stones.

43. **Strawberries** ↑ flavonoids, vitamins and minera ls, Boosts memory.
_____   Calms stress. ↓ inflammation, heart disease and cancer.

44. **Sweet potatoes** Native to Americas. ↑in antioxidants. "Antidiabetic
_____   carbs." Preserves eyesight. Lifts mood. Fights cancer.

45. **Tomatoes** ↑in lycopene, vitamins and pantothenic acid. Combats
_____   wide range of cancers. ↑skin's sun protection factor.

46. **Watercress** ↑ in vitamins, calcium and phosphorus. Great for salads.
_____   Prevents osteoporosis. Anticancer properties.

47. **Watermelon** ↑ in Lycopene. (red pigment) Promotes weight loss.
_____   ↓ cholesterol, blood pressure & stroke risk.

48. **Wheat germ** ↑ *octacosanol* and vitamin E. Sparks alertness. ↑ per-
_____   formance. Balances metabolism, regularizes bowels.

49. **Wild rice**   ↑in fiber, low in fat, rich in protein, minerals and B vita-
_____   mins. ↓ kidney disease. Normalizes blood sugar. ↓strokes

50. **Yams**   Staple in West Africa, Caribbean and Filipines. High in
_____   vitamins, carbohydrates and potassium.

\+ _____ % **TOTAL VQ #5**

The best *fitness foods* from all over the world are readily available at local the farmers' market or grocery. Explore new recipes and challenge your taste buds as you embark on that exciting journey toward vibrant health and natural weight control.

Chapter 17
Reversing Childhood Obesity

Obesity is on the way to becoming the leading preventable cause of death. Cutting physical activity and healthy nutrition programs is penny-wise and pound foolish... we're going to pay sooner or later.

David Satcher, M.D. former U.S. Surgeon General

John Stoessel of ABC's *20/20* once did a piece in which he asked first graders about their choice of friends. Would they rather have a friend who was fat, instead of a friend with one leg...or someone who was blind, or someone who was a criminal? Shockingly, each kid gave the same answer - anyone but a fatty! Another experiment simply showed silhouettes of an obese child. When students were asked what kind of person they thought this would be, the words most frequently used were, "stupid, lazy and ugly." The not-so-funny thing was that many of the kids expressing these opinions were themselves, well...you know.

Obesity rates among children have more than *tripled* over the past two decades. 50 percent of school children are overweight, fully 25 percent are obese. Children as young as 10 years old drop dead at school from heart attacks, as dramatically reported in *People Magazine*. Meanwhile, those who profit from the status quo contend that things are not that bad, the sky is not falling. On the other hand, reacting to these statistics, New York's health commissioner Dr. Thomas Freden warns that we have "a calamity in the making." Dr. Robert H. Eckel, president of the American Heart Association, describes these same statistics as "alarming." We are not talking about the occasional chubby child here or there, but an ever-growing trend that threatens to unleash monumental medical burdens in the near future. It is a challenge which begins in the cradle itself.

The good news is that we do not have to feel like hostages to inevitable societal changes. The solutions are not complex, but it does require some courage and commitment on the part of responsible adults. No doubt, you and I already put some of these measures into practice. We only need to do just this much more, in a coherent and consistent fashion, in order to see measurable results.

251

Bosom Babies

The rise of obesity is clearly linked to the global demise of breast-feeding. Having reviewed the impact on maternal weight in the previous chapter, it is very important that we now examine how human milk sets up the body's future metabolism. Even those who may not have been involved in breast-feeding either as a baby or mother, can benefit from a respectful discussion on the most helpful approach from this point forward.

Researchers at the Maximillian University in Munich, Germany have confirmed that the longer babies are breast-fed the less likely they are to be obese. Not only that, it is well-known that breast milk contains living antibodies which support the baby's immune system during the first critical months of development. Research proves that breast-fed babies have significantly fewer colds and ear infections and do better at school. Their mothers therefore end up wasting far less time and anxiety with added doctor visits. The American Academy of Pediatrics published it

> *Lactating mothers who consume coconut products increase levels of lauric acid in their milk. This helps burn fat and provides greater antimicrobial protection to their babies.*
>
> See: *American Journal of Clinical Nutrition*; 1998, 67: 301 - 308

"Breast-feeding and the Use of Human Milk" in *Pediatrics*, Vol. 100 No. 6, December 1997. The document points out that human milk helps prevent respiratory and abdominal illnesses, Sudden Infant Death Syndrome (SIDS), and later on, various allergic and immune-related diseases such as lupus and lymphoma.

Breast milk is always warm, always hygienic and *never* runs out. (Observe those heart-wrenching TV specials on hunger relief. Even starving mothers continue to produce milk to ensure their children survive them). Breast milk is cheaper too. The overall medical cost saving can be calculated in the billions. Instead we have a generation of grandmothers who cannot share from personal experience, the nuances of nursing a baby. On channels like *Animal Planet,* game wardens can be seen teaching the young of endangered species how to hunt and fend for themselves in the wild. Does it not appear equally unnatural that today we need "Lactation consultants" to coach young moms in this strange lost art?

The *pathogenesis* of obesity (the science of how the disease develops) reveals the lack of personal and cultural tradition to quit eating when full.

17. Reversing Childhood Obesity

From day one, the breast-fed baby learns when to stop. When baby gets full, that signals mother's milk to stop, sort of like a gas pump. How much milk did he get? We cannot know for sure, but it was enough. It is part of the magical feedback loop in that mother-child bond which a man can never fully understand.

The formula bottle has no such automatic shut-off valve. In fact, when baby tries to stop, watch what happens. Mother tends to sneak the bottle between his lips to drink more. According to the *American Journal of Public Health,* 44 percent of Hispanics kindergartners are overweight compared to 32 percent for Blacks and Whites. Why? Twice as many Hispanic kids were bottle-fed past age 1. Meanwhile mother takes perverse pride in her "little porker's" great appetite, boasting how many ounces he already drinks. Bottle-fed babies have been shown to consume up to 25 percent more calories. Such children are doomed to a lifetime of battling the bulge. Surely, all babies are soft, sweet and cuddly, but a breast-fed baby simply does not get overly fat.

Zero Food Waste

Double messages confuse our march toward wellness. A prime example is the YMCA Camps' approach to teaching the concept of not wasting food. I spent a couple exciting weekends with other parents of 4th graders roughing it with the kids at Camp Storer in Jackson, Michigan. The overall curriculum was quite impressive. A robust environmental ethic permeated all activities such as hiking, wildlife, composting, boating, archery and spooky stories. They instilled core values such as caring, respect, responsibility, putting God first, others second and self third. However, the major theatrics were reserved for when camp counselors ironically donned pig costumes and exhorted children to *eat all that you put on your plate.*

In theory, the message was powerful: Do not take more than you need out of respect for those who were hungry. In so doing we keep costs down, save energy and so on and so forth. However, using moral suasion to force down leftovers simply sounds like an airbrushed Great Depression admonition to "clean your plate." Given the current obesity crisis, I find this approach uniquely puzzling.

The rustic cabins averaged at least 50 yards from the camp cafeteria. Maybe for the first time in their lives, many of these little campers did not have the same easy access to a refrigerator as they did at home or when visiting family. Not surprisingly, their hands tended to be a bit heavy when

253

serving themselves at the buffet. If the child realizes that he is full, why compound one mistake with another? Come on, now. How can gorging oneself here help hungry children anywhere?

We see a number of grateful parents in the office who have taken the time to adjust the eating environment at home. A *sensible leftover policy* is fundamental to learning mastery over food. Listen to the stomach and it becomes second nature. Force-feed it and you know the result. We can only safeguard our children from the errors of our generation by making the message crystal clear. It is easier to keep the weight off in the first place than resorting to a parade of frustrating diets trying to unload the pounds later.

Child-Targeted Advertising

Some of us are old enough to remember when children's programming was primarily on Saturday mornings. This is indelibly etched in my mind from my first day on call as an intern on the Ob-gyn rotation. The nurse had paged me to evaluate an expectant woman in distress. I could hear the patient's screams as soon as I reached the floor. I raced to her room. By the time I arrived, the contractions had subsided. She was all alone - but not quite lonely.

"So. How're you doing this morning?" I breathlessly tried to clothe my voice with relaxed authority, but my insides were tied in anxious knots. After all, this was my first time making a clinical decision as a graduate physician.

I felt I was intruding. She was all wrapped up in the company of cartoon characters flashing across the screen. She giggled gleefully as Road Runner tricked Wiley Coyote, causing him to *pluuuunge* over the edge of that tall cliff - again! This was followed by an ad for some kiddie cereal. That was when it struck me how young my patient looked. It was magnificent weekend weather outside. The sheets bunched up at her feet glowed in a broad beam of radiant sunlight streaming through the window. I flipped through her chart. Age: 13! Okay. I remember deliberately walking around to engage her line of vision. She actually leaned to the right as if in a hypnotic trance blankly staring *around* me at the television. "Amazing!" I, thought, turning to the nurse who by then had caught up with me. Nurse simply smiled and shook her head. "You ain't seen nothing yet," she whispered wistfully.

Suddenly, the stillness was shattered by another shrill scream as

17. Reversing Childhood Obesity

waves of wicked contractions once again wracked my patient's bloated body. The poor child instantly grabbed my white coat, pleading for me to get rid of the pain.

Two decades later, with the advent of 24-hour cable TV, cartoon network, *Nickelodeon* and the *Disney Channel,* food manufacturers revel in vastly increased direct access to kids. If you have ever seen the child throwing a tantrum in the supermarket, it was most likely because mother dared to oppose his choice of snack placed in the grocery cart. It is estimated that the average child will see 10,000 television ads per year telling them that unhealthy food rocks.

Experts agree that young children are generally unable to distinguish between ads and regular programming. This prompted the World Health Organization / Food and Agriculture Organization (WHO/FAO) to urge all nations to place "restrictions on marketing of junk food to children." Many countries have moved in that direction with a few notable holdouts. Former Surgeon Generals Koop, Satcher, and Carmona (under the Reagan, Clinton and Bush administrations) jointly testified before Congress how their scientific initiatives were usurped by political interference. A prime example is how the junk food lobby has consistently deflected efforts for healthier eating claiming *parents are the ones making their kids fat,* not their food. Given that McDonald's alone spends $600 million on marketing, what chance does that poor supermarket mother have?

Where Are We Heading To?

School Boards in progressive districts have been boldly influencing the foods available to those under their care. The Federal government is playing catch up. Many dieticians see the National School Lunch program as still falling short. The program was introduced to level the nutritional playing field in the lean decade following World War II. President Harry Truman's goal was to produce students who were "well nourished...healthier and more alert" by fostering *good food habits.*

Until recently, the school lunch program was still heavy on foods that the US Department of Agriculture itself officially discouraged: Meat and cheese at the expense of fresh fruits and vegetables. The simple reason was conflict of interest. Remarks in the Congressional Record revealed that the USDA, headed by political appointees, seemed more responsive to the *surplus-removal programs* for farmers in key constituencies, rather than the well-being of the students who have little say. The same was the case with Women with Infant Children (WIC) program food packages that seldom included fruits and vegetables.

While students in other developed nations receive free fruit to encourage a more healthy diet, it was not until 2002 that Congress began funding a limited trial program for selected schools in a few states. As it turned out much of the fresh fruit deteriorated on the way from central locations to the school cafeteria. Very slowly, the idea emerged of permitting school systems to purchase produce directly from local farmers.

All that reminds me of Bo, one of my medical school classmates from the Bronx. One of his favorite stories was of a grade school field trip to the farm. The class had come across this enclosure in which there were big animals with horns.

"There's a moose! There's a moose!" He exclaimed.

"No Bo," counseled his buddy from country. "That's a cow... *that's where we get our milk from*," his country friend answered.

"Don't be silly. Our milk comes from cartons. That's a moose. See its horns? ...Here Moosie, Moosie."

Bo recounted how he tried to get the attention of his 'moose' by beckoning through the paddock. His friend kept warning him that he was getting the animal upset. He remained unconvinced until it charged, goring the post and missing them by inches. The teacher almost fainted. Bo jokes that to this day he can remember learning little else from grade school other than where milk really comes from!

The vast majority of children today likewise believe that real food comes in a can, a wrapper or carton. Excess processed foods load kids up with preservatives and give an addictive sugar buzz. Our mission must now be to teach children this basic precept: The closer the food to the hand of God, the better it is for us.

Grandparents are known for talking about having had to walk to and from school in the snow, barefoot, uphill...both ways! Would one risk sounding like that to say that there was hardly any talk of hyperactivity in times past? Today teachers spend more energy trying to keep order than focusing on the curriculum. Studies today show that obese kids are more than twice as likely to be diagnosed with attention-deficit and oppositional defiant disorder, depression, anxiety and related conditions. This has been directly linked to the doubling sugar consumption among teenagers to 20 percent of total calories consumed.

There was a time when candy was a treat. At Halloween, Christmas,

17. Reversing Childhood Obesity

Valentines and Easter, one could really splurge. Today, kids see candy as a daily right. Parents are frustrated when they send their children off with healthy snacks only to be brought back untouched or later hear of it used in food fights. We are up against junk food used as the currency of friendships at recess. Those with cool snacks rule. Left to their own devices, the average child would feast all day on HoHos, soda pop, candy and chocolate. According to *The Brown University Child and Adolescent Behavior Letter*, this has a direct impact not only on the obesity rate, but also on behavior problems. It is becoming evident that cutting back on the excess calories could mean cutting back on the Ritalin as well.

> *A plate of **nachos** is loaded with a cool 1500 calories.*

Junk-Free Zone

Food service managers at the schools and universities get caught in a dilemma. They respond to complaints by adding healthy choices to the cafeteria menu while students make a beeline for the nearest pizza shop. Leftovers are lost and budgets constraints discourage future efforts. We cannot force students to eat what they may not want to. At the same time, the school is the primary institution of learning. If there is no impediment to opting out of nutritious meals, then we are failing in our mission to "bring up a child the way he should go."

How can we combat this problem? There are no simple answers, but let us look at a couple different angles. Cigarette smoking in enclosed spaces has never left quietly into the night. Smokers generally believe they have the right to pollute the public air, but the public has no right to impose sharing fresh air with them. The following chapter (*Corporate Wellness*) expands on that. However, when society takes a deep breath and does the right thing, results have been consistently positive and unequivocal.

What are the parallels with food? What if students were limited to only eating off campus once a week? Would they not come to see *Fun Food Friday* as a treat rather than a way of life? We could rotate the days. For example, 7th graders and below should not be allowed to leave the school campus. 8th graders, eat out on Mondays, 9th graders on Tuesdays, 10th on Wednesdays and so forth.

Naturally, food controls should apply to all students, rather than just picking on the overweight. This would be accompanied by a concerted nutrition education campaign emphasizing that a steady diet of junk food is bad for every one of us. We need to always bear in mind that this is a battle in which we are massively outgunned by commercial interests. Their expensive ads will always be *spiffier* in comparison to anything do-gooders can come up with.

It is a delicate matter and has to be well thought out. We have to use our authority beginning in the classroom when introducing selected healthy choices. We have to dramatize it and make it fun. Teachers need to set the example by eating healthy snacks - again, not just the overweight teachers. This might be the only chance for children who have nutritionally-challenged parents at home.

Many schools have exclusive contracts allowing certain soda and other junk food companies the exclusive right to install their vending machines. In return they receive easy thousands of dollars in cash subsidies for team uniforms, band equipment and other sponsorships. In a time of tight school budgets, principals and superintendents feel hooked. However, the Federal government is finally following the lead of a number of vanguard school systems that have banned soda, candy and junk food on campus. They have changed their school vending machines to dispense bottled water, genuine fruit juices, smoothies, energy bars, and low-fat, low-salt chips. If you want to judge how progressive a school system is, just check out their nutrition policy.

Drastic and sudden nutrition make-overs can force junk food underground. Student dealers can be as imaginative as any drug ring in the community, smuggling in their backpacks what kids can no longer get from vending machines. Despite a manageable backlash, the equation is changing in our favor. Our job is to model our strategies on local school boards most successful in making the shift to healthy nutrition.

Video Games and Internet

A young man in South Korea played video games for 50 hours... non-stop! He called his mother to say that he would be home soon then collapsed from fatal heart failure. Most kids in the United States are not quite that extreme, but the consequences are adding up. The average American child spends approximately 24 hours each week watching television. By age 70, the average American will have spent the equivalent of *seven years for watching television*. One judge sentenced a gentleman to ten months house arrest without TV. Many bright, legal minds applauded this creative sentencing to keep non-violent criminals out of jail. Others condemned this approach as cruel and unusual punishment. Many of us would go into some serious withdrawals. God forbid that we miss a single episode of our favorite sitcom or soap opera.

Aside from that, video games are becoming increasingly more gory and suggestive. Hidden sex scenes were discovered in a few of the most popular versions. *Grand Theft Auto* and *Mortal Combat* indulge players with mayhem and Columbine-like wasting of police and innocent bystanders. That incites ordinary kids' horseplay to become rougher and more callous. This is a common prelude to gratuitous violence and grisly crimes such as the infamous X-Box murders in Florida. The Jaws of Life may not be strong enough to pry kids away from those modules. Many parents dread interrupting this digital world with reminders of homework or household chores.

The challenge is to encourage our children to be thinkers and doers rather than evolving into the spectator culture. They grow up to over-value celebrity athletes who are increasingly using performance-enhancing drugs to stay at the top of their game. Meanwhile, the gulf between the activity levels of athletes and regular people continue to widen.

Sociologists from another planet would be intrigued with *Homo sporticus* found in western societies. They would observe a flabby male painted in bright team colors going through the rather peculiar rituals of fired up fans. The brain is bursting with sport trivia, but devoid of a basic understanding of current affairs in the world around him.

> *All of us have to recognize that we owe our children more than we have been giving them.*
>
> Hillary Clinton

This particular species becomes extremely animated over professional sporting competition. His most intense exertion is from pumping his fists and cheering wildly as his favorite player returns a punt all the way for a touch-down.

Males produce small amounts of the female hormones as part of nature's balance. However fat cells also produce estrogen. As fat percentage increases, estrogen goes up and manliness goes down. *H. sporticus* retreats into the confines of his Lazy boy, glued to the TV, with the same fixation as my first patient's attention to Road Runner and Wily Coyote. Already, 17 percent of boys are overweight compared to 14 percent of girls. The athletic ideal of a lean, muscular and virile male is rapidly becoming an impossible dream. How do we protect our boys from growing up into what one western governor describes as *girlie men?*

259

Manna*fast* Miracle

Few countries can match with the US advanced investment in competitive sports. After all, NCAA football couches routinely earn more than ten times the salary of the more than the average tenured professor. The point is that while it is not possible for everyone to make a living as an athlete, each of us ought to learn early the importance of staying active. The playground quickly becomes a very hostile place for the inactive, husky student. They are frequently embarrassed and picked last for teams. The vicious cycle has to be broken. By age 12, parents and coaches have a good idea which kids are on track to become gifted athletes. Rather than just throwing in the towel on the rest, let us be quick to redirect their energies into regular, non-competitive, physical activities for enjoyment, relaxation and good health. Gym should offer a wide array of monitored fun options such as dodgeball, hula-hoop, volleyball, skipping and more.

Physical Education Optional?

Even with rising obesity, physical education (P.E.) nationwide decreased from 42 percent in 2000 to a startling 28 percent in 2005. The electorate, many on fixed or evaporating incomes, demonstrate increasing tax fatigue when faced with levies for funding local education. P.E. programs are often the first on the chopping block, fueled by the notion that it "is not on the same level with academic subjects in life's importance." (Illinois school board member, *American School Board Journal,* 2002). We must find ways to rectify this self-defeating trend.

As a student at the Dominica Grammar School on the island, I remember dressing in our all-white sports outfits at least once a week. We scrubbed and whitened our tennis shoes, which fostered pride in appearance. P.E. and lab classes always offered an exciting break from being cooped up in the classroom all week. Parents understood that their children could get hurt in sports, yet there was hardly any thought given to suing anybody. Apart from the major sports of cricket and soccer, *everyone* was involved in track and field. Participation was 100 percent and consistent and throughout the academic year, even among the disabled. Talented athletes were then selected through a series of heats to compete on Sports Day. We did not have much, but everyone participated according to their ability. The motto was *Mens Sana en Corpore Sano,* (Latin: a healthy mind in a healthy body). Not only did we get some fresh air, but we also learned much about character, about team spirit, about giving our best. We learned the value of "pressing forward toward the prize." These are intangibles costing little; and yet were so priceless.

The fact is that the overwhelming majority of parents and students support required physical education and do not believe that it undermines academic performance. Excluding overweight youth from intramural sports places them at risk for shunning structured exercise program for the rest of their lives. School Boards are beginning to find ways to make gym facilities available after hours with volunteer supervision and waivers to liability. Others are actually placing greater emphasis on grading physical education *effort* on the report card. Students should be encouraged to participate in the *Presidential Fitness Award* (www.presi dentschallenge.org) mentioned in Chapter 6. Just as we rank schools by SAT scores, so too we can compare average BMI's and the percentage of students earning Presidential Fitness Awards.

The solutions to childhood obesity are surprisingly straightforward. Some school systems in desperation are outsourcing their cafeteria management to national diet chains. This is nothing is but an expensive, timid, hands-off approach. We need instead to courageously act on our convictions and simply follow the formula of schools successful in reducing childhood obesity. We can begin by giving incentives to students who have less starches and sweets in favor of different colors on their plates: something green (lettuce, string beans), something yellow (carrots, squash), something red (tomatoes, radishes). Actively promoting healthy choices reduces our children's exposure to junk food in the learning environment. It is evident, that they get used to it to the extent that we are creative enough to make it fun.

Legal and budgetary barriers to *universal physical education* must be eliminated. Past generations worked hard preparing a better life for their children. An ominous, even sinister trend now points to our children's lifespans being shorter than ours. To quote Senator Chuck Hagel, (R) Nebraska, "It is unpatriotic not to question your government." Seeing the results of our nutrition policy, one has no choice but to be patriotic for the sake of our children. We must reverse childhood obesity now!

I was taught that the way of progress

is neither swift nor easy.

Marie Curie
French/Polish Physicist, discoverer of radioactivity.

REVIEW

1. Discuss why bottle-fed babies consume more and why.

2. How do limits on childhood advertising affect obesity rates?

3. Discuss strategies for improving nutrition in your school system.

4. What ways have you found helpful in improving childhood activity levels?

5. Discuss more nutritious options to candy-based treats on occasions like Halloween.

Chapter 18
Corporate Wellness Training

If a window of opportunity appears, don't pull down the shade.
Tom Peters, Management Guru

N
o smoking on the job, neither inside nor outside the building - not even at home! Speculation swirls as to what led Howard Weyers of Okemos, Michigan to clamp such a total ban on his insurance claims company. What is clear is that several workers quit rather than subjecting themselves to such far-reaching restrictions, especially after he began targeting overweight workers as well.

For those working at home, this chapter may not be of immediate interest. Nonetheless, one can easily see how the principles discussed here directly impact the family budget. In any event, press reports portrayed Weyers as a non-smoking, daily-jogging, fitness freak. His unwavering stance sent privacy advocates into a *hissy fit* with threats of lawsuits on behalf of those 'oppressed' workers. They contend that imposing his personal discipline on employees was patronizing, if not illegal. Critics seemed oblivious to a national death toll from smoking exceeding that from alcohol, AIDS, traffic accidents, narcotics, murders and suicides *combined*. The average household, smoking or not, subsidizes treatment of smoking related illnesses to the tune of about $600 annually. If that came as a separate bill in one's mailbox today, you can be sure that the government imposing such a tax would be tossed out in the next election. And to put it in perspective, as we saw in Chapter 3, the cost of obesity even exceeds that.

After crunching the numbers, Weyers boldly went beyond fuzzy theories and politically correct sentiments. He concluded that his workers have options. They could simply capitalize on the $35 incentive toward a health club fee and $65 for assistance in quitting smoking. If they exercised their freedom to continue the lifestyle of their choice, they should no longer expect his company to support their habits. As far as we know, Howard Weyers is not only still in business, but also quite the hero to many CEO's struggling under the crushing weight of burgeoning healthcare costs.

Can your workplace make you sick or force you to get well? Can your personal health influence your company's survival, especially in the face of increasing overseas sweatshop competition? How far can a company go in trimming its health benefits expenditure? Is there a right way or a wrong way to corporate wellness? What are the essential elements of a basic corporate wellness program?

Many of us now spend more waking hours with co-workers than with family members. It follows that health habits are as powerfully influenced by corporate culture as by the clinic, church or community. The mission of this chapter is to stimulate interest and outline the general format of a modern corporate wellness program. Responsible workers will learn how to take advantage of available healthcare benefits. It is blueprint for the rank and file to initiate such programs in cases where management may be slow to see the light. Just imagine what a credit it would be if you could approach your boss with sound ideas on how to decrease net spending on healthcare in your company!

From the management standpoint, given the fact that businesses are required to provide 'sickness' benefits for employees, it really seems to make sense to invest proactively in keeping them healthy...

"No way!" bellowed my college economics professor. "First of all the unions won't allow it. And corporations are not going to waste money on wellness programs. If workers want to exercise, they can do it on their own dime."

That was 1978 and we were discussing Japanese structured group exercises before workers began their shifts. The class consensus at the time was these were robotic *kamikazes* conditioned with a fanatic devotion to the glory of the corporation. That surely would not fly with your typical free-thinking, red-blooded American, or any union representing them.

Look at what is happening in the "Big Three" in Detroit. See who's laughing now. Even as we debated in class, the *Land of the Rising Sun* was already beginning to whip the West in industrial efficiency. That was well before smoking was almost universally banned from the American workplace. And that was well before American politicians began making pilgrimages to Japan offering competitive tax breaks to lure automotive factories to their constituencies. That was well before the spiraling health costs of obesity began to increasingly render American companies uncompetitive in the global marketplace.

But is the effort targeting the relevant sectors? According to Richard Wagoner, General Motors CEO, $1500 is added to the cost of each automobile produced in the US. Foreign manufacturers spend *one tenth* as much. We do not have to go far to drive home that point. I surveyed a Japanese auto plant in the Midwest that had authorized 75 gastric bypasses in 2002. Alarmed at their skyrocketing health costs, they instituted a stringent diet and exercise criteria for anyone applying for gastric bypass surgery. They also invested in well-equipped gym and professional support. In 2003, they authorized only 2 obesity surgeries. The net result is that their workers - in America - are not only better motivated, have fewer sick days, but overall health costs are measurably reduced as well. This situation is simply untenable. Brace yourself. Something has to give.

With millions of manufacturing jobs being outsourced to emerging economies, a surprising number of American workers still hold on to a selfish 1970's thinking. They expect to inherit good jobs with good benefits, but still demand that the company keep their hands off their bodies except to write a blank check for whatever their health needs. You cannot have it both ways. And saying, "Thank God I do not work in a factory," does not make one immune. Whether working in the arts, sports, service organizations, or even the ministry, few are untouched by unemployment in their midst. When a major factory closes, bread-earners have to settle for minimum-wage jobs, if any. Area physicians are forced to accept pennies on the dollar of outstanding medical bills. Taking the harsh step of sending such workers to collections mostly stirs up ill-will and a rash of bankruptcies.

In today's economy, even white-collar managers and professionals worry whether their job will be digitally hijacked tomorrow by someone halfway around the world. Many people have no idea that their prompt tax refunds may have been computed by overseas accountants and specially trained analysts at a fraction of the stateside cost. A growing number of hospitals find it cheaper to have x-rays and various scans read by radiologists in countries such as India. Studies done at night are transmitted electronically overseas and the readings often return cheaper and even faster compared to having a radiologist on call locally. At the present rate, Goldman Sacs forecasts that the economies of India and

China will overtake that of the US within our lifetime.

The May 29, 2006 issue of Time Magazine gave another stunning example of the far-reaching effects of global competition. It told of an uninsured, self-employed, Alabama chiropractor who was facing a $90,000 herniated disc surgery. He flew to Thailand and had the same procedure performed by a US-trained surgeon for just $10,000. As we saw in Chapter 9, elective surgeries are the major source of profits for hospitals. The fact that an increasing number of companies and health plans are encouraging patients to consider overseas options could revolutionize health care in America.

As a result, even the most conservative organizations and Republican lawmakers are taking a fresh look at universal health insurance and novel approaches to medical cost-containment. Many executives are still unsure where to start, concerned that this might end up being just another unnecessary expense.

Why a Wellness Program

In the plantation economy 200 years ago, the master paid no wages but was responsible for the feeding, clothing, housing and upkeep of his slaves, such as it was. In comparison, the modern manager wants little to do with employees beyond instructing his secretary to send out birthday cards and perhaps sharing eggnog at the company holiday party. The worker is free to quit at anytime and his health is his own affair. But to the extent that it impacts corporate profits, individual health has become very much the boss' domain and concern.

Analysts feel that we have come to a pivotal point in history. Society cannot long endure with half of our medical resources being siphoned off for the care of people disinclined to care of themselves. It is therefore the challenge of management to provide robust wellness programs to overcome the inherent weakness and predictable threats mentioned above.

Sitting on the board of a managed care health plan made me keenly aware of the cutthroat decisions regarding underwriting companies with poor safety or sickness profiles. It was intriguing to see how various industries were assessed. For instance, one would imagine that construction workers were more exposed to injury and would therefore have higher health premiums. As it turns out, in the short term, they tended to be rather low consumers of health care. They seldom sought medical attention except for job related accidents, which are covered by the worker's compensation anyway. In contrast, nursing homes and hospital staffs were considered high consumers of medical care. Whether more hypochondriac from being surrounded by so much disease; it is not clear. In any event, the system can be quite capricious. The dependent of an employee - someone never seen on the worksite - could unexpectedly incur major medical costs such as a liver transplant. This could easily saddle the entire company with substantially higher premiums the following year.

This is no different from how automobile insurance works. High-risk groups, such as teenage males and those with more speeding tickets or accidents pay steeper premiums. But when it comes to health, they average person thinks: "Oh, my insurance company was wonderful! They covered all the bills, no questions asked." For one thing, in the era of HMO pre-certification, such scenarios are becoming increasingly rare. Also, insurance companies stay in business by simply spreading the costs across the group. As in the gambling business, *the house always wins*. Insurance companies consistently remain among the most lucrative of businesses. Want to find the insurance headquarters in a new city? Just pick out the tallest building on the skyline and chances are you've found it. Their executives make tens of millions in annual *bonuses* while the worker and his caregivers have to beg for necessary tests or treatments. How do insurance companies remain so profitable? They are highly efficient at collecting premiums. However once an individual or company's health utilization profile rises, they simply impose exorbitant premium increases or decline to renew coverage the following year.

Employers generally use insurance benefits as a competitive advantage to lure quality workers. This, however, is in no way synonymous to a robust corporate wellness. In many ways, "good insurance" simply makes individuals choice targets for unscrupulous health care providers. Having an attractive health plan often entitles the bearer to undergo superfluous tests and referrals within a particular healthcare system to milk reimbursements. Providers in turn defend the practice by saying it makes up for uncompensated (uninsured/charity) care. It is a system that provides fodder for plaintiff attorneys who are in on the racket. Ideally, the state should be an honest broker. However, in practice, dependence on campaign contributions results in government policies lurching between these two main interest groups. Masses of workers and small businesses fueling the economy are generally left out in the cold. The way out of this bind is for workers to understand clearly that increases in health expenditure directly affects the company's ability to provide raises and bonuses.

Effectiveness of Wellness Programs

The awareness generated by a wellness program creates a certain kind of buzz. I cannot tell you how many times we come across workers who for the first time were finally confronted with the scale, or came face-to-face with some health concern which they had long postponed. The reasons for people not doing what they know they should do are sometimes so trivial. One worker admitted that she had not sought medical attention in 30 years because she felt (as a child) that a surgeon was too rough while checking for what turned out to be appendicitis. If her belly was already hurting, she complained bitterly, why should he still want to push on it? Until the corporate health fair we conducted, no knowledgeable family member or health professional had the opportunity to communicate to her the necessities of a physical examination. Another worker was scared to have any check ups because some rookie phlebotomist botched a blood draw over a dozen years ago.

Regardless of whether management feels that these may not be their choicest workers, each plays an important role in the organization. There may be the smoker whose only remaining reason for not quitting is fear of further weight gain. While pills, patches and gums have varying effectiveness, experience shows that inspiration, education and support are much more important in determining long-term success. Consider that worker with all kinds of red flags that he is about to crash and burn. On a personal level, managers have little choice but to respectfully keep their distance because this is a 'private matter,' a family issue or "something between him and his doctor" - whether or not any such relationship exist at all. This could be a key individual in the organization whose heart attack could disrupt production or tip next year's premium into the red zone.

A thoughtfully sponsored corporate wellness program is the moral equivalent of placing one's arm over his shoulder and saying "Hey, buddy. We're concerned about you. Let us know if we can help." Like picture day at school, a health fair is a refreshing break from the routine, a reprieve from the drudgery. The super-charged atmosphere and excitement of such programs offer the best chance for lifestyle change. The good-natured prodding and ribbing of co-workers can finally nudge someone into undergoing indicated tests where even loved ones may have failed for years.

Today in America, corporate healthcare expenditures now exceed corporate profits. Companies respond by making greater use of temporary workers while striving to keep their permanent workers healthy. Dr. Roy Shephard, past president of the American College of Sports Medicine found that work-site wellness programs can save companies as much as $700 per worker per year, more than enough to pay for the average wellness program. (*The Physician and Sports Medicine, 1999*). Coca Cola reported a reduction in health care claims with an exercise program alone. Swedish investigators found that mental performance was significantly better in physically fit workers (27% fewer errors) than in non-fit workers. (*Physical Fitness and Mental Performance During and After Work.* Sjoberg, Hans. *Ergonomics, 1983:23 977-987*). In a government study, the Canada Life Assurance Company experimental group realized a 4% increase in productivity compared to the control group, after starting an employee fitness program. Further, 47% of program participants reported that they felt more alert, had better rapport with their coworkers, and generally enjoyed their work more. (*The Canadian Employee Fitness and Lifestyle Project*).

Implementing a Wellness Program

Management is beginning to appreciate that attention to wellness is not to be confused with the many regulations that distract from productivity. Unlike the Weyco case at the beginning of the chapter, a sound approach to wellness should not be perceived as some new decree like Moses coming down the mountain with the Ten Commandments. Perhaps one of the single most important factor affecting the success and durability of a health project is tapping into worker initiative. In any firm there are usually a few individuals who are independently excited about wellness. Regardless of their position on the totem pole, input and energy from such *champions* help to drive the process long after management has refocused on new contingencies. They serve as catalysts for on-the-job wellness committees from different departments and the union, if indicated.

Ideally, sponsoring a planning retreat for these *change agents* affords both recognition and reward for their contributions. It is important to realize that we are dealing with a collection of human beings rather than just raw materials, units of production, or marketing trends. Workers must be persuaded to do something that would not only be good for themselves but also essential to the viability of the company. Such an approach contributes powerfully to an intangible called *corporate morale.*

At *Heartland Nutrition Institute,* we involve rank and file workers at an early stage by sending out carefully tailored medical questionnaires. This allows us to harvest preliminary data for analysis and provides a marker for assessing program effectiveness. We ensure that the entire process is HIPPA compliant in order to maintain individual privacy and confidentiality regulations. Simply put, iron-clad guarantees must be given that adverse health information garnered from such programs will in no way be used to victimize the worker.

That is precisely the weakness in the Weyco approach. It may seem expedient and cost-effective to utilize home-grown talent, but the downside is risking the potential appearance of individual persecution. And this does not just refer to drug testing, as even a sugar test for diabetes may be misused and cause legal problems down the road. For this reason it makes sense to at least kick off the program with an *outside consultant.* A motivational *keynote address* by a known expert provides a fresh, new voice to sell workers on buying into the program.

Program Mechanics

The Human Resources/Personnel department traditionally works with hospital occupational health departments in managing injured workers and facilitating timely return to active employment. That describes a *reactive* role. Large firms may have the advantage of in-house physicians, nurses and trainers who work in a coordinated and sustained fashion to help *proactively* reduce health costs. What about smaller firms? Lacking these kinds of resources they often times default to simply providing insurance, processing workers compensation claims and tabulating sick days. For such companies, Transformation Consulting has designed cost effective strategies to improve fitness and reduce total health expenditure.

Our approach to corporate wellness is a health fair format bracketed by important assessments both before and after the event:

18. Corporate Wellness Training

Pre-Health Fair

- Survey prevalence of at-risk populations
    - Smokers
    - Overweight
    - Sedentary
    - Substance abusers
- Industry specific occupational health and safety requirements
- Overview of worker's compensation claims
- Review of corporate sick time profile
- Medical history forms/hand-outs regarding health concerns
- Review of random drug testing policies and procedures

Health Fair

- Screening for
    - Blood pressure
    - Cholesterol
    - Diabetes
    - Body Composition
    - Cancer.
    - Fitness
- Prizes and recognitions
- Sign up interested participants

> *A man too busy to take care of his health is like a mechanic to busy to take care of his tools.*
>
> ### Spanish proverb

Post Health Fair

- Individual Health Risk Profile.
- Corporate Wellness Summary - Aggregate Report
- Schedule executive physicals
- Referrals to primary care physicians
- Track results, (1-month, 6 months and 1 year

The wellness consultant is primarily tasked with stimulating interest in fitness fundamentals and injury prevention. A concerted effort must be made to involve workers on all shifts and at all levels.

Tangible Benefits

Smoking cessation and weight management are the two most controllable variables in employee health. Companies choose different approaches based on a variety of workforce characteristics such as length of time with the company, and existing benefits. One option is covering the entire cost of certain programs as long as the employee responsibly attends sessions. Another is to reimburse the participant in part or in full upon successful completion. Those not challenged by nicotine or weight are often lulled into thinking that workplace wellness does not apply to them. In such these cases the program serves as a reminder for routine screening (Page 308). It also provides them the perfect opportunity to assert leadership by reaching out to others who need encouragement.

Corporate wellness should channel directly into the family physician or existing community medical programs. Hospitals and related organizations often sponsor community health fairs. To stimulate business, basic evaluations, cholesterol/blood pressure checks and diabetes screening are made available for free or at a discounted charge. This is an excellent resource for companies working with tight budgets. All that is left to be done is to provide incentives for employee participation and *passports* to track attendance. In so doing corporate wellness can be accomplished in quite a cost-effective manner.

In our consultations with small to midsize firms, we advise how to structure break-time to facilitate walking. This is becoming an increasingly popular practice. Like the teachers in schools discussed in the previous chapter, management itself must show leadership and model those healthy behaviors. Companies which are in tune with wellness are more likely to sponsor teams for community health events such as Relay for life, Race for the Cure, Easter Seals, March of Dimes, disaster relief and dozens of other very worthy causes. This makes for excellent public relations by raising the company profile in the community as well as advancing a sense of esprit-de-corps among its workers.

Industry and popular magazines rate companies in different spheres of worker friendliness. Having such a reputation in regards to healthcare is advantageous when it comes to retaining talent and reducing replacement costs for injured or sick workers. Taken together, these initiatives say to the workers, "We care." Studies show that use of fun prizes such as romantic getaway packages or direct cash bonuses has doubled over the past 20 years. Non-monetary incentives, however, such as *employee of the month* recognition and privileged parking spaces can be just as effective in supporting healthy lifestyle changes. Reasonably applied, such benefits do not break the bank, but rather go a long way in improving overall job satisfaction.

Statistics clearly show that obesity-related diseases now constitute a fat slice of health expenditure. These substantially impact our corporate job security and in turn the prosperity of our communities. Whatever the workplace setting, the ideas discussed above empower employees to engage constructively in their own healthcare.

We accept that at no time will everyone in society be 100 percent shipshape. To some extent, we will always bear each other's burdens. However, it is simply unacceptable that so many of us are just letting ourselves go. In an economy with escalating pressures on health budgets, the wise choice is to make a paradigm shift. When management decides to raise the bar to a new level of corporate wellness, we do not expect specimens of fitness like a football team or platoon of Army Rangers. However, despite all the whining and howls of protests, in due time, the average health surely begins to creep upward.

However bluntly, the Weyco story at the beginning of the chapter speaks directly to this issue. Being an insurance business itself probably had something to do with seeing clearly how worker health impacts profits. Workers not taking advantage were on their own. Corporations are in the business of maximizing returns on investment. In effect, a sound wellness program can set the example for the wider society of in regards to one's personal responsibility to improve overall health standards.

Do not go where the path may lead.
Go instead where there is no path
and leave a trail.

Ralph Waldo Emerson

273

REVIEW

1. Name two of the most important components in workplace wellness today.

2. What are the main differences between health insurance and workplace wellness?

3. What advantage does the workplace have in reaching individuals with health messages?

4. What are the best ways to improve worker participation in wellness programs?

5. How does corporate wellness in the United States compare to Canada, Britain and the Asian economies?

Chapter 19

Community Weight Loss

Friendship is born at that moment when one person says to another, "What! You too? I thought I was the only one!"

C. S. Lewis

Author, The Lion, the Witch and the Wardrobe

An American professor traveling through Europe described how his train made a stop at a station outside Paris. Boarding passengers struggled between the aisles, squeezing all their luggage into the overhead compartments. These newcomers really look a lot, lot heavier than everyone else, he mused. It was only upon hearing their familiar accents that it dawned on him where every single one was from.

Meanwhile, visitors stateside proudly pose for photos in front of the famous landmarks and towering testaments to American ingenuity. Yet, what they find most striking is that this is a land of really supersized people. In their countries, no effort is spared in attracting the US tourist dollar. However there is increasing annoyance at having to 'expand' their facilities specifically for the increasing girth of their guests. Global public accommodations were traditionally 18 inches wide. Now, even British parliamentarians are on record complaining over the need to replace seating in historic theaters. Reversing this dubious distinction among the community of nations is not a job for the individual.

Group Action

Geese flying gracefully overhead have long moved artists to reach for their brushes. This poetry in motion is also driving scientists to take a closer look. They have discovered that flying in this unique V formation actually *reduces* wind *resistance*. Flocks are therefore able to fly almost twice as far as each bird could do on its own! A wayward goose immediately feels the difference and quickly gets back with the program - if he wants to make it. Modern sports physiologists instruct their racers how use to this principle. Whether it is track, swimming, cycle or auto, *coast* behind competitors and let them break up the air ahead. Take advantage of this facilitated aerodynamics (or the "wake," in case of water sports), and then at some strategic point, make your move.

Humans tend to be more individualistic and competitive. Somebody has to win and somebody has to lose. Nature however, teaches teamwork. When the lead goose gets tired, it democratically drops back and another rotates up to become the "tip of the spear." No one gets burned out as the whole flock gets from point A to point B. This indeed, is the pattern for true community wellness!

Commercial weight management programs are propelled by pure profit motive predicated on the preferences of the *individual* buyer. On the other hand, those motivated by a higher calling see in the obesity epidemic a golden opportunity to pursue the common good. Like the flock in full flight, connecting like-minded people is essential in making a lasting impact. It would surprise you how many people share that exact, same desire percolating in your heart this very moment. Could it be that you are one of those called to provide leadership in this area? In order to do this, let us examine the main components of effective community weight loss programs. This will equip us to secure ongoing inspiration in order to maintain massive group action.

The Bucyrus Benchmark

"It only takes a spark to get the fire going." When a distinct group makes a concerted move toward fitness, it is like a tide that raises all ships. By joining forces, we create *synergy*. This is the marvelous math of doubling or tripling our effectiveness. 1+1 no longer is just equal to 2 or even 3, but 4 or more! Synergy and success come from support. When one person gets distracted and discouraged, another must be ready to step up to the plate.

Tammi Wolfe did just that. As manager of the Bucyrus Community Hospital Cardiopulmonary Rehab department, she landed a $25,500 state grant designed to help rural communities with healthy lifestyle changes. This was a big deal for this small northwest Ohio town and serves as a fine example of how far any community can go when working together. Ms. Wolf formed a team to plan and implement the program. The message was simple: it is virtually impossible for anyone walking a *total* of 10,000 steps or five miles a day to be obese. In our push-button/drive-through society, most of us do about 1000 to 3000, (thewalkingsite.com). It turns out that by doing just about an additional **mile a day** will keep us fit and trim. The committee distributed digital pedometers for participants to make up the deficit with purposeful daily walking. Grant money was also used in part to purchase T-shirts and packets explaining the program. The Chamber of Commerce joined in to kick off a *Buff-Up Bucyrus* afternoon lawn party.

The emphasis was on lifestyle modification, not just weight loss. When I interviewed Ms. Wolfe and her staff, she pointed to the small incentives used to stimulate interest. Participants keeping records of how much and how often they walked were eligible to win prizes from area businesses. The program generated a kind of excitement such as Bucyrus had never seen. As the word got out, so many more people wanted to come on board that organizers were forced to announce a moratorium to keep things manageable.

> *The best lack conviction while the worse is full of passionate intensity.*
>
> **William Butler Yeats**

Weight Loss Fundamentals

The format of community weight loss is simple and straightforward. Avoid the exotic features of different diets such as those based on imbalance of foods. Every major responsible health organization advocates the following principles:

1. Make time for personal exercise.
2. Renounce oversized portions.
3. Eat more fruits, vegetables and whole grains.
4. Cut your intake of saturated/trans fats and cholesterol.
5. Strive for healthy emotional responses to negative events.
6. Monitor total calories, not just "carbs."
7. Secure that critical ingredient of support.

Earlier chapters dealt with the first six points. Here is an example why point # 7 is so important:

72 year-old Grace R., a retired librarian from across the state, was bedridden at over 650 pounds. An only child who never married, she took pride in having cared for her parents at home. I

was consulted as a surgeon to treat her large leg ulcer. Healing took place over several weeks of debridement, special dressing changes and antibiotics. She shared with me some of her treasured books and bemoaned the general decline in reading among the youth. However, it soon became evident that no one had systematically tackled her weight problem. She definitely was not interested in obesity surgery; neither would she be considered a candidate at her age.

Using Manna*fast* principles, we worked with Grace in the obesity unit to shed 370-plus pounds. With intensive physical therapy, she developed the strength to care for herself and walk again. She said she felt 30 years younger, never having been close to that weight most of her adult life. Grace would weep with joy each time she reflected on what she accomplished. "I just wish my parents could see me now!" Those words flashed a light bulb in my mind. Grace knew I could not manage her case forever. Anyone could do this with the right help. She was longing for someone close to validate her progress. She was crying out for *a group in her own community setting* to help celebrate and secure her success.

Communal Weigh In

Out of control obesity thrives on denial. I can just hear the objections. "Come on, Doc. Are you kidding me! Even skinny people have problems getting on a scale in public; far less those with a little weight!" True, getting weighed is perhaps one of the more amusing dramas in the physician's office. Some flat out refuse. Others carry on as if it were a sacred right of privacy – such as confession or casting a secret ballot. Some try to hide the results even from the nurse! Several would excuse themselves to the bathroom. Upon their return, they would think for a few moments and remove their shoes, empty their pockets

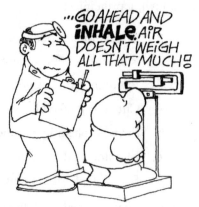

and ponder whatever else they could shed and still remain decent. On occasion, they vigorously argue that the result is different from their home scale or another physician's office.

19. Community Weight Loss

Granted, people are very finicky about their weight. In fact we make every effort to safeguard their dignity. That is precisely why the *Great American Weigh-In* sponsored by the American Cancer Society (ACS) is such a radical concept. As we saw in Chapter 4, ACS now clearly classifies obesity as a cancer risk. The weigh-in is therefore based on the *Great American Smoke Out.* Over the past 30 years, this highly effective campaign has given

> *Hand wash hand*
> *mek hand come clean.*
>
> Guyanese proverb
> (More is accomplished
> through cooperation).

smokers a unique opportunity to quit. Like checking on smoke detectors with changing of daylight savings time, each March 5th now serves as an annual reminder for every American to get on the scale.

Taking stock of health from a communal standpoint provides that much-needed reality check. It often triggers a renewed commitment to personal fitness. Take advantage of many helpful groups which are free or almost free. While neighborhood walking or cycling clubs may be available, *Covenant groups* go deeper. They are based on altruism rather that just self-interest. They are based on encouraging others and making our community a better place.

Starting a Community Program

Obesity is today's 'leprosy.' It is finally getting the amount of attention it deserves, though not always the right kind. TV reality shows like "The Biggest Loser" portray the drama of weight loss as entertainment. It also tends to be voyeuristic and demeaning. Producers go for the sensational. It ramps up ratings to get the viewer to say "Wow, did you see how huge that fat guy was!" Ironically, people hate being stared at, even when they get paid for their 15 minutes of fame. The proliferation of websites geared to obesity are helpful, but not a replacement. The internet is excellent at connecting people and transmitting information. However, it lacks oversight and professional accountability. An eager blogger cannot be prevented from transmitting lots of harmful information. Furthermore, these various media lack the personal warmth and caring that can only come from the physical presence of trusted human beings.

Anybody can start a community weight loss program. You certainly do not need a personal background in the field of health, athletics or social service. However, it is strongly advised to make connections with local professionals and agencies. Start with a small group of committed people who are willing to work and communicate. This is your *steering committee*. This group will draw up plans and identify resources. As you start having regular meetings, invite others who may be outside your circle of friends. Everywhere, people are feeling the pain of obesity. It often happens that those least expected to support community activities turn out to be your biggest assets.

Follow Up

Fully expect the response to be poor at first. It is important to try your level best at being inclusive. As you reach out, get telephone numbers and emails. Consider setting up an online bulletin board. Secure sponsors, but do not allow your idea to be hijacked by big businesses that may seek to profit more than they contribute. Remind yourself that you're doing this for the people. Service organizations such as Lions, Rotary and Kiwanis, Amvets, churches, newspapers and radio are generally quite supportive of genuine, non-profit community projects. Their public service announcements are excellent ways to get the word out.

A church initiative in Denver, Colorado used hymns to focus on walking. Lyrics such as "Show me how to *walk* in Thy Word," When we *walk*

> *If you run out of gas, everyone travelling with you is stranded.*
>
> Rev. T.D. Jakes

with the Lord" encouraged walking an additional 2000 steps (one mile) a day. That is equivalent to burning an extra 100 calories. It is no surprise therefore that Colorado takes first place in fitness by having a population that is only 14.9 percent obese. These good folks know it makes absolutely no sense to say, "I can't lose weight." They eventually come to the point of accepting, "For whatever reason, I cannot or have not been doing my mile-a-day."

Everybody Loves a Parade

This chapter is all about how we motivate people to do just that. To change society, we have to go public. All communities have parades. Nothing beats the pride of organized groups in sparkling uniforms marching to the beat of rousing music. Besides Independence Day, there may be a St. Patrick's, Heritage Festival or Thanksgiving parade. Your community wellness group can sign up marchers. If you put together a float, make sure you take turns walking. Your general theme is celebrating health. Make it a day for the handicapped who refuse to be sidelined, for families to celebrate their centenarians who can still get around, for the obese who are working on their weight. Every day, brave social workers, visiting nurses, and emergency personnel venture into depressed and dangerous neighborhoods. Highlight their work. Tie it in with a health fair after the parade. Contact vendors interested in providing free screenings in return for publicity. Select as grand marshal a newsworthy survivor or teacher, valedictorian or area sports champion, pharmacist or therapist, officer or firefighter, nurse or doctor, who has really made a difference. Anyone who has captured the hearts and minds of the community in the past year can help us gel around a common theme. Even your top weight loser could lay claim to this coveted honor to be an inspiration to others.

Putting Others First

Serving as Battalion Surgeon for this Army Reserve unit out of Toledo Ohio, afforded me a virtual field laboratory for observing human behavior. The 983rd Combat Engineers were a different breed from the medical professionals and clerical staff I traditionally worked with on the civilian side. These were blue-collar carpenters, masons, bulldozer operators, electricians, construction workers etc. The mission of our support unit was to enter a hostile theater of action to secure access roads, construct bridges and fortify defenses.

I soon came to appreciate a strict hierarchy among the various military services: Navy: adventure; Coast Guard: lifesavers; Air Force: above the rest. However, Army (infantry and armored cavalry) consider themselves the 'boots on the ground,' the gung-ho, 'real soldiers,' licensed to break things and kill people. They carried themselves with the bravado of the ancient gladiators' oath, "We who are about to die, salute you!" There was something deeply spiritual about caring for such warriors, who once pointed in a certain direction, did what they had to do. Yet I took pride in being associated with the part of the Army dedicated to *build things and heal people.*

I recall my first meal with my unit on annual training after officer boot camp. It was a long convoy out to this hot and dusty undisclosed location. Lunch was quite delayed, but unlike many others, I had followed orders and had not brought along any snacks. Chips and candy bars never looked so good.

I tried in vain to quell the rumbling in my stomach. When chow was finally ready, I was by no means the first in line, but I did not see any reason to be the last either. The troops were irritable. And others kept cutting ahead of me as I responded to impromptu medical concerns, setting up appointments for my field ambulance. From time to time, I cast an eager eye ahead, willing the process along. Suddenly, everyone was on their best behavior. It soon became clear - the Commanding Officer was approaching. And he was coming directly to where I was. I snapped a crisp salute.

"At ease, Doc." He placed his hand on my shoulder. It sounded important. He leaned over and whispered with a smile, "Enlisted men first."

It took several awkward seconds for it to register. Oops. I discretely followed him to the back of the line where all the officers were talking shop. Stomachs were distinctly rumbling back here too, but it was the privilege of being an officer to be in control.

From that vantage point I was able to observe how the tension in the air subsided as the troops were served. What a wonderful sedative food is! I guess that is why they say a hungry man is an angry man. Relaxed laughter replaced griping and fretting as the soldiers fanned out to mingle with buddies. Some sought solitude in the shade to savor their sustenance. Others poked fun at what Uncle Sam had to offer. Meals Ready to Eat (MRE's) preserved in handy olive-green plastic packets. Processed grub never comes close to Mom's cooking, but it definitely hit the spot. School cafeteria-like camaraderie blossomed as patriots traded mashed potatoes and gravy for rice 'n beans and swapped brownies for peanut butter and jelly sandwiches.

I also learned a very important leadership principle that day. Just as the captain of a ship is the last to bail out, put the welfare of those in your charge ahead of yours. During regular worship service, we have a separate ministry for children in the fellowship hall. Although there is no hint of starvation, kids pay serious attention to their snacks. As basic Bible lesson, each is afforded a unique opportunity. They get to serve the munchies, decide who will ask the blessing and to have *the privilege of being the last to eat*. Maybe someday, someone will look back and say, "All I needed to know about how to live, I learned in Junior Church!" What a talent to be able to calm those digestive secretions and exaggerated fears that the goodies may be gone before your turn comes around!

As Chief Medical Officer of my unit, a major task was to monitor the fitness of our troops. Many had grown accustomed to the security offered by the Department of Defense. Overweight soldiers really wanting to qualify for those good retirement benefits simply do what it takes to shape up or ship out. Not once did I hear, "I just can't lose weight." Not once. In contrast, civilian life offers certain rewards. Without the challenge of periodic fitness checks, the super obese end up on disability. Society steps in with motorized scooters and aids for household help. Thereafter, they never walk again. Without the substantive accompanying programs to treat the condition, obesity consumes an ever larger portion of the health care pie. The weight-challenged are in effect enabled and subsidized by the taxes of those making the effort to take good care of themselves.

Military weight loss programs work because there are real consequences to failing. Another important reason is the knowledge that whether officer or enlisted, we are all in it together. We are very much a community. Leaving no soldier behind is not just a slogan. This is the sense of interdependence that I strive to infuse in all my patients. They leave my office consultation motivated to connect with others in their own communities. This must be their source of sustaining support till our next appointment, or until such time that they can soar on their own.

Ancient Rome imploded under the sheer weight of its own excesses. The Latin phrase: *Nobis fabula narratur,* translates into "Their story is our story." History provides ample indicators of our collective fate if we as a people neglect the opportunity to take corrective action. It is no longer just about you or me individually. Many in society have allowed themselves to grow more out of shape than ever thought possible. The experience of the traveling professor left him no doubt what was needed to reverse the way we are perceived overseas.

In the clash of cultures, we are encumbered by our own weight. What one accomplishes in a private fitness program is all well and good. However, in a season of tightening budgets, the health of our fellow citizens directly impacts our own. A candle lighting another loses nothing; rather all gain more light. Military, corporate and church programs show impressive success when working collectively. The call today is for true *Christian Soldiers*, unlike the conquistadors of old or religions today that impose conformity under threat of sword or bomb. Instead, they nurture integrity by covenanting together to bring their appetites under subjection. What a rush it is inspiring others to achieve the same! Like that flock of geese at the beginning of the chapter, this just may be your time to be the "tip of the spear" for your community.

It don't mean a thing

if it ain't got that swing!

Duke Ellington

283

REVIEW

1. How would you compare community weight loss activities to efforts to reduce smoking?

2. What did Buff-Up Bucyrus and the Denver Church Initiative have in common?

3. What would be the advantage of combining a health fair with a wellness parade?

4. Give one example of group action for a common goal with which you have been or can be involved.

5. Name two issues targeted by community weight loss programs

Chapter 20

One Love

In the presence of hope, faith is born.
In the presence of faith, love becomes a possibility.
In the presence of love, miracles happen!

Rev. Robert Schuller
The Hour of Power

A total waste of time, Phyllis thought, as she and Jessica approached the duplex. With all the two had gone through with their weight problems, she seriously doubted that there was much else this Covenant Group thing could offer that they had not already heard. To be perfectly honest, they were a bit uneasy as to what was in store for them. More tasteless recipes, laying on of hands or some kind of whiny singing of *Kumbaya?* Jessica, at least, was somewhat intrigued. Whatever it was, these meetings sure seemed to be doing Felicia a lot of good. People at work could not help but notice those changes. That girl was really pumped!

Transformations

The door boasted a lovely arrangement with a seasonal theme to it. As Jessica reached for the buzzer, it swung open.

"Guys they're here! Let's get started."

Excited faces crowded the door: Nicole and Daphne from church, Jenny from work and someone else, the one in front, whom she could not quite place. Her T-shirt sported a faded photo of this really swollen, sad-looking woman. Below the picture was printed 2001.

"Hi, I'm Vicki. Glad y'all could come!"

"Oh, Vicki! I heard so much about you."

"All good I hope!" With a grand flourish, she waved them into the modest but elegant residence. Pictures of Vicki's family were everywhere. Her sons' pennants and other sports artifacts gave the home a distinct macho image. Four other women and two men rose to greet the newcomers, exchanging names and gentle hugs. Fresh-cut flowers adorned the table neatly set with embroidered place mats and fine china. The treadmill folded up in the corner looked somewhat out of place.

"Everything looks so nice!" Phyllis observed approvingly.

"You know what, these were wedding gifts. Can you believe this is the first time we're using them?"

"Really?!"

"Oh yeah, I am so into tea these days. I am having camomile this evening; how about you? We also have peppermint, Lipton, Countrytime, orange pekoe, green tea, Earl Gray - take your pick."

"Hmm. I think I'll try green tea," Phyllis flashed her million-dollar smile. "It has lots of antioxidants, right?"

"That it does," replied Vicki eagerly. Phyllis glanced at the T-shirt again. There was some resemblance. But before she could say anything, Vicki turned to her other guest. "How about you, Jessica?"

"Choices, choices, choices," Jessica sang softly. "That camomile - I heard something special about it; can't remember..."

"Well, it's supposed to settle the stomach, but it's also a relaxer. I like that. It helps me sleep."

"Sounds great! Think I'll try it."

Larry and Brandon were the only males there. They had reconciled themselves to the fact that in any program dealing with weight, women would win by a landslide. And you know what? They didn't seem to mind all the attention. Brandon walked over to Phyllis with a tag and marker to write her name.

"Welcome Ma'am! Brandon's the name. What's yours?" He had this deep drawl with a hint of a Southern accent.

"Hey watch it! Makes me feel old." She elbowed him jokingly. He shrugged, stammered and smiled. "Anyway, I'm Phyllis. And this is my friend Jess."

"Nice green outfit," Brandon bounced back, "If I remember correctly, one of the actresses had on something like that at the Oscars just last week. Can't remember her name, do you?"

Phyllis shook her head slowly, blushing. "Some line there...Brandon. Thank you anyway."

"Oh, come on. I didn't mean it that way. It's the color that struck me... Okay, how would you call it?"

"Well, if you have to know it's *chartreuse*."

"Chartreuse? What's that?"

"Just something between a yellowish teal and lime green." Phyllis teased. "Got to know your colors, Brandon. See that blouse she's wearing? Would you call that pink or mauve?"

"Don't even go there, my brother!" It was Larry to the rescue. "You know, that's the problem with them gals. They just don't know how to call something red or green or blue. Know what I'm saying?!" The guys roared with laughter, high-fiving and punching each other's clenched fists.

"Tell me about it!"

Jessica definitely was not the *I'm-here!-Let-the-party-begin*! kind of person. She eased her arm around her friend's shoulder, trying to think of something witty to throw into the ring. That's Phyllis for you, she thought. She was hardly there five minutes and already she had the guys going!

Just then, Vicki plopped down into the cushy sofa and called the meeting to order. The chatter quickly quieted down. "Larry, why don't you open in prayer?" Larry paused. Vicki continued. "While you're thinking about it, here goes: Lord, help us to be what we know we should be. Amen."

"Hey! I didn't say I was not going to pray."

"Like I said guys; we don't need a sermon. Snooze you lose - chop chop!" Laughter erupted across the room. Jessica was not sure what Phyllis was thinking, but there was an unmistakable atmosphere of friendliness, sincerity, and focus in this group. Already, she was feeling quite comfortable, part of something bigger than her shakey efforts at self-improvement.

Vicki tapped briskly on her pad. "Alright folks, this is our fourth weekly meeting and we have many good things to report. As you know, I teach at Washington Elementary. The boys're in the basement doing their homework - I think...and Dave, well, he's not back from work yet. Anyway, he reminded me to tell you how much he enjoys having you guys over. That makes the boys and me pick up the house!" This elicited knowing smiles all around.

Vicki paused to sip her hot tea, sticking out her pinky with an air of sophistication. She talked briefly of how she ballooned out of control after the birth of her second son. She mentioned something about undiagnosed post-partum depression and how she snapped out of it after her closest cousin went down on United Flight 93. The newcomers listened with rapt attention to how she was able to overcome her weight problem and committed herself to helping others do the same. This lean, take-charge, dynamo of a woman sitting there, hardly looked anything like that picture on the T-shirt.

As others worked on their juice, coffee or bottled water, Vicki introduced the remainder of the group. First was Shirley, a bank manager.

A recently diagnosed diabetic, Shirley brought homemade low-cal chocolate chip cookies. They were so delightfully scrumptious that she found herself getting defensive about the recipe and the hospital website where she downloaded it. It was a compliment, but Shirley was taking it the wrong way. Vicki explained to the newcomers that they usually had some fun with this part of the meeting: the practical tip for the week. There was always something new from the Cleveland Clinic, Mayo Clinic, Web MD, etc. In any case, a cookie here or there was not going to ruin one's weight program, she opined.

"Hi, I'm Daphne." Like some A.A. meeting, the group chorused back encouragingly, "Hi Daphne!" She hesitantly described her week. She was a very private person, timid even. However, she felt the meetings were useful in keeping her on track. She stuck to the basic script: controlling snacks, exercise, pounds lost; thank you. Vicki took the opportunity to remind them to dwell on the optimism of overcoming, rather than going on and on the negativity of their former condition.

Jessica felt eager to tell her story. Phyllis, on the other hand, dreaded having to open up about her surgery. People always seemed to react in a jealous way. They would look at her as if she was so lucky, cheated or took the easy way out. If only they knew. In any case, they were the new kids on the block. Perhaps it was best waiting to get a good sense as to how much people were saying, (or not saying) about themselves. There was definitely more to this meeting than the typical group therapy session. Whatever happened during the rest of the meeting, she was happy they made the effort to attend.

More Blessed to Give

"Hi, I'm Jennifer." She was a part-time nurse, mother of two, who worked third shift. From what she said, there was little doubt that she was perhaps the one making the biggest sacrifice. This was the time she would normally be taking her nap before heading to work. She was the group's medical advisor responsible for facilitating seamless communication with their associate physician. Quite the talker, Jenny told of the fun she was having with her *Mannameter.* It reminded her of grading her own tests at school. She also proudly reported having lost 8 pounds since the start of the program and how people were already making positive comments. Dr. Pellegrino was a perfect example. A prosperous-looking orthopedist working on her surgical ward, he just blurted out one day, "You're too energetic and contented these days. Tell me, something happened last weekend?!" The unit secretary stifled a giggle. When she ventured to ask him what made him say that, he conceded that he could not quite put his finger on it.

An aggressive surgeon, Dr. Pellegrino was known for his motto, "We get all the breaks." He was given to boasting to any who would listen about his yacht at Hilton Head and his timeshare on the slopes of Aspen, Colorado. Recovering from a recent angioplasty, he must have seen something in her that he himself was lacking. As far as she could recall, those were actually the kindest words she had ever heard from his mouth. So she took that as a big positive. For her part, Jennifer made a very interesting comment: After working so hard taking care of others, it was nice finally focusing on her own self for a change.

"Hi, I'm Larry..." At 48 years of age, with the last 15 stuck in the shipping office, he had given up on many of his life's fondest dreams. Larry did not talk much about his wife except to say that she was always nagging him about seeing the doctor. The best life insurance for the kids is having him around, was her constant refrain. One day she wanted him to go walking, another day she was trying out some exotic vegetarian recipe. When he finally broke down and kept the appointment that she made for him, the doctor's warning strangely echoed hers. As far as he was concerned, since he was started on just one pill, he was fine. He went along his merry way, even taking pride in the fact that there were many others in worse shape than he was. He never paid his wife any mind until one of his friends at work suddenly keeled over at his desk - just like that!

Larry told of how he cut back on surfing the net and TV late at night and starting setting his alarm one hour earlier. He never thought he would be able to make that sacrifice, but after a while it was not like pulling teeth anymore. Before, he barely had time to jump from his warm bed into the shower, grabbing a bite as he rushed out of the door. Now he started off with exercise and writing down his plans for the day. After all, his son was on a rigid high school sports training schedule and was only too proud to give the old man some fitness pointers. Having smoked all his life, Larry did not feel quite ready to deal with that. He did start rolling his own cigarettes because of expense. He found that it actually slowed him down some, making him more aware of the habit. He did quit though, drinking so much soda.

Since the incident at work, everyone seemed to be talking about whether management would finally put together that wellness program. Larry knew he had a lead on them. It did not bother him one bit when his co-workers would tease him about the bottled water he carried all the time. All he knew was that he was feeling so much better about himself. With his 4 ½ pound weight loss, he laid claim to the 'loser of the week' prize. It was just a little gag gift from his Covenant Group, but had so much meaning for him. Now here he was inviting guys to the meeting. Apart from Brandon, others had promised to check it out

> *You make a living by what you get, you make a life by what you give.*
> Tennis star, Arthur Ashe

but none had shown up yet. Anyway, he took that opportunity to caution against nagging people because, at least for him, it seemed to build up more resistance.

"Hi, I'm Brandon. You know me. I'm the quiet one." Jessica and Phyllis gave each other that 'Yeah right look.' However, they soon found his contribution to be more than just interesting. Attending a meeting like this was part of a larger effort to re-define himself. All his life, he worked in this rural factory making bathroom fixtures where his father and grandfather had worked before. Now the company was downsizing and suddenly he found himself on unemployment. Naturally, that caused a lot of resentment. He began paying a lot more attention to what was going on in the world nowadays. At one time he ate, slept and dreamed NASCAR, but now he was channeling more of his time and energy into retraining and adult education classes. The local university really helped him appreciate and learn how to get along with folks from different backgrounds. Although few people would believe it a couple months before, he had succeeded in giving up drinking a case of beer each week. He would be the first to say that switching to a low carb brand did nothing for his belly.

Brandon was the one who came up with the idea of donating a dollar for each pound lost. He collected the subscription and led the discussion as to which charity or disaster relief the group would donate to each week. He called it *Pound for Pound*. Ironically, the more one lost, the more one gave. It was just a few more bucks to part with, but they did so cheerfully. The winner earned special stickers, bragging rights and kudos from those he inspired. Brandon topped off his remarks by throwing out for discussion a question he would get asked from time to time: "If I regain the weight, do I get my money back?!"

Recipe for Romance

"Hi, I'm Marcia..." She was anxious about not being left behind. Her breakup with her boyfriend had done a number on her. "Maybe he just wasn't the right guy for me," she sighed. For the first time the visitors felt a little bit like strangers. It was obvious that they had come in the middle of something. "Better find out now than later, honey," Cleo chipped in. As the more mature, divorced mother with a couple kids out of college, Cleo would come up with some seasoned words of wisdom which always seemed right on time. She reached over and hugged Marcia. Everyone went: "Ohhhhh."

Marcia dabbed her eyes, smiling bravely. Larry fiddled with the handout, leaned back, waiting out this touchy-feely segment. Whatever she was going to say just smacked of guy-bashing. Brandon supported his jaw with his arm propped up on the side of the sofa. He found that kind of soap opera mush rather boring. It would be hard picturing his former drinking buddies sitting still for all that stuff.

Nevertheless Marcia had piqued the group's interest. She related how, before, in a situation like this, she would just buy a tub of her favorite butter pecan ice cream. It would be gone in one sitting while listening to Gloria Gaynor's *I will Survive,* over and over again. "This time I picked up a couple books from the library and hit the treadmill - something like this."

It was her turn to do the exercise demo. She got up and unfolded the treadmill, leading the group in a few minutes of stretching. She set the machine to a gentle trot and resumed her story of love lost.

"Go Marcia, Go!" The group cheered.

"Ain't nobody gonna stop me now..." She huffed between breaths. "...I did this for about 20 minutes." She fixed her headband, her face now glistening with sweat. "Then I had a nice long bath...scented candles... a good romance book...the works...I kept telling myself...I'm not the first...to go through this...girlfriend...that workout felt...soooo good." She got a warm round of applause as she dismounted. "I never felt so motivated to exercise in my life!"

Marcia knew she was on a roll. "I don't know what I'd do without these guys," she whispered to the newcomers as she patted her brow. As the group weighed-in and recorded their waist and hip measurements, they discussed their cholesterol reports (they actually had copies!) There was talk about planned Covenant health screenings and new ways to cooperate with physicians to save on health costs.

Marcia could tell that the visitors would soak up her story. In hushed whispers she shared how she had met this guy Mark, online. She really thought he would have been different. When filling out the part of the dating form requesting body size information, she had clicked 'rather not say.' She knew it would be a fib to check 'athletic' or even 'average.' But with a good man so hard to find, she said there was no way she would wreck her chances by admitting she was 'ample.'

Whatever, something in her unfinished profile had attracted this interesting response. She could not believe she found a match so compatible in her own zip code. She herself was a bit 'gun shy' at first, holding back when he kept asking her to email him a picture. She claimed she did not know how to add an attachment. And even when he took the time to explain in detail, she kept putting it off by saying she wasn't a geek. She reminisced on the last wedding she attended. She even dared to think that she should have joined the girls clamoring to catch the bouquet.

Marcia was virtually holding her breath at the thought that she had finally met someone for whom weight was not an issue. Mark himself had boasted that he did regular sit-ups since his stint in the military and that he had six pack abs. According to her, he still had something of a gut on him, but hey, who's perfect? Apart from that, everything else he said seemed right on the money. She did get a good dose of reality, however, during their first date. He just did not seem to have the enthusiasm that simply oozed out of his e-mails. More disturbing, she could not help but notice how his eyes would wander away when a slimmer, more attractive woman walked by. She might as well have been talking to a fly on the wall.

She came to the conclusion that perhaps that kind of behavior came from just having a Y chromosome. One of her favorite Broadway musicals came to mind. In *The King and I*, Yul Brynner as the King of Siam expounded, "A man is like a bee going from flower to flower." Was Mark just being a typical male? In any case, they continued to meet and would have a decent time. Each date, though, seemed to end with that familiar quick peck on the cheek, and empty promises to call the next day. He was always the perfect gentleman, yet deep down she wondered, perhaps a little too perfect for her liking.

It did not take long for her to figure out the pattern. She developed her own pattern as well after a while. Despite his inducements to eat up when they went out for dinner, she stuck to her Caesar salad. The moment the door closed behind him though, she would hit the refrigerator. When at last she decided to confront him about the size issue, she was pleasantly surprised when he replied that it did not bother him one bit. He told her with a straight face that he had fallen in love with who she was as a person and what the scale said had nothing to do with it. That question seemed to bring out more warmth and caring in him. She was so relieved to get this out of the way. It was like a dream come true: A working man who did not smoke, do drugs or experiment with other lifestyles. At first she was excited to diet and exercise. Gradually she gave that up as there just did not seem to be enough hours in the day. As soon as she was convinced that he was no longer looking at her through wide-angled lenses, she once again became casual about her size.

However, one evening he did not call as promised. After hours of worrying, she decided to go to a grocery store a little further from her neighborhood which was having a really good sale. As she was unloading her shopping cart in the parking lot, she happened to notice a couple casually strolling on the other side of the row of vehicles. They were laughing playfully with each other. As she got behind the wheel, something about the way the man moved caught her attention.

She nervously circled around. Cars behind her searching for parking spots honked impatiently as she slowed to a crawl. Her eyes pierced the subdued lighting. Oh no! Sure enough, it was Mark - and on his arm was this thing: someone with a carefree, girlish figure. The revealing tank top and belly-button ring did not help matters. Marcia stumped on the pedal and sped off angrily. It was all a blur as frightened shoppers scattered at the sudden screech of burning rubber. It just wasn't like her to be such a green-eyed monster. She always prided herself as being cool, calm and collected. Her reaction was scary. But this was too much. It really hurt.

Marcia told of spurning his emails and screening his calls. He even left a couple messages for her at work. In the weeks that followed she just felt numb. The walls seemed to be closing in on her. She knew that she needed to get out of her apartment. Perhaps a little shopping therapy at the mall would shake her from this funk. She always had a weakness for clothes, but even there a shock awaited her. Even the plus sizes that she once wore were way too tight. Marcia couldn't believe how much weight she had gained. The tears welled up as the fashionable outfits that beckoned her from the rack, now mocked her in a rumpled pile on the fitting room bench. Vicki's Covenant Group meeting invitation a few weeks before could not have come at a better time. She was so ready to lose this weight. This time she was not doing it for a man, but for herself.

Marcia had thought better of publicly burdening the group with all these sordid details. The pulsating rhythms of their theme song filtered softly in the background. She just could not get it out of her mind since that Caribbean cruise a couple years ago and had recommended it to the group. The lyrics of *One Love* by Reggae icon Bob Marley seemed to resonate with everything that she was going through:

> *Give thanks and praise to the Lord...*
> *Let's get together and feel all right.*

This covenant group was her lifeline. That was all she wanted - friends that she could count on. Friends who were not waiting for insurance plans to fix their health problems. Friends making the best of the Internet to take control of their own health. Her thoughts were interrupted by the chimes of the doorbell. They looked at each other in eager anticipation. Whose friend would it be to enter with a better-late-than-never story? Vicki skipped out of her chair to see who it was. She hesitated briefly. Could it be another Girl Scout cookie sales pitch or fund-raiser for the local volunteer fire department? It's so hard to turn them down, but this would really be bad timing...

"Support group? Sure! That would be right here!"

Everyone strained to see who it was. Marcia's heart nearly jumped out of her chest. It was Mark - and that other woman! How could he?!

"Hey Marcia, this is my sister, Angie," he announced, walking right up to her. "She insisted that I try meeting you here!"

No Turning Back

The proceedings of a Covenant Group meeting are as diverse and as fascinating as the individuals who attend. It is beyond what a physician, health club, or commercial diet program can offer. It is a magnet for real people, dealing with everyday issues, supporting each other's fight to overcome food addictions. It is a structured forum for exchanging weight loss tips on how to be a "Lasting Loser." A variety of ice-breaking games and fun activities can be used to balance the profound nature of its mission. It is a safe place for people to get out of their shell and share what is on their heart. Covenant Groups are based on the premise that a lonesome coal soon burns out, but together with others sustains a roaring fire. The only agenda is putting faith into action while keeping up with the latest that proven science has to offer.

The premise of this book is that anyone can achieve the level of self-control to transform his stomach for lasting weight loss. These Mannafast precepts pre-existed our indulgent generation by thousands of years. They surely will endure for eons to come. It may not have the splashy appeal of the fad diets, but it works. It will always be available as a sensible alternative for people of faith and reason.

The main challenge is how we get to the point of wanting to. *Planes of Progress* showed this to be an inherently spiritual process, a willingness to submit to the cosmic Wisdom as it sparks that desire in our hearts. From there, we analyzed the anatomy of the stomach, how it works and how to use it for us, not against us. We celebrated the marvelous talents of chefs who produce delightful delicacies to fan our gourmet appetites. At the same time we concluded that to the extent that we regularly consumed fruits, vegetables and less processed foods, the leaner and healthier we would be. We cannot indefinitely gulp down chemical sodas instead of water and natural juices and reasonably expect our body to be fountains of wellness. This is a message that we have to instill in our families, especially our children who are most at risk.

What Jesus Did

It is all well and good to speculate *what would Jesus do* in a particular situation, but perhaps it would be more useful to reflect on what He actually did. In His own words: "The Spirit of the Lord is upon me, because he has anointed me to preach the good news to the poor, He has sent me to heal the brokenhearted, to preach deliverance to the captives, to open the eyes of the blind, and to set at liberty those who are bruised." (Luke 4:18). It is also written that He "went about all Galilee, teaching in their synagogues, and preaching the gospel of the kingdom, and healing all manner of sickness and all manner of disease among the people" (Matthew 4: 23).

We see therefore that Jesus' ministry essentially involved preaching, teaching and healing. This is the example for every believer, not just ministers or physicians. *Preaching* is not limited to the wearing of ecclesiastic robes and pontificating behind a pulpit or in front a TV camera. In its most basic form, it is the simple act of communicating the Good News to those who would listen. More importantly it is responding to the quiet cries for help that each of us hear every day. A kind word of encouragement may be all it takes.

Not everyone will respond. Some of those who need it most are the ones more likely to set you up and break your heart. That was the case even in Jesus' ministry. The Lord Himself had twelve apostles - one sold out. That ratio: 11 out of 12 or little more than 90 percent turns out to be perhaps the best result that one can realistically expect. There are good people who will be warned, encouraged, begged to do something about their health to no avail. No doubt, you can think of a person like that right now. We are all on our way to meeting our Maker, but in our right minds, we all would all like to postpone that as long as possible. Yet, as a physician I am well-reconciled to the fact that regardless of my successes, I will lose some patients 'before their time.' It is consoling to say, "Those whom God loves die young." It is quite a different story when a life is cut short by self-inflicted disease. The sad fact is that in the race for wellness, the Devil takes the hindmost.

Your Mannafast Ministry

At no time should we burden ourselves with the notion that it is our sole responsibility to save the world. All that is expected of us is to share the Word without infringing on the rights of others for self-determination. Understand that we cannot do it alone. The Apostle Paul put it this way, "One planted, another watered, but God gave the increase" (I Corinthians 3:6). Just give it your level best with all your God-given grace and charm. Even the scoffers cannot help but come away with a little mustard seed of message. It's alright if someone else gets to see that seed finally land on fertile ground, take root, and bring forth much fruit. Indeed, we worship a God of second chances. Even when one makes a life-changing decision, that commitment must be nurtured and shielded from the negative influences seeking to overcome it. This is the *teaching* from which comes the *healing*.

Jesus taught that "Whatsoever things you ask when you pray, believe that you receive them and you will have them. (Mark 11:24). God always answers. When we pray for material and *external* things, His answers may not necessarily be the way we want. We cannot all have the perfect figure anymore than we can all be homecoming queen, MVP, valedictorian, employee of the month or CEO or American Idol. However, when we pray for *internal* or personal change, the outcome is likely to be 100 percent unless we stand in the way. Whenever we send out words of encouragement and wholeness, be assured that every single person is moved in a direction of improved health. Everybody wins. Those ministered to, get their physical lives turned around. The one doing the ministering is blessed by the fruits of his ministry. Just hearing someone say, "Thank you for helping me turn my life around," is simply priceless!

As we have seen, the obesity epidemic is a very real and present danger in today's society. Those overly challenged by weight suffer discrimination and depression, leading ultimately to disability and dependency. Many stop going out - even for medical care, because they are made to feel uncomfortable by those who should be helping them. One patient related to me how a doctor actually came out to the waiting room and ordered him to leave. When he asked why, she replied that he would break her chair. The patient protested that he had been to the office several times and never had problems with the chairs. But the doctor was adamant and discharged him from her practice anyway. Not surprisingly, it was not until admission to intensive care with advanced medical problems did this patient have any further contact with the health-care system.

It is a huge red flag when someone no longer goes out on account of weight. The time comes when even electric scooters cannot help with visits to family, church, shopping or other social functions. The morbidly obese disappear under radar, filling the dungeons of modern society faster than imaginable. One gentleman from about over 500 miles away grew so large that he became permanently confined to his living room sofa. When EMT's extracted him for the trip to our facility, he promptly went into respiratory distress. The doors had to be broken down so he could be transported *in his own sofa* - all the way to Ohio via semi. As soon as he was transferred into the bariatric bed, the same thing happened - he could not breathe. He required a tracheostomy for weeks of treatment in the ICU. Today, he has a new life after losing several hundred pounds.

Jesus was "moved with compassion" at the plight of the afflicted. So should we. What a ministry awaits the faithful when it dawns on them the needy mission field exists right on their own doorstep! The hospitality of opening one's home to Covenant Group meetings directly serves the needs of those who feel uncomfortable in settings that would otherwise be therapeutic. Privacy is respected and the aptitude of those with medical experience is cherished

In generations past, believers viewed the church as a spiritual emergency room. It was a place not only to find quiet time for their souls, but also refuge from the pressures of life. There, they would chance upon a man of the cloth for confession and counseling. For many who cannot afford a club membership, a personal trainer, a therapist or other committed health care professional, the church today is in a position to offer both prayerful support and holistic health exhortation. The church today longs for those who are persuaded that fitness and health of the temple of the Holy Spirit is a moral obligation. Society will look back and wonder why it took us so long to take the faith option, free of the risk, the pain and the expense.

That day begins as each church equips itself with the basics: a first aid kit, a blood pressure cuff. Larger congregations will also be equipped with high-tech devices like defibrillators now commonplace in public places like airports, concert halls and stadiums. As we accept the notion that dietary indiscretions and overweight is the leading cause of illness in our communities, we will want to add something radical like...well - a scale! What a testimony it is for a church to be known as one that offers not only a path to spiritual rebirth, but also to rebirth of health and vitality as well.

The Anointing

You probably heard about the three successful men raised by a single pious mother. They got to talking about how they had chosen to honor her for Mothers' Day. The first announced that he had built Mama a mansion. Not to be outdone the second boasted he provided Mama with a fully-loaded Mercedes complete with a chauffeur.

Feeling a bit self-conscious, the third son explained his gift this way. "You know Mama enjoyed reading Scripture. But her eyesight's bad now so I sent her a parrot that memorized the entire Bible. It took the Gideons 10 years to train it. All she has to do is just say the chapter and verse and the parrot recites it."

Having always taught her boys to be grateful, it was not long before Mama's thank you cards were in the mail.

"Jesse," she wrote, "I feel like a queen in a castle! However I only live in one room and I have to maintain the whole house."

To Dwayne she raved about how proud she felt in her Mercedes but confessed, "I'm too old to travel much and that driver does not even greet me. He just talks on his cell phone all the time."

But to her baby Tayshaun, Mamma wrote, "You're always the most thoughtful. *That little chicken you sent me was delicious!*"

As we have seen, throughout life, food rules center stage. Like fire, it is a wonderful servant but a terrible master. Mankind has been plagued by horrible scourges throughout history, but none as frustrating as the stronghold of obesity. Patients come to the doctor anticipating lectures to quit smoking, watch cholesterol, lose weight etc. Often they arrive solidly in pessimist mode, resentful about being herded through an increasingly impersonal assembly line. Their defenses are up. After being poked and prodded, they would rather just grab that prescription and call it a day. That is why a family member or friend is in such a better position to influence them in the right direction of fundamental lifestyle changes. Compared to the few minutes with the physician, loved ones have tons more time to keep on persuading through example and prayerful, gentle words.

20. One Love

Few concepts presented here are really new. All we claim to have done it to use the latest technology to apply the wisdom of the ages to a very modern and unique problem. We are now convinced that it is well within our ability to put food in its place and so transform our bodies back to what God intended. Beyond this, Manna*fast* fosters genuine, vibrant, self-reliance and the deep satisfaction of having contributed to the goodness in this world. From our results it is evident that we have not yet begun to see, to hear or to imagine, what can be accomplished by a dedicated group of believers committed to shaking up the world of healthcare as we know it.

We are now equipped to claim health and happiness as our inalienable right as children of the Kingdom. We are indeed "a chosen generation, a royal priesthood, a people set apart" (I Peter 2:9). It is not about an endless struggle to maintain, flapping our wings so hard to stay airborne. It is about simply spreading our wings out wide like the eagle and soaring on divine air currents. We come in different shapes and sizes, but today and henceforth, we come together against obesity.

The typical commercial vanity diet promotes a selfish attitude that says, "Look at me, don't I look good?!" It a one-size-fits-all approach that ignores individual medical/emotional history and pervasive eating disorders. Manna*fast* is tailored to you. It says, "With God's help, I'm unstoppable...and you can do it too!" Jessica and Phyllis learned how to use *Mannameter* to step up to higher planes of progress. Brad too, rough-and-tumble as he was, finally came to realize that being a man meant more than just bringing home a paycheck. He had to be there for his family. Their secret was finding reliable back-up. It's all about the Covenant.

Truly, in the presence of love, miracles happen. To the extent that we believe, we achieve. Many now sense the same stirrings that you and I now feel in our hearts. Let us find them. Christ proclaimed: "My food is to do the will of Him who sent me to finish His work" (John 4:34). Manna*fast* issues that same personal and powerful challenge to you. First secure your own anointed and abundant health. Then reach out. Touch the lives of others, and so fulfill the mission of our times.

May the Lord bless you and keep you:
May the love of God embrace you,
May He cause His face to shine upon you,
Be gracious unto you and give you peace.

Adapted from Numbers 6:24-26

Mannafast Miracle Order Form

May I Help?

Dear Dr. Sam,
I would like to help someone with *Mannafast Miracle*. Please send your elegantly packaged, personally autographed copy with the following inscription:

To: _____

Remarks: _____

_____

From: ☐ (Your name)   _____

☐ Someone who cares

☐ Blank

☐ Other   _____

Your email address _____

Delivery Address:

_____

_____

_____

Please copy and fill out the above information. Enclose a check for $25 (includes shipping and handling) with the order form and mail to:

Heartland Nutrition Institute
478 West Market Street,
Tiffin OH 44883

Shipments generally arrive within 2 weeks. For faster service, and further ideas on how to we can more effectively assist a loved one, or to start the professionally supervised program, log on to:

www.mannafast.org
or call 419 447-9313

Appendix

Target Weight for Healthy Females			
Height	Frame		
	Small	Medium	Large
4' 10"	101	116	131
4' 11"	104	119	134
5 feet	107	122	137
5' 1"	110	125	140
5' 2"	113	128	143
5' 3"	116	131	146
5' 4"	119	134	149
5' 5"	122	137	152
5' 6"	125	140	155
5' 7"	128	143	158
5' 8"	131	146	161
5' 9"	134	149	164
5' 10"	137	152	167
5' 11"	140	155	170
6 feet	143	158	173
6' 1"	146	161	176
6' 2"	149	164	179
6' 3"	152	167	182
6' 4"	155	170	185

Target Weights for Healthy Males			
Height	Frame		
	Small	Medium	Large
4' 10"	99	114	129
4' 11"	103	118	133
5 feet	107	122	137
5' 1"	111	126	141
5' 2"	115	130	145
5' 3"	119	134	149
5' 4"	123	138	153
5' 5"	127	142	157
5' 6"	131	146	161
5' 7"	135	150	165
5' 8"	139	154	169
5' 9"	143	158	173
5' 10"	147	162	177
5' 11"	151	166	181
6 feet	155	170	185
6' 1"	159	174	189
6' 2"	163	178	193
6' 3"	167	182	197
6' 4"	171	186	201

Heartland Nutrition Institute

Contact Information

Name_____ Date of Birth_____

Today's Date_____

Referring or Family Dr._____ Dr's Tel. #_____

Your street address_____

City_____ State, zip_____

Telephone #'s: Home_____ Cell_____

Employer or school_____ Work/school # _____

Email_____

Medical History:

Height_____ Weight_____ BMI_____

Waist_____ Hip_____ W/H ratio_____

How did you hear about this program?_____

Your main goals for this program: (1)_____

(2)_____(3)_____

What role does faith play in your personal healthcare?_____

_____

Appendix

(Please list any additional information on separate sheet).
Hospitalizations (year / diagnosis)

_____
_____
_____

Surgeries (date / type)

_____
_____
_____

Current **Medications and Doses**:

Medication_____ Doses_____

Medication_____ Doses_____

Medication_____ Doses_____

Medication_____ Doses_____

Medication_____ Doses_____

Allergies   □ Yes   □ No
If yes, please list:_____
_____

Describe your present **activity level / exercise program**
□ Inactive / Sedentary   □ 30 minutes a week
□ Occasional   □ 30 minutes 2-3 times a week
□ Busy at home / work   □ 30 minutes more than 3 times a week

Do you have any **injury, joint pain, or other impediment** to normal exercise?
□ Yes   □ No
Explain_____
_____

Any difficulty doing activities of daily living? (Self-care, putting on shoes, going to mail box, grocery shopping, climbing stairs)

_____
_____

Do you use any of these **assistive devices?**
□ Oxygen   □ Walker   □ Wheelchair   □ Cane
□ Bi-Pap or C-Pap for sleep apnea   □ Joint replacement   □Prosthesis

Appendix

How does your weight affect you?

- □ shortness of breath
- □ diminished energy
- □ urine leak
- □ joint pain
- □ trouble finding clothes
- □ trouble fitting into chairs
- □ skin fold rash
- □ vein problems
- □ poor self-esteem

How long have you been overweight?

- □ from childhood
- □ after marriage
- □ after pregnancy
- □ after depression
- □ after menopause or hysterectomy
- □ after injury, illness, surgery, or trauma
- □ after medicines eg. hormones, steroids, etc.
- □ weight at high school graduation_____lbs.

Weight loss efforts tried:

- □ Atkins
- □ Zone
- □ Diet or exercise programs
- □ Laxatives
- □ Appetite suppression drugs
- □ Weight Watchers
- □ TOPS
- □ Hypnosis
- □ Tapes
- □ Fat blockers
- □ Jenny Craig
- □ Protein Power
- □ Support groups
- □ Purging
- □ Others

Do you, or did you, have any of the following medical conditions?

- □ heart disease
- □ depression
- □ breathing problems
- □ leg swelling
- □ leg inflammation
- □ skin condition
- □ muscle or joint pain
- □ high cholesterol
- □ sinusitis
- □ hypertension
- □ bleeding disorders
- □ colitis
- □ anorexia
- □ discharge
- □ diabetes
- □ sleep apnea
- □ thyroid disorder
- □ breast condition
- □ headaches
- □ sex'l dysfunction
- □ constipation
- □ bulimia
- □ ulcer
- □ other

Do you think you have signs of an eating disorder, (anorexia, bulimia or bingeing?) Describe any problem or weakness for particular food.

_____
_____
_____

Year of most recent:

physical_____   pap smear_____

mammogram_____   prostate check_____

Have you ever had a cholesterol or lipid test?

□ No   □ Yes (approximate date performed)_____

Was your cholesterol in the good range or bad range?

□ Good   □ Bad   □ Don't know

Appendix

HABITS: (optional)

Do you drink alcohol?   □ No   □ Socially   □ Regularly
    (What kind, how much, how often?) _____

Do you smoke?   □ No   □ Yes
    If Yes: Packs / Day_____   Number of years_____

Do you wear a seatbelt?   □ Sometimes □ All the time
Do you take a baby aspirin daily?   □ Yes   □ No
Do you eat fruits and vegetables daily?   □ Yes   □ No
Do you do monthly breast self exams?   □ Yes   □ No
Do you eat fish twice a week or take fish oils? □ Yes   □ No
Do you take vitamins and or antioxidants?   □ Yes   □ No

Hobbies / Things you enjoy doing in your free time_____
_____

Type of work (manual, office, sedentary, professional, work at home, disabled, unemployed) and amount of physical energy expended_____
_____

FAMILY WEIGHT GENETICS
For each first degree relative, fill out the approximate age, any major medical conditions and weight status - NL: Normal, OW: Overweight, MO: Morbidly Obese (over 100 pounds above normal body weight). The first three in the table below are examples.

RELATIVE	AGE	WEIGHT STATUS	MEDICAL PROBLEMS
Mother	52	NL	none
Father	54	OW	Diabetes, Heart dz.
Bro/Sis	25	MO	Sleep apnea
Mother			
Father			
Bro/Sis			
Bro/Sis			
Bro/Sis			
Bro/Sis			
Child			
Child			
Child			
Child			

A Powerful Root

When Mom would treat our stomach upsets with **ginger beer**, we had no idea the extent of its medicinal properties. Ginger is really a rhizome (root) *Zingiber officinale.* Its active ingredients have been identified as pungent volatile oils which include zingerone, shoagoles and gingerols.

Wendell Christian, LSM
Southern Caribbean Forces
British Army, WWII

Albertha Christian, O.M.
Caribbean nurse, 1964
Under a *yampère* (breadfruit) tree

The remarkable benefits of ginger has been validated by numerous studies conducted by pharmacologists and herbalists in various countries.

Its use was first documented over 500 years ago during the Qing Dynasty in the Guagdong province of China. Over the centuries, it spread overland to India then carried by the British to Africa, the Caribbean and from there to the rest of the New World.

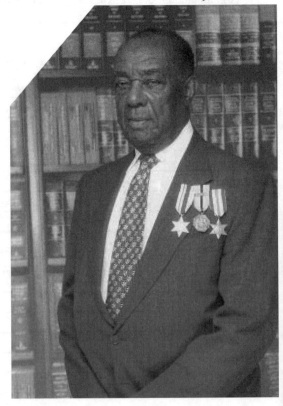

Clinical uses for ginger:

- To treat gastroenteritis, indigestion, morning sickness, motion sickness, nausea after surgery and chemotherapy.
- Carminative (prevents intestinal gas).
- Cardiotonic (thins blood and lowers cholesterol). Improves cardiac output accounting for its improved sense of well being.
- Anti-inflammatory; minimizes joint pain. Helps prevent scurvy.
- Antibacterial and antipyretic (lowers fever).
- Expectorant; used in teas for upper respiratory tract infections
- Sedative and aphrodisiac.

Ginger is a commonly used spice by top chefs. International indigenous cuisine generate a variety of unique beverages. The relatively low incidence of stomach problems and obesity among Caribbean people may be attributed in part, to the popular consumption of ginger beer. This is a non-alcoholic beverage tasting somewhat like regular ginger ale but without the fizz. It has a more fruity bouquet and a little more of a bite to it. Islanders frequently serve honored guests their own home-made version especially on festive occasions. I remember relatives and friends raving about my mother's recipe. It was one of the first things she taught us how to make.

Ginger beer recipe

Ginger roots are readily available from your neighborhood supermarket. Scrape of the thin tan-gray skin using a short knife. Chop and finely grate or blend the ginger root. Add a quart of water, 2 tablespoons of rice, 1 tablespoon lemon juice, a pinch of clove, and cure overnight. Strain through a muslin cloth and sweeten to taste. Served chilled.

It does not take long to feel the difference when one replaces soda pop with 100% vegetable or fruit juices and natural home-made beverages. Moreover, ginger beer is highly effective in helping to facilitate *stomach conditioning* as described in Chapter 5. Drink ½ glass before your customized meal 3 times a day. The beverage has a profound toning effect, helping to decrease actual stomach size. Continue based on targets established in *Jumpstart*, Chapter 1. This is a refreshing and delicious way to achieve lasting weight loss.

Appendix

Recommended Common Screening Tests for Healthy Adults
Executive Physical

Your name: _____   Date: ___/___/___

TESTS	Age 18-24	Age 25-39	Age 40-59	Age 60-74	Age 75+
BLOOD PRESSURE	Every 6 months - more often if abnormal				
CHOLESTEROL (Less than 200)	Depending on M.I. risk	At least annually			
FITNESS CHECK	Body mass index, resting pulse, review of nutritional weight and waist/hip status, personal exercise program				
FASTING BLOOD GLUCOSE / HgbAIC	Every 5 years	Every 2-5 years, depending on weight and diabetes family history			
CHEST X-RAY	As required for employment, preparation for surgery, medical condition and exposure to smoke, radon, etc.				
HEMATOCRIT (Blood count)	Every 5 years	Every 2 years or as indicated by periods, pregnancy or medical condition			
URINALYSIS	Every 5 years			Every 2 years	
	Whenever indicated by symptoms				
SIGMOIDOSCOPY Consider family history of polyps, colitis, and cancer.	If indicated by rectal bleeding, change in bowel habits, etc.		Every 3-5 years Age 50 +		
BREAST EXAM (Monthly self-examination)	By health care provider				
	About every 3 years or as indicated	Every 1-2 years	Annually age 50 + (post-menopausal)		
MAMMOGRAPHY / ULTRASOUND	Baseline at age 35-40, then every 1-2 years. Earlier and/or more often with breast mass symptoms or family history.				
PELVIC / PAP	Annually; less frequently after total hysterectomy per physician discretion				
PROSTATE EXAM	As indicated		Annually – *reminders helpful*		
PSA, CEA, CA 27 29 (Tumor Markers)			Every 1-3 years, depending on risk		

"Prevention is better (and cheaper) than cure"
Heartland Nutrition Institute